T0231749

BIOMARKERS AS TARGETED HERBAL DRUG DISCOVERY

A Pharmacological Approach to Nanomedicines

BIOMARKERS AS TARGETED HERBAL DRUG DISCOVERY

A Pharmacological Approach to Nanomedicines

Edited by

Mahfoozur Rahman, PhD
Sarwar Beg, PhD
Mazin A. Zamzami, PhD
Hani Choudhry, PhD
Aftab Ahmad, PhD
Khalid S. Alharbi, PhD

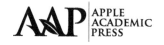

AAP | APPLE ACADEMIC PRESS

First edition published 2022

Apple Academic Press Inc.
1265 Goldenrod Circle, NE,
Palm Bay, FL 32905 USA
4164 Lakeshore Road, Burlington,
ON, L7L 1A4 Canada

CRC Press
6000 Broken Sound Parkway NW,
Suite 300, Boca Raton, FL 33487-2742 USA
2 Park Square, Milton Park,
Abingdon, Oxon, OX14 4RN UK

© 2022 Apple Academic Press, Inc.

Apple Academic Press exclusively co-publishes with CRC Press, an imprint of Taylor & Francis Group, LLC

Reasonable efforts have been made to publish reliable data and information, but the authors, editors, and publisher cannot assume responsibility for the validity of all materials or the consequences of their use. The authors, editors, and publishers have attempted to trace the copyright holders of all material reproduced in this publication and apologize to copyright holders if permission to publish in this form has not been obtained. If any copyright material has not been acknowledged, please write and let us know so we may rectify in any future reprint.

Except as permitted under U.S. Copyright Law, no part of this book may be reprinted, reproduced, transmitted, or utilized in any form by any electronic, mechanical, or other means, now known or hereafter invented, including photocopying, microfilming, and recording, or in any information storage or retrieval system, without written permission from the publishers.

For permission to photocopy or use material electronically from this work, access www.copyright.com or contact the Copyright Clearance Center, Inc. (CCC), 222 Rosewood Drive, Danvers, MA 01923, 978-750-8400. For works that are not available on CCC please contact mpkbookspermissions@tandf.co.uk

Trademark notice: Product or corporate names may be trademarks or registered trademarks and are used only for identification and explanation without intent to infringe.

Library and Archives Canada Cataloguing in Publication

Title: Biomarkers as targeted herbal drug discovery : a pharmacological approach to nanomedicines / edited by Mahfoozur Rahman, PhD [and five others].
Names: Rahman, Mahfoozur, 1984- editor.
Description: First edition. | Includes bibliographical references and index.
Identifiers: Canadiana (print) 2021010953X | Canadiana (ebook) 2021010970X | ISBN 9781771889025 (hardcover) | ISBN 9781003045526 (ebook)
Subjects: LCSH: Herbs—Therapeutic use. | LCSH: Biochemical markers. | LCSH: Nanomedicine. | LCSH: Alternative medicine.
Classification: LCC RS160 .B56 2021 | DDC 615.3/21—dc23

Library of Congress Cataloging-in-Publication Data

CIP data on file with US Library of Congress

ISBN: 978-1-77188-902-5 (hbk)
ISBN: 978-1-77463-787-6 (pbk)
ISBN: 978-1-00304-552-6 (ebk)

About the Editors

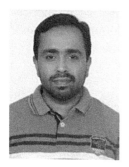

Mahfoozur Rahman, PhD
Assistant Professor, Department of Pharmaceutical Sciences, Faculty of Health Science, Sam Higginbottom University of Agriculture, Technology & Sciences (SHUATS), Allahabad, India

Mahfoozur Rahman, PhD, is an Assistant Professor in the Department of Pharmaceutical Sciences, Faculty of Health Science, Sam Higginbottom University of Agriculture, Technology and Sciences (SHUATS), Allahabad, India. His major areas of research interest include development and characterization of nanosized drug delivery systems for inflammatory disorders, including psoriasis, arthritis, neurodegenerative disorders, cancer, etc. In addition, he is also working on amalgamation of herbal medicinal plants with modern therapeutics in order to deliver scientifically acceptable therapies for various diseases management. To date he has published over 130 publications in peer-reviewed journals, such as *Seminar in Cancer Biology, Drug Discovery Today, Nanomedicine*, etc. He has also published 40 book chapters, five international books, and three articles in international journals. Overall, he has earned highly impressive publishing and citation record in Google Scholar (H-index of 28 and total citation over 2000 to date). Dr. Rahman has received travel grants from various international congresses, such as IAPRD, MDS, Nano Today Conference, KSN 2019, etc. He is also serving as an editorial board member and guest editor for several journals.

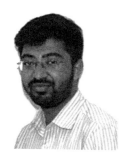

Sarwar Beg, PhD
Assistant Professor, Department of Pharmaceutics, School of Pharmaceutical Education and Research, Jamia Hamdard, New Delhi, India

Sarwar Beg, PhD, is an Assistant Professor in the Department of Pharmaceutics, School of Pharmaceutical Education and Research, Jamia Hamdard, New

Delhi, India. He has over a decade of teaching and research experience in the field of pharmaceutics and biopharmaceutics, especially in the development of novel and nanostructured drug delivery systems using Quality-by-Design paradigms. Before joining Jamia Hamdard, Dr. Beg worked as a Research Scientist at Jubilant Generics Limited, Noida, India. He has authored over 150 publications, 48 book chapters, 10 books, three Indian patent applications and served as a guest editors of several international journals. He has a Google Scholar H-Index of 26 and over 2800 citations to his credit.

Mazin A. Zamzami, PhD

Associate Professor in Clinical Biochemistry,
Chairman of the Biochemistry Department,
Faculty of Science at King Abdulaziz University,
Jeddah, Kingdom of Saudi Arabia

MazinZamzami, PhD, is an Associate Professor in Clinical Biochemistry and the Chairman of the Biochemistry Department, Faculty of Science at King Abdulaziz University, Jeddah, Kingdom of Saudi Arabia. Dr. Zamzami joined the KAU family in 2002 as a Lecturer in Biochemistry in the Faculty of Health Sciences. Previously, Dr. Zamzami directed the Serology Department as well as worked as a senior laboratory technician in the Clinical Biochemistry Department at Al-Thagher Hospital, Jeddah, Saudi Arabia, for approximately five years. His clinical research interest is in the molecular basis of disease, particularly nucleotide metabolic diseases, and pharmacogenetics. He has several published articles and has presented papers at international and national scientific conferences.

Hani Choudhry, PhD

Assistant Professor of Cancer Genomics and the
Head of Cancer and Mutagenesis Unit at the King
Fahd Center for Medical Research in King Abdulaziz
University (KAU), Saudi Arabia

Hani Choudhry, PhD, is an Assistant Professor of Cancer Genomics and the Head of Cancer and Mutagenesis Unit at the King Fahd Center for Medical Research at King Abdulaziz University (KAU), Saudi Arabia. He is also a Visiting Assistant Professor at the NIH Center of Excellence in Genomic Science, Center for Personal Dynamic Regulome, School of Medicine, Stanford University, California, USA. Dr. Choudhry has received a number of international and prestigious awards, including two AACR Scholar-in-Training Awards, the Susan G. Komen for the Cure Award and Proffered Paper Award for Non-coding RNA in Cancers at the EACR Annual Meeting. He has published over 40 research articles in high-impact and respected scientific journals.

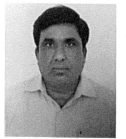

Aftab Ahmad, PhD
Associate Professor of Pharmacology,
Health Information Technology Department,
Jeddah Community College, King Abdulaziz University,
Jeddah, Kingdom of Saudi Arabia

Aftab Ahmad, PhD, is an Associate Professor of Pharmacology in the Health Information Technology Department at Jeddah Community College of King Abdulaziz University, Jeddah, Kingdom of Saudi Arabia. He had completed numerous research projects as a principle investigator (PI) funded by the deanship of scientific research (DSR) of King Abdulaziz University. He has contributed more than 100 full-length research articles to reputable national and international journals and is also an expert reviewer for several journals. His current h-index is 13, and he has been cited over 1,400 times to date.

Khalid S. Alharbi, PhD
Assistant Professor of Pharmacology and Toxicology;
Head of the Pharmacology Department,
College of Pharmacy, Jouf University, Sakaka,
Saudi Arabia

Khalid S. Alharbi, PhD, is an Assistant Professor of Pharmacology and Toxicology and the Head of the Pharmacology Department, College of Pharmacy at Jouf University, Sakaka, Saudi Arabia. He obtained both his BSc (Pharmaceutical Sciences, 2002) and MSc (Toxicology, 2009) from the College of Pharmacy at King Saud University (KSU), Riyadh, Saudi Arabia. He was awarded his PhD (Pharmacy and Biomedical Sciences, 2016) from Stathclyde University, United Kingdom. Dr. Alharbi's

Contents

Contributors

Mohd. Abid
Faculty of Pharmacy, IFTM University, Lodhipur Rajput, Delhi Road (NH-24), Moradabad – 244102, Uttar Pradesh, India

Muhammad Afzal
Department of Pharmacology, College of Pharmacy, Jouf University, Sakaka, Kingdom of Saudi Arabia, E-mail: afzalgufran@gmail.com

Sanjay Agarwal
Formulation Research Lab., Advance Nanomeds, Plot No. 142/20A, NSEZ, Noida – 201305, Uttar Pradesh, India

Farhan Jalees Ahmad
Nanomedicine Research Lab., Department of Pharmacy, School of Pharmaceutical Education and Research, Jamia Hamdard, New Delhi – 110025, India

Iqbal Ahmad
Formulation Research Lab., Advance Nanomeds, Plot No. 142/20A, NSEZ, Noida – 201305, Uttar Pradesh, India; Nanomedicine Research Lab., Department of Pharmacy, School of Pharmaceutical Education and Research, Jamia Hamdard, New Delhi – 110025, India

Shakeeb Ahmad
Nanomedicine Research Lab., Department of Pharmacy, School of Pharmaceutical Education and Research, Jamia Hamdard, New Delhi – 110025, India

Farhan Jalees Ahmed
Department of Pharmaceutics, School of Pharmacy, Glocal University, Saharanpur – 247121, Uttar Pradesh, India

Syed Salman Ali
Assistant Professor, Faculty of Pharmacy, IFTM University, Lodhipur Rajput, Delhi Road (NH-24), Moradabad – 244102, Uttar Pradesh, India, Phone: 8936935838, E-mail: salmanali.ali32@gmail.com

Sultan Alshehri
College of Pharmacy, King Saud University, Riyadh, Saudi Arabia

Kumar Anand
Department of Pharmaceutical Technology, Jadavpur University, Kolkata – 700032, West Bengal, India

Mohd. Aqil
Department of Pharmaceutics, School of Pharmacy, Glocal University, Saharanpur – 247121, Uttar Pradesh, India

Sandeep Arora
Department of Pharmacology, Chitkara College of Pharmacy, Chitkara University, NH-64, Jansla, Rajpura, Punjab – 140401, India

Mohammad Atif
Department of Pharmaceutical Sciences, Shalom Institute of Health and Allied Sciences, Sam Higginbottom University of Agriculture, Technology, and Sciences, Allahabad, Uttar Pradesh, India

Sarwar Beg
Department of Pharmaceutics, School of Pharmaceutical Education and Research,
Nanomedicine Research Lab, Jamia Hamdard (Hamdard University), New Delhi – 110062, India

Snigdha Bhardwaj
ITS College of Pharmacy, Delhi-Meerut Road, Murad Nagar, Ghaziabad – 201206, Uttar Pradesh, India

Rudranil Bhowmik
Department of Pharmaceutical Technology, Jadavpur University, Kolkata – 700032,
West Bengal, India

Sabya Sachi Das
Department of Pharmaceutical Sciences and Technology, Birla Institute of Technology, Mesra – 835215,
Ranchi, Jharkhand, India

Syed Azizullah Ghori
Department of Pharmacy Practice, College of Clinical Pharmacy,
Imam Abdulrahman Bin Faisal University, P.O. Box 1982, Dammam – 31441, Saudi Arabia

Sadaf Jamal Gilani
College of Pharmacy, Jouf University, Aljouf, Sakaka, Saudi Arabia

Monalisha Sen Gupta
Department of Pharmaceutical Technology, Jadavpur University, Kolkata, West Bengal, India

Chowdhury Mobaswar Hossain
Bengal School of Technology, Chinsurah, Hooghly, West Bengal, India

Syed Sarim Imam
Associate Professor, Department of Pharmaceutics, College of Pharmacy, King Saud University,
Riyadh, Saudi Arabia; School of Pharmacy, Glocal University,
Delhi-Yamunotri Marg (State Highway 57), Mirzapur Pole, Saharanpur – 247121,
Uttar Pradesh, India, E-mail: sarimimam@gmail.com

Mohammed Jafar
Assistant Professor, Department of Pharmaceutics, College of Clinical Pharmacy,
Imam Abdulrahman Bin Faisal University, P.O. Box 1982, Dammam – 31441,
Saudi Arabia, Mobile: +966502467326, E-mail: mjomar@iau.edu.sa

Mohammed Asadullah Jahangir
Department of Pharmaceutics, Nibha Institute of Pharmaceutical Sciences, Rajgir, Nalanda – 803116,
Bihar, India

Chandra Kala
Glocal School of Pharmacy, The Glocal University, Delhi-Yamunotri Marg (State Highway 57),
Mirzapur Pole, Saharanpur – 247121, Uttar Pradesh, India

Sanmoy Karmakar
Department of Pharmaceutical Technology, Jadavpur University, Kolkata – 700032, West Bengal, India,
Tel.: +91-8017136385, E-mail: sanmoykarmakar@gmail.com

S. M. Kawish
Nanomedicine Research Lab., Department of Pharmacy, School of Pharmaceutical Education and
Research, Jamia Hamdard, New Delhi – 110025, India

Imran Kazmi
Glocal School of Pharmacy, Glocal University, Mirzapur Pole, Saharanpur, Uttar Pradesh, India,
E-mail: kazmiimran2005@gmail.com

Najam Ali Khan
Faculty of Pharmacy, IFTM University, Lodhipur Rajput, Delhi Road (NH-24), Moradabad – 244102, Uttar Pradesh, India

Ruqaiyah Khan
Department of Pharmacology, Chitkara College of Pharmacy, Chitkara University, NH-64, Jansla, Rajpura, Punjab – 140401, India

Abdul Muheem
Department of Pharmaceutics, School of Pharmaceutical Education and Research, Jamia Hamdard, New Delhi – 110062, India

Himani Nautiyal
Siddhartha Institute of Pharmacy, Dobachi, Dehradun, Uttarakhand, India

Mahfoozur Rahman
Assistant Professor and Researcher at Department of Pharmaceutical Sciences, Faculty of Health Sciences, Shalom Institute of Health and Allied Sciences, Sam Higginbottom University of Agriculture, Technology, and Sciences (SHUATS), Allahabad, Uttar Pradesh – 211007, India, Mobile: +91-8627985598, E-mail: mahfoozkaifi@gmail.com

Subhabrata Ray
Dr. B. C. Roy College of Pharmacy and Allied Health Sciences, Durgapur, West Bengal – 713206, India

Suma Saad
Nanomedicine Research Lab., Department of Pharmacy, School of Pharmaceutical Education and Research, Jamia Hamdard, New Delhi – 110025, India

Ankit Sahoo
Department of Pharmaceutical Sciences, Faculty of Health Sciences, Shalom Institute of Health and Allied Sciences, Sam Higginbottom University of Agriculture, Technology, and Sciences (SHUATS), Allahabad – 211007, Uttar Pradesh, India

Shakir Saleem
Department of Pharmacology, Chitkara College of Pharmacy, Chitkara University, NH-64, Jansla, Rajpura, Punjab – 140401, India, E-mails: shakirsaleem@gmail.com; shakir.saleem@chitkara.edu.in

Md. Adil Shaharyar
Bengal School of Technology, Chinsurah, Hooghly, West Bengal, India; Department of Pharmaceutical Technology, Jadavpur University, Kolkata – 700032, West Bengal, India, Tel.: +91-9748902723, E-mail: adil503@yahoo.co.in

Alankar Shrivastva
Faculty of Pharmacy, IFTM University, Lodhipur Rajput, Delhi Road (NH-24), Moradabad – 244102, Uttar Pradesh, India

Sandeep Kumar Singh
Department of Pharmaceutical Sciences and Technology, Birla Institute of Technology, Mesra – 835215, Ranchi, Jharkhand, India, E-mail: dr.sandeep_pharmaceutics@yahoo.com

Md. Taleuzzaman
Faculty of Pharmacy, Maulana Azad University, Jodhpur, Rajasthan, India

P. R. P. Verma
Department of Pharmaceutical Sciences and Technology, Birla Institute of Technology, Mesra – 835215, Ranchi, Jharkhand, India

Sobiya Zafar
Nanomedicine Research Lab., Department of Pharmacy, School of Pharmaceutical Education and
Research, Jamia Hamdard, New Delhi – 110025, India

Abbreviations

AA	arachidonic acid
AB	aortic banding
AD	Alzheimer disease
ADR	adriamycin
AG	andrographolide
Ag-CurNCs	silver-curcumin nanoconjugates
AIA	adjuvant-induced arthritis
ALD	anti-leishmanial drugs
ALP	alkaline phosphatase
ALT	alanine aminotransferase
AMA	antimalarial activity
AMD	age-associated macular degeneration
AMI	acute myocardial infarction
AmP B	amphotericin B
API	apigenin
APP	amyloid-β precursor protein
ARM	Artemisinin
ASSOCHAM	Associated Chambers of Commerce and Industry in India
AST	aspartate aminotransferase
AzA	azelaic acids
Aβ	amyloid-β
BAL	bronchoalveolar lavage
BA-SLN	solid lipid nanoparticles of baicalin
BA-SOL	baicalin ophthalmic solutions
BBD	Box-Behnken design
BGs	bioglass
BITC	benzyl isothiocyanate
BMDCs	bone marrow-derived dendritic cells
BP	blood pressure
BS	*Boswellia serrata*
BW	body weight
C. decidue	*Capparis decidue*

CAA	caffeic acid
CA-CNP	calceinlabeled CNP
CA-NP	calceinlabeled NP
CAT	catalase
CAT	Committee for Advanced Therapies
CBER	Center for Biological Evaluations and Research
CBGA	cannabigerolic acid
CCBs	calcium channel blockers
CCD	central composite design
CCRD	central composite rotatable design
CDER	Center for Drug Evaluation and Research
CDRH	Center for Device and Radiological Health
CHA	carbonated hydroxyapatite
CHF	congestive heart failure
CIA	collagen-induced arthritis
CN	curcumin-stacked nanocatalysts
CNT	carbon nanotubes
COA	coumaric acid
COMP	Committee for Orphan Medicinal Products
CPL	cephaeline
CS	chitosan
CSIR	Council of Scientific and Industrial Research
CSLN	cationic solid lipid nanoparticles
CTnI	cardiac troponin I
Cu	copper
CUR	curcumin
CUR-NEM	curcumin-loaded nanoemulsion
CurNisNp	curcumin and nisin loaded polylactic acid nanoparticle
Cur-PLGA-NPs	curcumin-encapsulated PLGA nanoparticles
CV	capillary vascularity
CVDs	cardiovascular diseases
CVF	cobra venom factor
CVM	Center for Veterinary
CVMP	Committee for Medicinal Products for Veterinary Use
CXCR4	chemokine receptor 4
CYPs	cytochrome P
DBT	Department of Biotechnology

DENA	diethylnitrosamine
DL	drug loading
DLPC	1,2-dilinoleoyl-sn-glycero-3-phosphocholine
DM	diabetes mellitus
DMARDs	disease modifying anti-rheumatic drugs
DMBA	7,12-dimethylbenz anthracene
DMSO	dimethylsulfoxide
DOX	doxorubicin
DPPC	1,2-dipalmitoyl-sn-glycerol-3-phosphocholine
DQ	quaternization
DRDO	Defense Research and Development Organization
DSC	differential scanning calorimetry
DST	Department of Science and Technology
ECG	electrocardiogram
ECM	extracellular matrix
EDHF	endothelium-dependent hyperpolarizing factor
EE	encapsulation effectivity
EGCG	epigallocatechin gallate
EMA	European Medicines Agency
EO	essential oil
ESF	European Science Foundation
FA	ferulic acid
FDA	Food and Drug Administration
Fe	iron
FFR	fructose-fed rats
FGF	fibroblast growth factor
FICCI	Federation of Indian Chambers of Commerce and Industry
FP6	six framework programme
FPF	fine particle fraction
Fpn	ferroportin
GA	gambogic acid
GAE	gallic acid
GCs	glucocorticoids
GEH-RGD NPs	gelatin/EGCG self-assembly nanoparticles
GJIC	gap-junctional intercellular communication
GP	genipin
GSE	*Gleditsia sinensis* extract
GTE	green tea extract

H_2O_2	hydrogen peroxide
HA	hyaluronic acid
HA-PLA	hyaluronate-polylactide
HCC	hepatocellular carcinoma
HCS	high content screening
HFCD	high-fat cholesterol diet
HMPC	Committee on Herbal Medicinal Products
HTN	hypertension
HTS	high throughput screening
HUVEC	human umbilical vein endothelial cells
I.M	intramuscularly
I.P	intraperitoneal
I.V	intravenously
ICMR	Indian Council of Medical Research
ICP	isocephaeline
IDE	insulin-degrading enzyme
IFN	interferon
IL-1Ra	IL-1 receptor antagonist
ILO	International Labor Organization
IMQ	imiquimod
iNOS	inhibits nitric oxide synthase
IR	ischemia-reperfusion
ISG	*in situ* gels
ISO	International Organization for Standardization
ITCs	isothiocyanates
IV	intravenous
IVIC	*in vitro-in vivo* correlation
KIM-1	kidney injury molecule-1
KVL	klaivanolide
LAL	limulus amebocyte lysate
LBL	layer by layer
LDH	lactate dehydrogenase
LDH	layered double hydroxides
LDL	low-density lipoprotein
LH	luteinizing hormone and estradiol
LNs	lymph nodes
LOX	lipoxygenase
LPO	lipid peroxidation
LPS	lipopolysaccharide

LRP1	lipoprotein receptor-related protein 1
MA-chitosan	myristic acid-chitosan
MBG	mesoporous bioglass
MC	methylcellulose
MCL	mucocutaneous leishmaniasis
MCT	monocrotaline
MDA	malondialdehyde
ME	marigold extract
MetS	metabolic syndrome
MMAD	mass median aerodynamic diameter
MMP	matrix metalloproteinase
MPO	myeloperoxidase
NCL	neocryptolepine
NCLN	nano-sized clinoptilolite
NCs	nanocapsules
NDA	new drug application
NE	nano-emulsion
NF-Kβ	nuclear factor-Kβ
NHANES	National Health and Nutrition Examination
NIPAAM	N-isopropyl acrylamide
NLC	nanostructured lipid carriers
NMG	N-methylglucamine
NMs	nanomaterials
NNI	National Nanotechnology Initiative
NO	nitric oxide
NPs	nanoparticles
NS	nanosphere
NS	*Nigella sativa*
NSAIDs	nonsteroidal anti-inflammatory drugs
NSET	nanoscale science, engineering, and technology
NSO	*N. sativa* oil
NSSEO	*N. sativa* L. seeds essential oil
NTF	nanotechnology task force
NTQ	nanothymoquinone
NV	neovascularization
OA	oleanolic acid
OECD	Organization for Economic Co-operation and Development
OHT	ocular hypertension

OII	ocular irritation index
ORA	office of regulatory affairs
OSI	oxidative stress index
OVX	ovariectomized
OZ	oryzalin
PA	phosphatidic acid
PAG	p-aminophenyl-1-thio-β-D-galactopyranoside
PB	penta block
PC	phosphatidyl choline
PCL/Cur/GLE-Ag NPs	poly (-caprolactone)/curcumin/grape leaf extract-Ag hybrid nanoparticles
PCNA	proliferating cell nuclear antigen
PDCO	pediatric committee
PE	pomegranate extracts
PEG	polyethyleneglycol
PEITC	phenethyl isothiocyanate
PEN	pentalinonsterol
PEO	poly (ethylene oxide)
PGI_2	prostacyclin
PKs	pharmacokinetics
PLA	polylactic acid
PLGA	poly lactic-co-glycolic acid
PMA	premarket approval
PN	papillary or nodular
PONT	partial optic nerve transaction
PS	phosphatidylserine
PSEN1	processing, γ-secretases of presenilin 1
PTL	parthenolide
PUE	puerarin
PUFAs	polyunsaturated fatty acids
PVEF	*Prunella vulgaris* ethylacetate fraction
PVP	polyvinylpyrrolidone
QA	quercitin
QBD	quality by design
QCT	quercetin
QNAR	quantitative nanostructure-activity relationships
QN-NLC	NLC loaded with quercetin
QN-NLC-Gel	QN-NLC based hydrogel
QSAR	quantitative structure-activity relationship

RA	rheumatoid arthritis
RAGE	receptor for advanced glycation end products
RES	reticulo-endothelial system
RF	rheumatoid factors
ROS	reactive oxygen species
RP	reducing power
RSM	response surface methodology
RSV	resveratrol
RV	right ventricular
SCU	scutellarin
SEM	scanning electron microscopy
SGOT	serum glutamate oxaloacetate transaminase
SGPT	serum glutamate pyruvate transaminase
SLN	solid lipid nanoparticle
SMA	styrene-maleic acid
SMCS	sulfur S-methyl cysteine
SNEDDS	self-nano emulsifying drug delivery system
SOD	superoxide dismutase
STZ	streptozotocin
TAC	total antioxidant capacity
TET-CNP	tetrandrine-loaded cationic solid lipid nanoparticles
TET-SOL	tetrandrine occular solutions
THC	tetrahydrocurcumin
TIMPs	tissue inhibitor metalloproteinase proteins
TMC	N-trimethyl chitosan
TNF	tumor necrosis factor
TNF-α	tumor necrosis factor-α
TOS	total oxidative status
TP-1	topoisomerase I
TPA	trypanocidal activity
TQ	thymoquinone
TQNE	thymoquinone nanoemulsion
TQ-NLC	TQ loaded nanostructured lipid carrier
TQRF	thymoquinone rich fraction
TQRFNE	thymoquinone rich fraction nanoemulsion
TQ-SLN	TQ-loaded solid lipid nanoparticles
TWH	*Tripterygium wilfordii* Hook F
UA	ursolic acid
UANL	UA nanoliposomes

UDL	ultra-deformable liposomes
UN	United Nations
US-FDA	United States-Food and Drug Administration
VAP	vitamin A palmitate
VAPL	VAP-loaded liposomes
VEGF	vascular endothelial growth factor
WHO	World Health Organization
ZnPcAL	zinc phthalocyanine

Preface

Conventional medications have limited efficacy and high toxicity. Herbal drug discovery based on biomarkers emerging as complementary and alternative medicine have tremendous potential with wide structural diversity, which is not usually seen with conventional/synthetic drug molecules. Recognition of various herbal constituents such as terpenoids, fatty acids, flavonoids, and steroids has been well explored in the management/treatment of various disorders. These agents target various biomarkers such as nitric oxide (NO), cytokines, chemokines, adhesion molecules, NF-kβ, lipoxygenase (LOX), and arachidonic acid (AA).

The second part of this book is on nanomedicine; the word *nano* is a buzz word today in the era of the twenty-first century. With the advent of nano-technology, the world has witnessed a significant momentum in exploring the precepts and perspectives of this evolutionary technology for diverse applications in various fields.

Importantly, nanotechnology applications in the healthcare sector have benefited a lot for their application in providing benefits to the patient community by serving unmet medical needs. In this regard, the physico-chemical properties of herbal drugs and vehicles are considered to be highly significant for drug absorption. These factors restrict the site-specific action and limited penetration through site. To avoid these shortcomings, nano/submicromedicines have been developed to improve the absorption of such bioactives via optimizing the physicochemical properties of herbal drugs, vehicles, and barriers.

The present book, *Biomarkers as Targeted Herbal Drug Discovery: A Pharmacological Approach to Nanomedicines*, focuses on their use in targeting various biomarkers and what is involves in various dreadful disorders, including arthritis, cardiovascular, ocular disorders, cancers, etc.

Nanomedicines in particular focus on their use in the treatment of diseases. Notwithstanding the benefits of nanotherapeutic devices, the healthcare sector has tremendously benefited in terms of reducing the mortality rate beyond the expectations.

A total of thirteen chapters encompassed in this book have been contributed by eminent scientists, researchers, and nanotechnologists across the globe with the primary goal of highlighting the key advancements, challenges, and opportunities in the area of application of herbal drug discovery based on biomarkers and their delivery by nanomedicines for disease treatment and regulatory guidelines. The book, therefore, carries a lot of potential as a repertoire of knowledge and package of information for herbal scientists, pharmaceutical scientists, nanoscientists, and nanobiotechnologists.

A succinct account of the key highlights of each of the chapters included in the book has been discussed in the below-mentioned text.

Chapter 1, which is entitled *Inflammatory Biomarkers: An Important tool for Herbal Drug Discovery,* provides a comprehensive remark on the finding of biomarkers, which played a key role in inflammatory disorders and the emergence of herbals in targeting on biomarkers for the management of Inflammatory disease.

Chapter 2, which is entitled *Herbal Anti-Arthritic Drug Discovery Tool Based on Inflammatory Biomarkers,* discusses the inflammatory biomarkers for specific arthritis and their targets by herbals for effective management of the said disease.

Chapter 3, which is entitled *Curcumin Nanomedicines and Their Application in the Management of Disease,* highlights the uses of curcumin from the kitchen to clinics. The chapter will also serve as a guide for clinicians and researchers in working on the development of curcumin-loaded nanomedicines as novel nanotherapeutic strategies for management of dreadful disorders.

Chapter 4, which is entitled *Ursolic Acid: A Pentacyclic Triterpene from Plants in Nanomedicine,* discusses the perspectives of ursolic acid and its delivery by nanomedicine for treatment and management of several threatening disorders.

The Chapter 5 of this book is entitled as *Phytoconstituent-Centered Byproducts and Nanomedicines as Leishmanicidal Scavengers.* Almost 1.6 million of new individual cases of cutaneous leishmaniasis (CL) and more than half a million of new individual cases of visceral leishmaniasis (VL) ensue every year all over the world. The natural products, chiefly plant-originated phytoconstituents and their by-products of varied structural groups and classes, display the anti-leishmanial activity (ALA). This chapter emphasizes some biopharmaceutical nanotechnologies for designing varied drug delivery approaches, including nanoparticles (NPs), nanocapsules (NCs), liposomes, micelles, cochleates, and nanotubes that are effective in its delivery.

Chapter 6 of this book is entitled as *Delivery of Herbal Cardiovascular Drugs in the Scenario of Nanotechnology: An Insight.* According to WHO, about 80% of the population still believes that drugs from natural sources have the potential for advancement on the clinical platform. Nanotechnology bears much hope for the development of many of these poor bioavailable herbal drugs. Therefore, the present chapter converting herbal drugs to the nanoscale delivery system using various fabrication approaches can result in the improvement of many pharmacokinetic profiles as well as *in vivo* stability and controlled absorption of the drug at the desired site.

Chapter 7, which is entitled *Nigella sativa Encapsulated Nano-Scaffolds and Their Bioactivity Significance,* has its active constituent thymoquinone, which has a wide potential to shows anti-tumor, anti-microbial, immuno-modulatory, anti-inflammatory, and anti-oxidant effects. The present book chapter highlights the encapsulation of herbal drug into the nano-scaffold that makes them more effective than the traditional dosage form. The drug nano-scaffold is able to enhance the therapeutic potential by enhancing bioavailability and targeting in the management of various disorders.

Chapter 8, which is entitled *Phytoconstituent-Loaded Nanomedicines for Arthritis Management,* addresses the available anti-arthritic synthetic treat-ment for the management of arthritis that are found to have multiple disad-vantages, such as serious side effects, high costs of treatment, the requirement of parenteral administrations and incomplete relief to the patient in respect to pain intensity and joint movements. Therefore, the present chapter highlights the research conducted, in recent years, using nanomedicines in combina-tion with herbal drugs as an effective therapy in arthritis and concludes with several important investigations with promising results for the treatment of chronic disease in an efficient way.

Chapter 9, which is entitled *Phytoconstituent-Based Nanotherapeutics as Ocular Delivery Systems,* discusses the popularity of herbals all over the globe because of their natural origin and lesser side effects. The application of nanoformulation opened the door in a disease like glaucoma, eye cancer, and other anterior ocular diseases by significantly modifying the properties of drugs and their carriers. This chapter summarizes the latest research reports regarding the possible administration of phytoconstituent-loaded nanoformulations for different ocular diseases.

Chapter 10, which is entitled *Rosmarinic Acid: A Boon in the Manage-ment of Cardiovascular Disease,* discusses the therapeutic application of rosmarinic acid in cardiovascular disease. Several research reports have demonstrated the therapeutic effects in said disease management.

Chapter 11, which is entitled *Long-Term Toxicity and Regulations for Bioactive-Loaded Nanomedicines,* summarizes the incorporation of natural bioactives into nanomedicines; their applications and evaluation have aggressively been put forward during the last couple of decades. The enormous ability of nanocarriers in enhancing the bioavailability, targeting, and efficacy of natural molecules have been well documented. This chapter outlines the suitability of various bioactive-loaded nanocarriers in therapeutics, their toxicity, and regulatory considerations.

Chapter 12, which is entitled *Resveratrol-Loaded Phytomedicines for Management of Cancer*, discusses the therapeutic application of resveratrol in cancer, and the role of nanomedicines in optimizing pharmacokinetics (PKs) and pharmacodynamics in cancer disease.

Finally, the last chapter of this book, i.e., Chapter 13, which is entitled *Thymoquinone-Loaded Nanocarriers for Healthcare Applications*, summarizes the occurrence of thymoquinone in nature, their traditional uses, and modern uses on the basis of various research that have done in various healthcare.

CHAPTER 1

Inflammatory Biomarkers: An Important Tool for Herbal Drug Discovery

MAHFOOZUR RAHMAN,[1] ANKIT SAHOO,[1] MOHAMMAD ATIF,[1] and SARWAR BEG[2]

[1]*Department of Pharmaceutical Sciences, Shalom Institute of Health and Allied Sciences, Sam Higginbottom University of Agriculture, Technology, and Sciences, Allahabad, Uttar Pradesh, India*

[2]*School of Pharmaceutical Education and Research, Nanomedicine Research Lab, Jamia Hamdard, New Delhi, India*

ABSTRACT

The conventional pharmacotherapeutics are more often restricted to non-targeted action, reducing safety, and effectiveness in the treatment of immune-related disorders, cancer, and other disorders. While the herbal benefits provided by conventional dosage forms are only suboptimal, complexities and obstructions are present. The increased interest in herbal medicines clearly shows that they are more safe and effective. Herbals are natural and have enormous potential and a wide range of structures, which are not common with synthetic/semisynthetic medicament molecules. Herbal medicinal drugs have lately received a wide range of treatments for various conditions including autoimmune immune disorders and other terrible conditions, including Alzheimer's, diabetes, cancer, etc. To date, there are various available phytoconstituents for treating the above-mentioned disease by targeting various inflammatory biomarkers including terpenoids, flavonoids, fatty acids, and steroids. All these products are very effective in the management by taking intervention on specific biomarkers including nitric oxide (NO), cytokines, chemokines, adhesive molecules, NF-Kβ, interleukins (ILs), lipoxygenase, and arachidonic acid (AA).

1.1 INTRODUCTION

Inflammation is a biological response which is very complex and derived from the Latin word 'inflammationem.' It is a response triggered by the damaged body tissue such as irritants pathogens or injured cells (Abbas, 2009), and is a defensive response involving molecular mediators, immune cells, and blood vessels. The primary function of inflammation is the location and removal of the original cell injuries and the removal of the tissue element harmed to enable the body to start repairing the tissue. The main inflammation symptoms are redness, heat pain, swelling, and loss of function (Abbas, 2009). Inflammation is regarded as an innate immunity system compared to adaptive immunity, since inflammation is a generic response and is unique to each pathogen (Abbas, 2009). Minor inflammation could lead to rapid tissue loss by stimuli (e.g., bacteria), and could affect organism growth and in chronic inflammation leads to hay fever, rheumatoid arthritis (RA), periodontitis, atherosclerosis, and sometimes cancer (e.g., gall bladder carcinoma). The word biomarker, a portmanteau of biological marker, relates to a wide subcategory of medical signs that can be corrected and measured reproducibly-that is, an objective indication of medical condition observed from outside the patient. Regarding medical signs and symptoms, signs of health are restricted or disorder perceived by patients themselves. In the literature, there are many accurate definitions of biomarkers and they're certainly significantly varied. In 1998, the NIH described a biomarker as "a characteristic that is objectively measured and measured as an indicator of normal biological and pathogenic processes or pharmacological responses to therapeutic intervention" (Abbas, 2009). A joint project on chemical safety, the International Chemical Safety program, headed by the World Health Organization (WHO) and in collaboration with the United Nation and the International Labor Organization (ILO), defined a biomarker as "any process, structure, or substance, that can be measured and influencing or predicting the effect or outcomes or disease in the body or its products" (Abbas, 2009). A much wider concept requires into consideration not only the incidence and result of disease, but also the impacts of procedures, medicines, and even unintended access to the environment, such as chemicals or nutrients. In its research on biomarkers' efficacy in financial risk assessments, the WHO has stated that almost every measurement of a true notion of biomarkers involves an exchange between the prospective danger and a biological system that may be either physical, chemical, or biologicals. The assessed reaction can be operational and biochemical, physiological at the molecular interaction, or the cellular level (Ferrero-Miliani, 2007). Biomarker examples include everything from pulse and blood pressure (BP) through fundamental chemistries to more complicated blood and other tissue laboratory tests. Medical indication has a wide history of use in clinical practice, the most significant quantifying medical signs modern laboratory science enables us to reproductively assess, as well as medical instruction itself and biological manufacturers.

From the ancient time, medicinal plants are globally used to prevent and to treat disease. The early manuscripts of herbal drugs data back to 5,000 years in India and China, gives the importance of plants in the management of health. According to the WHO more, than half of the world population uses the medicinal plant-based system for the primary healthcare and medicinal plant to contribute near about 80% of the raw material in the traditional medicinal system. The demand of herbal drug is increasing day by day as the side effect and toxicity of the allopathic drug cause increase in the use of an herbal drug which leads to the drastic development of herbal drug industry. The demand of herbal medicines has been constantly rising every year (Vishal, 2014; Mishra, 2016). In developing countries, peoples use herbal drugs for the treatment of disorders and diseases as it is a part of their culture in those communities. Now researchers gave more attention to plants to discover new leads, thereby fulfilling the health care needs and reducing the number of deaths due to untreatable infections. In the development of various human diseases, inflammation plays an essential role including Asthma, inflammatory bowel disease, RA, Crohn's disease, and tendonitis. Chronic inflammatory response, however, is a driving force for the advancement of cancer, atherosclerosis, Alzheimer's disease, diabetes, and obesity. When inflammatory is under control, it is helpful to protect the organ against complete collapse, while uncontrolled treatment leads to unwanted physical decay.

1.2 ANTI-INFLAMMATORY HERBS HAVE PROVEN BENEFICIAL BY COMBATING INFLAMMATORY RESPONSE THAT LEAD TO SEVERE ABNORMALITY IN BODY SYSTEM

Herbal medicine used for the treatment or preventing diseases like inflammatory diseases and indeed a priceless source of valuable chemical compounds that developed into indispensable drug medical practice and their valuable effects in inflammatory diseases have not been thoroughly studied. Herbal medicine is a valuable part of traditional medicine and modern medicine, and it will be the same as in the future. There are now over 100 natural drug products being clinically tested and at least 100 compounds or molecules at the preclinical stage of development (Harvey Al, 2008). Most of these molecules are derived from a lead from plant and microbial sources and are in the developmental stage. The cancer and infection medication discovery program are based on natural products but a number of other therapeutic areas, such as inflammation, cardiovascular, gastrointestinal, neurosciences, and metabolism, are also targeted. Among 108 different therapeutic projects, indicate that 46 are in pre-clinically active and 14 in phase-1, 41 in phase-2, 5 in phase-3, and 2 are in the pre-registration phase (Harvey Al, 2008). There are generally six categories for the NCEs class. However, botanical sources, fungi, bacteria, and marine sources are the four major classes. In addition to these four classes of substances, the modern pharmaceutical chemistry includes two different classes of manufactured substances, synthetic chemistry, and combination chemistry from these natural sources.

1.2.1 DIRECT USE OF BIOACTIVE COMPOUNDS

Bioactive lead compounds with structure may act as more potent compounds, e.g., paclitaxel for Taxus species.

A new chromophore that can be transformed with/without chemical analogs into a drug compound. Pure phytochemicals are used for standardization of crude plant extract or material as a marker for compounds. Pure phytochemicals can be used as pharmacological tools.

1.3 CHALLENGES WITH HERBAL DRUG DEVELOPMENT

Globally about 422,000 plant species have been identified, of which 12.5% plant species have been used for medicinal purpose and 8% of the medicinal plants are under the threatened' category (Schippmann et al., 2002). Still the biological activities of many plants are not explored, and few of the plants are well recognized in official pharmacopeias, such as the Ayurvedic pharmacopeia of India and Japanese pharmacopeia. Indian Ayurvedic Pharmacopeia contains 540 plant monographs and 976 compounds formulations (Joshi et al., 2017). Japanese, 14th edition Pharmacopoeia lists 165 herbal and 16th edition 276 crude drugs such as herbal medicines and extracts that approved for use in kampo remedies (Pan et al., 2014). The pharmacological actions and the concentration in plants depend on their phytoconstituents and on the plant habits. The plant habit has a major impact on the concentration of phytoconstituent and this factor plays an important role in the medicinal importance of any plant. Approximately, 90% of the medicinal herbs in the Indian medicinal are collected from natural and wild sources. The unsuitable collection (stage of maturity, dried haphazardly, and stored for a long time) is rapidly depleting the resource and many species are under threat (Lalitha, 2013).

1.4 BIOMARKERS TARGETED HERBAL DRUG THERAPY

1.4.1 ALZHEIMER'S DISEASE (AD)

In 1906, German Physician Aloes Alzheimer, who first describe brain disorder and named after its Alzheimer's disease (AD). AD is a neurodegenerative and progressive disease that mainly affects an aged over 65, and reported for 50%–60% of dementia cases (Francis et al., 1999). Alzheimer's condition is characterized by a decrease in speech function, increased apathy, and deterioration of virtually all intellectual functions, progressive loss of memory, disorientation, and gait irregularities.

The loss of memory is due to the scarcity of the neurotransmitter acetylcholine. Inhibiting the action of the enzyme acetylcholine esterase which breaks up the neurotransmitter can improve the acetylcholine transmitter concentration in the brain. Drugs that prevent messenger breakdown or acetylcholine stop the disease's growth (Jayaprakasam et al., 2010). Herbs for antioxidant and anti-inflammatory activities which could be used to treat Alzheimer's disease have been investigated. The herbal herbs that inhibit AchE contain COX-2, which are used for the indication of AD as a herbal medicine. Some Indian herbs used in the Ayurvedic preparations which are excellent for slowing down the brain degeneration caused by Alzheimer's like Padma (Nelumbo nucifera), Kataj, Galo Satva, Musta Arjun, Guduchi, Ashwagandha, Amalaki, Pancha-TiktaGhrutaGugguli, Vacha, etc.

1.4.1.1 CURCUMA LONGA L. (ZINGIBERACEAE)

It is a source of an orange-yellow pigment called curcumin, (diferuloylmethane), compound of turmeric. Studies have shown that curcumin has antioxidant and anti-inflammatory activity and that it aids in the fight against AD (Jayaprakasam et al., 2010).

1.4.1.2   BOCOPA MONNIERI (SCROPHULARIACEAE)

The herbal nutraceutical *Bocopa monnieri* (Brahmi), also recognized as memory enhancement in patients with Alzheimer's disease, is defined in the Ayurveda system as memory improvement and concludes that it can be useful in those patients but further research is required (Goswami et al., 2011).

1.4.1.3   GINKGO BILOBA L. (GINKGOACEAE)

Ginkgo biloba L. is the herb most renowned for its capacity to improve circulation systematically. BP is reduced and the aggregation of platelets is inhibited. Ginkgolides are the main chemical constituent of *Ginkgo biloba* and are a relevant antioxidant, with neuro-protective, and cholinergic activities in AD management. Scientific studies showed its promise on cognition-enhancement, if used during the early stage of the Alzheimer's disease. Extract of *Ginkgo biloba* showed therapeutic benefits in similar, too prescribed medicines like Donepezil or Tactrine with minimally unwanted side effect in the controlled clinical trials of a control and placebo groups (Elias et al., 2010).

1.4.1.4   GLYCYRRHIZA GLABRA (FABACEAE)

Aqueous extract of licorice on A25-35 induces apoptosis in PC12 cells. The result suggests that GWE exerts a protective effect against a fragment-induced apoptotic neuronal cell death. Extract from the root of licorice is reported to treat or even prevent the death of brain cells in disorders such as Alzheimer's and its related symptoms (Ji et al., 2011).

1.4.1.5   LIPIDIUM MEYENII WALP (BRASSICACEAE)

Lipidium meyenii Walp is also known as maca. Maca shows a profitable improvement in learning and memory. *Lipidium meyenii Walp* improves experimental memory impairment, induced by ovariectomy, due in part to its AchE inhibitory and antioxidant activities. Results showed that *Lipidium meyenii Walp* can improve learning and memory in ovariectomized (OVX) mice and this impact may be linked to its capacity to reduce lipid peroxidation (LPO) and AchE in OVX mice (Kumari et al., 1995).

1.4.1.6 *PANAX GINSENG (ARALIACEAE)*

The root of Ginseng has been used since ancient times in folk medicine in countries such as Korea and China to boost Qi. The medicinal use of Ginseng goes back to thousands of years. Panax Ginseng (Ren-Shen) contains propanetriol, oleanolic acid (OA), and saponins protopanaxadiol, reported having memory-enhancing action for learning impairment generated by scopolamine. The use of ginseng extract claims to attain and retain both physical and mental well-being (Sheela et al., 1992).

1.4.1.7 *ACORUS CALAMUS* L. *(ARACEAE)*

In the Ayurveda medicine system, *Acorus calamus* has been used for the treatment of behavior changes, memory loss, and for learning performance. *Acorus calamus* L. inhibits the AChE. It contains a majority of asarone (Karunanayaka et al., 1984). *Acorus calamus* also shows anti-inflammatory, cardiovascular, immune-suppressive, antioxidant, anti-spasmodic, hypolipidemic, antimicrobial, antidiarrheal, anthelmintic, and cytoprotective.

1.5 DIABETES MELLITUS (DM)

It is a chronic metabolic disorder of carbohydrate, protein, and fat, which is a lifelong condition affecting the person's blood glucose and insulin level in the body. In diabetic condition, pancreases either do not produce enough insulin or the body does not use it properly. It is estimated that the world-wide prevalence of diabetes will increase from 4% in 1995 to 5.4% by 2025. According to WHO prediction, the major burden will occur in developing countries?

A study in India over the last decade has shown that the prevalence of diabetes is not only high, but also rapidly increasing in the urban population. An estimated 33 million adult with diabetes is living in India. By 2025, the number is expected to rise to 57.2 million.

Symptoms for diabetic conditions may include:

1. High level of blood sugar level;
2. Unusual thirst;
3. Frequent urination;

4. Loss of weight and extreme hunger;
5. Blurred vision;
6. Extreme weakness and tiredness;
7. Irritability, mood changes.

Many people use herbs and supplements to cure diabetes, but they are not effective and stand-alone, but they may use herbs to relieve symptoms and reduce the risk of complications.

1.5.1   ACACIA ARABICA (BABULS)

Acacia is growing throughout India, particularly in the wild. The extract of this plant acts as an anti-diabetic agent by acting as a secretagogue to secrete insulin. In the experiment, it induces hypoglycemia in control rats. In powdery seeds of Acacia administered to normal rabbits at a weight of 2, 3, and 4 g/kg, the hypoglycemic effect is caused by insulin-releasing in the pancreas cells (Wadood et al., 1989).

1.5.2   AEGLE MARMELOS (BENGAL QUINC, OR BEL)

Blood glucose and serum cholesterol and urea are reduced by aqueous leaf extract and reduced relative to controlled alloxanized rats. The hypoglycemic activity also occurs through the injection and avoided a maximum blood sugar growth at a 1-hour oral tolerance test (Karunanayake et al., 1984).

1.5.3   ALLIUM CEPA (ONION)

Dried onion powder fraction either soluble or insoluble compound show anti-hypoglycemic activity in diabetic rabbits. Onion also has hypolipidemic and antioxidant activity. Administration of the amino acid sulfur S-methyl cysteine (SMCS) in alloxan-driven diabetic rats for 45 days has significantly controlled blood glucose, serum, and tissues lipids and normalizes liver glucose activities 6-phosphatase, hexokinase, and HMG Co-A reductase activity (Roman-Ramos et al., 1995; Kumari et al., 1995). When a single oral dose of allium cepa juice was given to diabetic patients, the level of postprandial glucose was significantly controlled.

1.5.4   ALLIUM SATIVUM (GARLIC)

Garlic is a herb grown throughout India. It has allicin, a compound that contains sulfate that gives a smooth odor and has significant hypoglycemic activity (Sheela et al., 1992). The hypoglycemic impact is supposed to be attributed to enhanced hepatic metabolism, enhanced beta-cell glucose discharge, or insulin-sparing (Zacharias et al., 1980). Garlic aqueous homogenate (10 ml/kg/day) orally administered to rabbits for 2 months 10 g/kg/day in the water, hepatics glycogen and amino acid, rapid sugar, and serum triglycerides decrease, as opposed to sucrose controls (Augusti et al., 1996). S-allyl cysteine is oxidant-controlled sulfur that contains the amino acid, a precursor of garlic oil and allicin, rather than insulin and glibenclamide that controls the lipid by oxidation (Al-Awadi et al., 1987). Garlic also exhibits anticancer, antimicrobial, and cardioprotective activities.

1.5.5   ALOE VERA AND ALOE BARBADENSIS

Aloe vera is a popular house decorative plant and a multipurpose folk remedy. Aloe has two basic products: latex and gel. Aloe gel is commonly known pulp or mucilage as aloe juice, and aloe latex is a bitter yellow exudate of per cycle tube below the outer skin of the leaves. Aloe gum extract effectively increases glucose tolerance in common rats as well as in diabetic ones (Aiabnoor et al., 1990). Treatment of chronic have no single dose of *Aloe barbadenis* exudates in alloxan diabetic rats indicates a hypoglycemic impact. The hypoglycemic action was also demonstrated in the diabetic rat, together with a chronic amount of the bitter principle of the same plant. This action of Aloe vera is through stimulation of synthesis and/or insulin release from pancreatic beta cells (Devis et al., 1989). This plant has anti-inflammatory activities that depend on the doses and improves the wound healing in diabetic mice (Chattopadhyay et al., 1987).

1.5.6   AZADIRACHTA INDICA (NEEM)

Hydro-alcoholic extract from this plant reported anti-hyperglycemic effects in treated streptozotocin rats and this effect is due to increased absorption of glucose in isolated rats and glycogen deposition (Chattopadhyay et al., 1987; Biswas et al., 2002). Apart from this neem having anti-diabetic activity, antimaterial, anti-bacterial, hepatoprotective, and antioxidant effects (Chattopadhyay et al., 2003).

1.5.7   CAPPARIS DECIDUA

This is commonly found in arid regions throughout India. In alloxanized rats, the hypoglycemic effect occurs when 30% extract from *Capparis decidua* (*C. decidua*) fruit powder was given to rats for three decades. In erythrocytes, kidney, liver, this extract also reduces alloxan-induced lipid peroxidation significantly. *C. decidua* has also been found to change super-oxide dismutase (SOD) and enzyme catalase (CAT) concentration in order to decrease oxidative stress (Agarwal et al., 1988). Additionally, decidua demonstrated hypolipidemic activity (Kamble et al., 1998).

1.5.8   EUGENIA JAMBOLANA (INDIAN GOOSEBERRY, JAMUN)

Eugenia jambolana in India is used to treat diabetes in households. This is also an important component of many herbal medicines for diabetes formulations. Aqueous, alcoholic, and lyophilized powder extracts have anti-hyperglycemic effects and a drop in blood glucose levels. It depends on the level of diabetes. It indicates 73.51% decrease in mild arthritis (plasma sugar >180 mg/dl), compared to 55.6% and 17.62% reduced in moderate (plasma glucose >280 mg/dl) and severe diabetes (plasma sugar >400 mg/dl). In streptozotocin-induced mice, the extract of Jamun pulp exhibited hypoglycemic activity within 30 minutes, whereas seeds of the fruit needed 24 hours. The oral administration of extract has led to an increased serum insulin level in diabetic rats. The incubation of plant extract with the isolated islet of Langerhans from both normal and diabetic animals stimulated insulin secretion. These extracts also inhibited liver and kidney insulins activity (Aderibigbe et al., 1999).

1.5.9   MOMORDICA CHARANTIA (BITTER GOURD)

Momordica charantia is used as an antidiabetic and antihyperglycemic agent in both India and other Asian countries. Extract of the pulp of fruits, seed, leaves, and entire plants were shown in various animal models as having a hypogly-cemic activity. Polypeptide p, isolated from fruits and tissue of *M. charantia*, has a significant hypoglycemic impact on langurs and humans when administered subcutaneously (Shibib et al., 1993). Ethanolic extract of *M. charantia* (200 mg/kg) had an anti-hypoglycemic and hypoglycemic impact in ordinary diabetic rats and STZ rats. This can be due to inhibition of glucose-6-phosphatase in the liver and stimulation of hepatic glucose-6-phosphate dehydrogenase activities in addition to fructose-1,6-biphosphatase (Vats et al., 2002).

1.5.10 MILK THISTLE

Milk thistle may have anti-inflammatory characteristics that may be helpful to people with diabetes. People have been using thistle as a tonic for the liver and many different ailments since ancient times. Silymarin is a compound that has been given the greatest attention by scientists with antioxidant and anti-inflammatory properties. These are the properties which can make milk thistle a useful herb for diabetes patients. Many of the silymarin studies are promising but, according to one review published in 2016, the research is not strong enough to recommend the herb or extract alone for diabetes. No side effect report appears and as a supplement, many people take milk thistle. However, it is best to talk to a doctor first before using any supplement.

1.5.11 URSOLIC ACID STEAROYL GLUCOSIDE

New stearoyl glucose of ursolic acid, urs-12-en-3-ol-28-oic acid 3-D-gluco-pyranosyl-4'-octadecanoate, and other compound were isolated from Latana camera L leaf. By the standard spectroscopic method, the structure of this new glycoside was elucidated and established. It showed a reduction in blood glucose levels in streptozotocin-induced diabetic rats.

1.6 CANCER

Cancer is mainly responsible for the abnormal and uncontrolled division of cells. Cancer with abnormal cell growth that invades or spreads to other parts of the body. Signs and symptoms include an abnormal bleeding, unexpected weight loss, prolonged cough, lump, and a change in bowl movement. These symptoms may indicate cancer or may be due to other causes. Many plant species are already used for cancer treatment or prevention. Researchers have identified new plant species that have proven anti-cancer properties with a high emphasis on herbal medicines used in developing countries. The 5th most common cause of death in carcinoma is primary liver cancer in the world and the 3rd leading cause of mortality. Hepatocellular carcinoma (HCC) cause for 85% to 90% of main liver cancer. The HCC has several interesting epidemiological characteristics, including dynamic temporal trends; considerable differences between geographical regions, racial, ethnic, and male and female; and several well-documented environmental variables that could possibly be avoided. In addition, there is an increasing knowledge of the molecular mechanism that causes hepatocarcinogenesis that almost rises significantly in reaction to chronic liver injury at the cirrhosis stage.

1.6.1 GLEDITSIA SINENSIS

Thorns of *Gleditsia sinensis* have historically been used in Chinese medicine and were considered one of the most important herbs for treatment. There is currently an investigation of the effect of *Gleditsia sinensis* on cancer. New drug development still necessary for the therapy of HCC, the most prevalent form of main liver cancer, with greater effectiveness. The beneficial impact of *Gleditsia sinensis* extract (GSE) and its regulatory effects on the miRNAs were determined by the use of the rat HCC model implanted with cancerous Walker-256 cells. GSE improves liver morphology significantly and dramatically induced HCC rat cell apoptosis. Furthermore, miR-21/181b/183 was up-regulated in HCC liver and both sorafenib and GSE reduced the elevation of these miRNAs. Down-Regulation PTEN/TIMP3/PDCD4 was consistent with the HCC liver target of miR3621/181b/183 and both GSE and Sorafenib altered the target genes. Also determined were the impacts of TIMP3 on MMP-2/9' expression. The results show the potential of GSE in HCC treatment and increase the understanding of miRNA-related mechanisms in GSE cancer (Lopez-Lazaro, 2008).

1.6.2 CURCUMIN

Curcumin (diferuloylmethane), obtained from *Curcuma aromatica* widely used as coloring and spice agent in food, possesses potent anti-inflammatory, antioxidant, and anticarcinogenic properties. The anti-carcinogenic property of curcumin has been reported different cancer (Chuang et al., 2000). Three important curcumin properties were studied with respect to HCC: Anti-HCC; anti-metastatic; and anti-angiogenesis activity. Chuang et al. checked the effect of curcumin on HCC mice model; cancer induced by N-diethylnitrosamine (DEN) and reported that curcumin inhibits effectively DEN-induced HCC in the C3H/HeN mice. Mice treated with DEN show a remarkable increase in the level of p21 (ras), expression of proliferating cell nuclear antigen (PCNA) and CDC2 protein, while curcumin inverted the level of all these biological markers. The effect of curcumin and tetrahydro-curcumin on tumor angiogenesis of HCC mice is also found in a study conducted by Joysungnoen et al. Human HCC cell line (HepG2) was inoculated with tetrahydro-curcumin orally injected into a dorsal peeling chamber of male BALB/v nude mice at 300 and 300 mg/Kg^{-1} per day. A fluorescence video microscopy and capillary vascularity (CV) were observed to measure tumor microvasculature. They found a substantial reduction in the curcumin and tetrahydrocurcumin (THC) in the CV. THC and curcumin have a dose-dependent anti-angiogenic effect and represent a common mechanism for their action against cancer (Yoysungnoen et al., 2005, 2006).

1.6.3   RESVERATROL

Resveratrol has been shown to have a strong growth inhibitory effect on various human cells, including HCC, as a compound of polyphenol found in peanuts, grape skins, red vine, and berries.

It rapidly absorbed by the liver and accumulates in it. Lancon et al. studied the resveratrol absorption and efflux in HepG2 cells. Resveratrol has been rapidly combined and fully metabolized to form two major resveratrol metabolites in eight hours: disulfate and monosulfate. In order to assess the inhibitory effect of hepatocarcinogenesis resveratrol, the HCC rat model is used by Bishayee et al. A single intraperitoneal (I.P) injection of diethylnitrosamine (DENA) produced the HCC, followed by promotion in drinking water with phenol barbital. Resveratrol has been discovered to have an important chemoprotective impact on hepatocarcinogenesis initiated by DENA through inhibition of apoptosis and cell proliferation. They found that a feasible mechanism could be that the apoptogenic signal induced by resveratrol is mediated through Bcl-2 down-regulation and Bax up-regulation (Bishayee et al., 2008). The inhibitory impact of resveratrol on apoptosis and cell proliferation in HepG 2 cells also were demonstrated by an *in vitro* study by Stervbo et al. resveratrol has been found to inhibit the synthesis of DNA and to increase the nuclear scale and granularity of HepG 2 cells in G1 and S phases. Resveratrol also activated apoptosis in HepG 2 cells, which was concentration-dependent. Resveratrol has been found that it interferes with distinct phase of cycle inhibiting cell proliferation and triggers apoptosis stimulation. The HepG2 cells were also used by Notas et al. to examine the effects of resveratrol on cell growth. They show that stilbene resveratrol inhibits cell proliferation, decrease ROS production by cell-cycle detention in the Phase G1 and G2/M, and induces apoptosis. They also discovered that stilbene resveratrol modulates the NO/NOS system by raising eNOS and iNOS expression, NOS activity, and nitric oxide (NO) production (Notas et al., 2006). Yan et al. studied the impacts of resveratrol in HepG2 cells on proliferation and gap-junctional intercellular communication (GJIC). They found that HepG2 cell stop development in S stage, to inhibit DNA synthesis and to cause cell apoptosis. After treatment with resveratrol, the GJIC level increased sharply implying an increased level of GJIC could play a role in the effect of resveratrol in cancer chemopreventative activity (Yan et al., 2006).

1.7   RHEUMATOID ARTHRITIS (RA)

Rheumatoid (RA) is the autoimmune inflammatory joint disease that affects nearly 1% of the world's population. It is connected with a special inflammation of continuous particular in synovial tissues leading to the gradual degradation of joint and bone cartilages. Different causative agents engaged in RA advancement include genetic and environmental factors that alter the shape of immunological event. RA can because of unusual immune response, eventually leading to synovial inflammation and devastation of the bone. For the development of RA, the etiology of RA was not fully explained. However, T-cell activation is mainly involved in retaining the differentiating community (CD) in T-cells and also in improving output of various cytokines including IL-1, IL-3, IL-6, and the migration of TNF-a macrophage (Rout et al., 2012). All these inflammatory mediators elicit synovial tissue functions such as proliferation, expression of metalloproteinase, and adhesion molecules, secretion of other chemokines, and prostaglandins. The matrix metalloproteinase (MMP) cartilage and bone by restructuring and degradation abnormally. Expression of adhesion molecular leads the T-cells to be excessively attached to synovial-type B cells, which produces a high level of MMP (Ekor, 2014). Neoangiogenesis is also induced by other variables, such as cyclooxygenase activation, NO synthase, and neutral proteases. The autoantibodies cluster, including IgM, IgG, and IgA, were established to exacerbate and are regarded as rheumatoid factors (RF). Different ailments, including inflammatory diseases of the immune system, have been researched widely for late and herbal pharmacotherapy as supplementary and alternative medicines for the optimum functioning of the body, over several decades. The pharmacotherapeutic delivered presently accessible through conventional dosage form offers therapeutic advantages only to the suboptimal extent, thus possess difficulties and obstructions in the treatment of RA. This required the design of novel drug delivery approaches to develop efficient, targeted, and safe drug delivery systems with enhanced therapeutic performance. Nanomedicines could work as drug carriers in order to effectively manage RA in current centuries. It has also been proved. Nanomedicines have distinctive features for the delivery of drugs and are treated remarkably promising options to conventional drug therapy. The topical nanomedicines are more useful due to greater skin retention ability, specific targeted action, drug dose reduction, lower adverse effects, and higher patient compliance among the various routes of drug administration accessible for RA. Although these therapies have several worthy characteristics, but the main difficulties linked with their wider acceptance include higher cost of production, lower long-term stability, lack of evidenced-based clinical data for their safety.

1.7.1   HERBAL PHARMACOTHERAPY IN RA

It is strongly recommended by the American College of Rheumatology that currently available medicine for RA have high toxicity and limited efficacy. In addition, people are dissatisfied with the treatment available and almost 60%–90% of RA patient's depends on complementary and alternative medicines obtained from the herbal source. Herbs with huge potential and broad structural diversity, which are not often observed with synthetic drug molecules. Many phytoconstituents, including as terpenoid flavonoids, fatty acid, and steroids have therefore been explored for their anti-RA action. Their ability for various inflammatory mediators like cytokines, chemokines, NO, adhesion molecules, NF-k, lipoxygenase (LOXs), and arachidonic acid (AA). Details concerning different phytoconstituents were addressed below.

1.7.2   THYMOQUINONE

A bioflavonoid obtained from the *Nigella sativa* seeds. It has been commonly used as a conventional drug in treatment of multiple diseases in the Middle and Far East Nations. Many literatures have also been reported about TQ, which shows beneficial effects in various inflammatory disorders like IBD, RA, and Osteoarthritis. Tekeoglu et al. demonstrated equal therapeutic advantages, including MTX, for administering TQ by I.P injection in adjuvant-induced arthritis (AIA) in rats. Another study has shown that the inhibition of the serum concentrations of IL-1 band TNF-a in RA by daily TQ dosing of 5 mg/kg per day.

1.7.3   RESVERATROL (RSV)

Resveratrol (RSV) is a polyphenolic compound that occurs naturally and is mostly derived from the skin of the grapes (*Vitis vinifera*). Various literatures have found that the root of polygonum cuspidatum is used as popular medicine in Japan and China, apart from grape skin. It includes enriched resveratrol. An effective action against arthritis is shown by the intra-articular injection of resveratrol by delaying in the IL-1, ROS, tumor protein (p53)-induced apoptosis, LTB-4, PGE2, and MPPs in animal models. Furthermore, it is also summarized in Table 1.1.

1.7.4   HESPERIDIN

Hesperidin is a citrus flavonoid reported for its wide variety of pharmaco-logical effects. The therapeutic effect of hesperidin is well investigated in the adjuvant rat arthritis model. At the 80, 160 mg/kg dose of hesperidin inhibits significantly the secondary paw swelling and down regulates production of IL-1, IL-6, and TNF-a in RA rats. Another research has shown that hesperidin has a significant impact of suppressing synoviocytes' proliferation in rat adjuvant arthritis model.

1.7.5   CURCUMIN

Curcumin obtained from *Curcuma longa*. The effect of anti-inflammatory, antioxidant, and anti-cancer behavior are commonly known. Limited bioavailability impeded their clinical use when orally administered. In addition, it has been investigated recently for its potential in RA to depress catabolic mediators and inflammatory, such as Il-b, stimulated NO, PGE2, COX-2, IL-8, MMP-3, MMP-9, when I.P administration of 23 mg of total curcuminoid/kg per day is given. It also inhibits mediators' processes in human chondrocytes, such as JNK, NF-kb, and JAK/STAT.

TABLE 1.1 It Shows Therapeutic Applications of Bioactive in Dreadful Disorders

Sl. No.	Phytoconstituents	Source	Arthritis	References
1.	Thymoquinone (TQ)	TQ is obtained from the black caraway seed (*Nigella sativa*)	It exerts anti-arthritic action in rats against carrageenan-induced paw edema by inhibiting inflammatory mediators	Abbas, 2009
2.	Resveratrol (RSV)	Resveratrol is a polyphenolic compound that occurs naturally, mostly obtained from the skin of the grapes (*Vitis vinifera*)	Intra-articular resveratrol injection shows effective action against arthritis by retarding the Ros, IL-1, tumor protein (p53)-induced apoptosis, PEG2 LTB-4 and MPPs in the animal models.	Abbas, 2009
3.	Gambogic acid	Gambogic acid (GA) is polyprenylated xanthone containing resin which is derived from *Garcinia hanburyi* and Garcinia Morella	GA can be regarded as promising anti-arthritic molecules that restrict the secretion of Il-1β and TNFs. Intraperitoneal administration of GA in the early and late stage of arthritis at a dose of 4 1g/g body weight each day to AIA rats can lead to full removal of inflammatory infiltration and cell proliferation.	Abbas, 2009
4.	*Gleditsia sinensis* Extract (GSE)	GSE is obtained from a *Gleditsia sinensis*, which is a flowering deciduous tree from Asia. Locust is common name (Fabaceae or Leguminosae family).	The effect of GSE on cancer is presently under investigation. The therapeutic impacts of *Gleditsia sinensis* extract (GSE) and its legislative impacts on miRNAs were evaluated using rat Hepatocellular carcinoma (HCC) model implanted with cancerous Walker-256 cells. In HCC rats, GSE recovered considerably the liver morphology and dramatically induced cell apoptosis. Our results currently show the ability of GSE in HCC therapy and broaden the knowledge of MiRNA-related processes for the impact of GSE against cancer	Singh, 2005
5.	Curcumin (diferuloylmethane)	Curcumin (diferuloylmethane), a compound isolated from *Curcuma longa* (Zingiberaceae).	Its anti-cancerous property has been researched extensively in different cancers. Three significant characteristics have been studied with respect to HCC: anti-HCC; HCC anti-angiogenesis; HCC anti-metastatic action.	López-Lázaro, 2008

TABLE 1.1 *(Continued)*

Sl. No.	Phytoconstituents	Source	Arthritis	References
6.	Silibinin (Milk Thistle)	*Silybum marianum* is from the Asteraceae family. The significant biological active compound of milk thistle is Silibinin, Polyphenolic flavonoid.	Studies have shown that silibinin has an inhibitory effect on several cancer cell lines including HCC. They found that both HEpG2 and Hep3B cell were strongly inhibited by silibinin. Silibinine also cause G1 arrest in HepG2, and G1 and G2-M arrests in Hep3B cells.	López-Lázaro, 2008
7.	*Ginkgo biloba* L. (Ginkgoaceae)	Extract is obtained from *Ginkgo biloba* L. also known as the Maidenhair three (Family Ginkgoaceae)	*Ginkgo biloba* enhances the protection against oxidative damage caused by Aβ protein (degrading hydrogen peroxide, preventing lipids form oxidation, and trapping the reactive oxygen species). *Ginkgo biloba* is best known for its capacity to improve circulation systemically. Their action is directly linked to vaso relaxation. Thus, *Ginkgo biloba* can inhibit platelets aggregation and lower blood pressure. When used during the premature phase of Alzheimer's disease, it promises cognition enhancement (booster).	Goswami, 2011
8.	*Salvia officinalis* (Lamiaceae)	This herb is obtained from *Salvia officinalis* commonly known as sage (family Lamiaceae)	Sage as it is referred more frequently for the treatment of Alzheimer's Disease. Assisting the brain in fighting against AD has been reported. Sage contains the carnosic acid and rosemary acid antioxidants. It is thought that these compounds protect the brain from oxidative damage.	Francis, 1999
9.	*Rosmarinus officinalis* (Lamiaceae)	This herb is obtained from *Rosmarinus officinalis* commonly known as Rosemary Mediterranean region (Family Lamiaceae)	The following natural COX-2 inhibitors are present in rosemary (Satapatrika): apigenin, carvacrol, eugenol, oleanolic acid, thymol, and urisolic acid. According to Duke 2007, if synthetic COX-2 could prevent AD, then natural COX-2 inhibitor could prevent Alzheimer's. Rosemary also includes almost two dozen antioxidant and a dozen more anti-inflammatory compounds.	Harvey, 2008

Sl. No.	Phytoconstituents	Source	Arthritis	References
10.	*Coccinia indica*	The dried extract is derived from Cocciniagradis, the Ivy gourd, also called scarlet gourd, tindora, and kowai fruit is a tropical vine (Family Cucurbitaceae).	*Coccinia indica* (*C. indica*) dried seeds (500 mg/kg body weight) had been used for 6 weeks in diabetic patients. The extract restored reduced lipoproteins and glucose-6-phosphatase and lactate dehydrogenase activity in untreated diabetic enzyme (LPL).	Kamble, 1998
11.	*Eugenia Jambolana* (Indian gooseberry, Jamun)	Extract from *Phyllanthus emblica* also known as emblic, emblic myrobalan, Indian gooseberry or Amla (family Phyllanthaceae).	73.51% reduction, whereas it is decreased respectively to 55.62 and 17.71% for moderate (plasma sugar>280 mg/dl) and severe (sugar>400 mg/dl) diabetes. The extract from jamun pulp demonstrated hypoglycemic activity within 30 minutes after administration for streptozotocin-induced diabetic animals whereas the seed of the same fruit took 24 hours. Diabetic rats have increased the level of serum glucose by oral administration of the extract. Insulin secretion was found to be stimulated on incubation of plant extract with isolated islets of Langerhans from normal as well as diabetic animals. These extracts also inhibited liver and kidney insulinase activity	Karuna-nayake, 1984
12.	*Momordica charantia* (bitter gourd)	Extract is obtained from *Momordica charantia* commonly known as bitter melon, bitter gourd is a tropical and subtropical vine of the family Cucurbitaceae.	Fruit pulp, seed, leaves extracts, and entire extract. Polypeptide p. isolated from *M. charantia* fruits, seeds, and tissues, show considerable hypoglycemic effect when administered subcutaneously given to langurs and human beings.	Karuna-nayake, 1984

1.7.6   GREEN TEA EXTRACT (GTE)

The presence of non-toxic epigallocatechin-2-gallate (EGCG), in green tea extract (GTE), oral administration at 200 mg/kg, has anti-arthritic effect. It delays IL-1 glycosaminogly by preventing NF-kB activity from being released into chondrocytes. It inhibits NO, IL-1 stimulated NO synthase (iNOS) and JNK action, which mediate destruction of the cartilage.

1.7.7   CELASTROL

Celastrol is pentacyclic triterpene obtained and used in Chinese traditional medicine. It has anti-tumor and anti-inflammatory properties. During the daily administration to AIA rats of celastrol I.P administration, shows anti-inflammatory action possibly through the inhibition of caspase-1 and inhibits the activation of NF-JB, and downregulation of the IL-1b and TNF secretion in an AIA rat model.

1.7.8   GAMBOGIC ACID (GA)

Gambogic acid (GA), which derives from *Garcinia hanburyi* and *Garcinia morella*, is a polyprenylated xanthone containing resin. It is used as a complementary and alternative medicine in South-East Asia. GA can be seen as successful anti-arthritis molecules that restrict the secretion of IL-1b and TNF. Intraperitonial GA administration in early and late stage of arthritis to AIA rats at 4 Ig/g body weight (BW) every day may result in the total removal of inflammation and cellular proliferation.

1.7.9   TRIPTERYGIUM WILFORDII HOOK F (TWH)

In the old Chinese medical documents TWH a plant grown mostly in South China is commonly used in the treatment of joint pain. Several patients with active symptoms who have not active against nonsteroidal anti-inflammatory drugs (NSAIDs) for at least 2 months have been given random TWH 60 mg/day or three months of placebo pills that have an identical appearance. At the end of the therapy, patients receiving TWH experienced significant progress compared with placebo in all parameters: tenderness score, swelling count, morning stiffness, and grip strength.

1.8   CONCLUSION

Herbs can perform a significant role in the initial therapy of Alzheimer's and other diseases, including Diabetes, Cancer, and RA. One of the herbs' main merits is that they are less toxic than pharmaceutical ingredients. There is no justification for not being able to use herbs side by side with synthesized drugs or other complementary approaches such as vitamins, antioxidants, SAME, and fish oil. It shows that earlier the therapy begins; the faster the result will be. Consequently, if the clients have family members who have a history of the disorder or other states with a poor memory, they can start taking such remedies before symptoms start delay or stop the advent of the symptoms. AD therapy with herbal medicines should be linked to the pharmacological therapy currently being used. In order to enhance the validation of the clinical trial, these trials should include the finding of an effective concept. Multicenter studies are needed to determine the efficacy of this drug on a further big scale. Until then this study showed how many herbs in the Indian medicine system, the Chinese medicine system, the European Medicine system, etc.), have benefited in therapy.

KEYWORDS

- **adjuvant-induced arthritis**
- **Alzheimer's disease**
- **arachidonic acid**
- **capillary vascularity**
- *Capparis decidua*
- **diabetes mellitus**

REFERENCES

Abbas, A. B., & Lichtman, A. H., (2009). Chapter 2: Innate immunity. In: Saunders (Elsevier) (ed.), *Basic Immunology. Functions and Disorders of the Immune System (3rdedn.)*. ISBN:978-1-4160-4688-2.

Aderibigbe, A. O., Emudianughe, T. S., & Lawal, B. A., (1999). Antihyperglycemic effect of *Mangifera indica* in rat. *Phytother Res., 13*, 504–507.

Agarwal, V., & Chauhan, B. M., (1988). A study on composition and hypolipidemic effect of dietary fiber from some plant foods. *Plant Foods Human Nutr., 38*, 189–197.

Al-Awadi, F. M., & Gumaa, K. A., (1987). Studies on the activity of individual plants of an antidiabetic plant mixture. *Acta Diabetologica., 24,* 37–41.

Augusti, K. T., & Shella, C. G., (1996). Anti-peroxide effect of S-allyl cysteine sulfoxide, an insulin secretagogue in diabetic rats. *Experientia., 52,* 115–120.

Bever, B. O., & Zahnd, G. R., (1979). Plants with oral hypoglycemic action. *Quart. J. Crude Drug Res., 17,* 139–146.

Bishayee, A., & Dhir, N., (2008). Resveratrol-mediated chemoprevention of diethyl-nitrosamine-initiated hepatocarcinogenesis: Inhibition of cell proliferation and induction of apoptosis. *Chemico-Biological Interactions, 179,* 131–144.

Biswas, K., Chattopadhyay, I., Banerjee, R. K., & Bandyopadhyay, U., (2002). Biological activities and medicinal properties of neem (*Azadiracta indica*) *Curr. Sci., 82,* 1336–1345.

Chakrabarti, S., Biswas, T. K., Rokeya, B., Ali, L., Mosihuzzaman, M., Nahar, N., Khan, A. K., & Mukherjee, B., (2003). Advanced studies on the hypoglycemic effect of *Caesalpiniabonducella* F. in type 1 and 2 diabetes in long Evans rats. *J. Ethnopharmacol., 84,* 41–46.

Chattopadhyay, R. R., Chattopadhyay, R. N., Nandy, A. K., Poddar, G., & Maitra, S. K., (1987). Preliminary report on antihyperglycemic effect of fraction of fresh leaves of *Azadiracta indica* (Beng neem) *Bull. Calcutta. Sch. Trop. Med., 35,* 29–33.

Chattopadhyay, R. R., Chattopadhyay, R. N., Nandy, A. K., Poddar, G., & Maitra, S. K., (1987). The effect of fresh leaves of *Azadiracta indica* on glucose uptake and glycogen content in the isolated rat hemi diaphragm. *Bull. Calcutta. Sch. Trop. Med., 35,* 8–12.

Chuang, S. E., Cheng, A. L., Lin, J. K., & Kuo, M. L., (2000). Inhibition by curcumin of diethylnitrosamine-induced hepatic hyperplasia, inflammation, cellular gene products, and cell-cycle-related proteins in rats. *Food and Chemical Toxicology,38*(11), 991–995.

Chuang, S. E., Kuo, M. L., & Hsu, C. H., (2000). Curcumin-containing diet inhibits diethylnitrosamine-induced murine hepatocarcinogenesis. *Carcinogenesis, 21*(2), 331–335.

Davis, R. H., & Maro, N. P., (1989). *Aloe vera* and gibberellins, Anti-inflammatory activity in diabetes. *J. Am. Pediat. Med. Assoc., 79,* 24–26.

Ekor, M., (2014). The growing use of herbal medicines: Issues relating to adverse reactions and challenges in monitoring safety. *Front Pharmacol., 4,* 177.

Elias, E. J., Anil, S., Ahmad, S., & Daud, A., (2010). Colon targeted curcumin delivery using guar gum. *Nat. Prod. Commun., 5,* 915–918.

Ferrero-Miliani, L., Nielsen, O. H., Andersen, P. S., Girardin, S. E., Nielsen, Andersen, & Girardin (2007). Chronic inflammation: Importance of NOD2 and NALP3 in interleukin-1-beta generation. *Clin. Exp. Immunol., 147(2), 061127015327006.*

Francis, P. T., Palmer, A. M., Snape, M., & Wilcock, G. K., (1999). The cholinergic chypothesis of Alzheimer's disease: A review of progress. *J. Neurol. Neurosurg. Psychiatry., 66,* 137–147.

Goswami, S., Saoji, A., Kumar, N., Thawani, V., Tiwari, M., & Thawani, M., (2011). Effect of *Bacopa monnieri* on cognitive functions in Alzheimer's disease patients. *Int. J. Collab. Res. Intern. Med. Public Health, 3,* 285–293.

Harvey, A. L., (2008). Natural products in drug discovery. *Drug Discov. Today, 13,* 894–901.

Jacobs, B. P., Dennehy, C., Ramirez, G., Sapp, J., & Lawrence, V. A., (2002). Milk thistle for the treatment of liver disease: A systematic review and meta-analysis. *American Journal of Medicine, 113*(6), 506–515.

Jayaprakasam, B., Padmanabhan, K., & Nair, M. G., (2010). Withanamides in *Withaniasomnifera* fruit protects PC-12 cells from beta-amyloid responsible for Alzheimer's disease. *Phytother. Res., 24,* 859–863.

Ji, Y. A., Suna, K., Sung, E. J., & Tae, Y. H. (2010). Effect of licorice (*Glycyrrhiza uralensis* Fisch) on amyloid-β-induced neurotoxicity in PC12 cells. *Food Sci. Biotechnol., 19,* 1391–1395.

Joshi, V. K., Joshi, A., & Dhiman, K. S., (2017). The Ayurvedic pharmacopeia of India, development and perspectives. *J. Ethnopharmacol., 197,* 32–38.

Kamble, S. M., Kamlakar, P. L., Vaidya, S., & Bambole, V. D., (1998). Influence of *Coccinia indica* on certain enzymes in glycolytic and lipolytic pathway in human diabetes. *Indian J. Med. Sci., 52,* 143–146.

Karunanayake, E. H., Welihinda, J., Sirimanne, S. R., & Sinnadorai, G., (1984). Oral hypoglycemic activity of some medicinal plants of Sri Lanka. *J. Ethnopharmacol., 11,* 223–231.

Kumari, K., Mathew, B. C., & Augusti, K. T., (1995). Anti-diabetic and hypolipidaemic effects of S-methyl cysteine sulfoxide, isolated from *Allium cepa* Linn. *Ind. J. Biochem. Biophys., 32,* 49–54.

Lah, J. J., Cui, W., & Hu, K. Q., (2007). Effects and mechanisms of silibinin on human hepatoma cell lines. *World Journal of Gastroenterology, 13*(40), 5299–5305.

Lalitha, N., (2013). Protecting traditional knowledge in Siddha system of medicine. *J. Intellec. Prop. Rights, 18*(3), 272–282.

Li, Q., Wang, Y., Feng, N., Fan, Z., Sun, J., & Nan, Y., (2008). Novel polymeric nanoparticles containing tanshinone IIA for the treatment of hepatoma. *Journal of Drug Targeting, 16*(10), 725–732.

Lieber, C. S., Leo, M. A., Cao, Q., Ren, C., & DeCarli, L. M., (2003). Silymarin retards the progression of alcohol-induced hepatic fibrosis in baboons. *Journal of Clinical Gastroenterology, 37*(4), 336–339.

López-Lázaro, M., (2008). Anticancer and carcinogenic properties of curcumin: Considerations for its clinical development as a cancer chemo preventive and chemotherapeutic agent. *Molecular Nutrition and Food Research, 52*(1), S103–S127.

Mathew, P. T., & Augusti, K. T., (1975). Hypoglycemic effects of onion, *Allium cepa* Linn. on diabetes mellitus-a preliminary report. *Ind. J. Physiol. Pharmacol., 19,* 213–217.

Mishra, P., Kumar, A., Nagireddy, A., Mani, D. N., Shukla, A. K., & Tiwari, R., (2016). DNA bar-coding: An efficient tool to overcome authentication challenges in the herbal market. *Plant Biotechnol. J., 14*(1), 8–21.

Momeny, M., Khorramizadeh, M. R., Ghaffari, S. H., Yousefi, M., Yekaninejad, M. S., & Esmaeili, R., (2008). Effects of silibinin on cell growth and invasive properties of a human hepatocellular carcinoma cell line, HepG-2, through inhibition of extracellular signal-regulated kinase 1/2 phosphorylation. *European Journal of Pharmacology, 591,* 13–20.

Notas, G., Nifli, A. P., Kampa, M., Vercauteren, J., Kouroumalis, E., & Castanas, E., (2006). Resveratrol exerts its antiproliferative effect on HepG2 hepatocellular carcinoma cells, by inducing cell cycle arrest, and NOS activation. *Biochimica et Biophysica Acta, 1760*(11), 1657–1666.

Pan, S. Y., Litscher, G., & Gao, S. H., (2014). Historical perspective of traditional indigenous medical practices: The current renaissance and conservation of herbal resources. *Evid. Based Complement Alter Med.,* 525340.

Roman-Ramos, R., Flores-Saenz, J. L., & Alaricon-Aguilar, F. J., (1995). Antihyperglycemic effect of some edible plants. *J. Ethnopharmacol., 48,* 25–32.

Rout, J., Sajem, A. L., & Nath, M., (2012). Medicinal plants of North Cachar Hills district of Assam used by the Dimasa tribe. *Indian J. Tradit. Knowl., 11*(3), 520–527.

Ryu, S. Y., Lee, C. O., & Choi, S. U., (1997). *In vitro* cytotoxicity of tanshinones from *Salvia miltiorrhiza. Planta Medica., 63*(4), 339–342.

Schippmann, U., Leaman, D. J., & Cunningham, A. B., (2002). Impact of cultivation and gathering of medicinal plants on biodiversity: Global trends and issues. In: *Biodiversity and the Ecosystem Approach in Agriculture, Forestry, and Fisheries* (pp. 142–167). FAO.

Sheela, C. G., & Augusti, K. T., (1992). Antidiabetic effects of S-allyl cysteine sulphoxide isolated from garlic *Allium sativum* Linn. *Indian J. Exp. Biol., 30*, 523–526.

Shibib, B. A., Khan, L. A., & Rahman, R., (1993). Hypoglycemic activity of *Coccinia indica* and *Momordica charantia* in diabetic rats: Depression of the hepatic gluconeogenic enzymes glucose-6-phosphatase and fructose-1,6-biphosphatase and elevation of liver and red-cell shunt enzyme glucose-6-phosphate dehydrogenase. *Biochem. J., 292*, 267–270.

Singh, R. P., & Agarwal, R., (2005). Mechanisms and preclinical efficacy of silibinin in preventing skin cancer. *European Journal of Cancer, 41*(13), 1969–1979.

Singh, R. P., & Agarwal, R., (2006). Prostate cancer chemoprevention by silibinin: Bench to bedside. *Molecular Carcinogenesis, 45*(6), 436–442.

Stervbo, U., Vang, O., & Bonnesen, (2006). C Time-and concentration-dependent effects of resveratrol in HL-60 and HepG2 cells. *Cell Proliferation, 39*(6), 479–493.

Tang, Z., Tang, Y., & Fu, L., (2003). Growth inhibition and apoptosis induction in human hepatoma cells by tanshinone II A. *Journal of Huazhong University of Science and Technology Medical Science, 23*, 166–8, 172.

Varghese, L., Agarwal, C., Tyagi, A., Singh, R. P., & Agarwal, R., (2005). Silibinin efficacy against human hepatocellular carcinoma. *Clinical Cancer Research, 11*(23), 8441–8448.

Vats, V., Grover, J. K., & Rathi, S. S., (2002). Evaluation of antihyperglycemic and hypoglycemic effect of *Trigonellafoenum-graecum* Linn, *Ocimum sanctum* Linn and *Pterocarpus marsupium* Linn in normal and alloxanized diabetic rats. *J. Ethnopharmacol., 79*, 95–100.

Vishal, V., Sharma, G. N., Mukesh, G., & Ranjan, B., (2014). A review on some plants having anti-inflammatory activity. *J. Phytopharmacol., 3*(3), 214–221.

Wadood, A., Wadood, N., & Shah, S. A., (1989). Effects of *Acacia arabica* and *Caralluma edulis* on blood glucose levels on normal and alloxan diabetic rabbits. *J. Pakistan Med. Assoc., 39*, 208–212.

Wang, X., Yuan, S., & Wang, C., (1996). A preliminary study of the anti-cancer effect of tanshinone on hepatic carcinoma and its mechanism of action in mice. *Zhonghua Zhong Liu Za Zhi, 18*(6), 412–414.

Wang, X., Yuan, S., Huang, R., & Song, Y., (1996). An observation of the effect of tanshinone on cancer cell proliferation by Brdu and PCNA labeling. *Hua Xi Yi Ke Da XueXue Bao.,27*, 388–391.

Wellington, K., & Jarvis, B., (2001). Silymarin: A review of its clinical properties in the management of hepatic disorders. *Bio Drugs, 15*, 465–489.

Wu, W. L., Chang, W. L., & Chen, C. F., (1991). Cytotoxic activities of tanshinones against human carcinoma cell lines. *American Journal of Chinese Medicine, 19*(3/4), 207–216.

Yan, F., Tian, X. M., & Ma, X. D., (2006). Effects of resveratrol on growth inhibition and gap-junctional intercellular communication of HepG2 cells. *Nan Fang Yi Ke Da XueXue Bao, 26*(7), 963–966.

Yoysungnoen, P., Wirachwong, P., Bhattarakosol, P., Niimi, H., & Patumraj, S., (2006). Effects of curcumin on tumor angiogenesis and biomarkers, COX-2 and VEGF, in hepatocellular carcinoma cell-implanted nude mice. *Clinical Hemorheology and Microcirculation, 34*(1/2), 109–115.

Yoysungnoen, P., Wirachwong, P., Bhattarakosol, P., Niimi, H., & Patumraj, S., (2005). Antiangiogenic activity of curcumin in hepatocellular carcinoma cells implanted nude mice. *Clinical Hemorheology and Microcirculation, 33*(2), 127–135.

Yuan, S. L., Wei, Y. Q., Wang, X. J., Xiao, F., Li, S. F., & Zhang, J., (2004). Growth inhibition and apoptosis induction of tanshinone II-A on human hepatocellular carcinoma cells. *World Journal of Gastroenterology, 10*, 2024–2028.

Zacharias, N. T., Sebastian, K. L., Philip, B., & Augusti, K. T., (1980). Hypoglycemic and hypolipidaemic effects of garlic in sucrose fed rabbits. *Ind. J. Physiol. Pharmacol., 24*, 151–154.

Zhao, B. L., Jiang, W., Zhao, Y., Hou, J. W., & Xin, W. J., (1996). Scavenging effects of Salvia miltiorrhiza on free radicals and its protection for myocardial mitochondrial membranes from ischemia-reperfusion injury. *Biochemistry and Molecular Biology International, 38*(6), 1171–1182.

Zhong, Z. H., Chen, W. G., Liu, Y. H., Li, Q. X., & Qiu, Y., (2007). Inhibition of cell growth and induction of apoptosis in human hepatoma cell line HepG2 by tanshione IIA. *Zhong Nan Da XueXue Bao Yi Xue Ban, 32*, 99–103.

CHAPTER 2

Herbal Anti-Arthritic Drug Discovery Tool Based on Inflammatory Biomarkers

MAHFOOZUR RAHMAN,[1] ANKIT SAHOO,[1] and SARWAR BEG[2]

[1]Department of Pharmaceutical Sciences, Faculty of Health Sciences, Shalom Institute of Health and Allied Sciences, Sam Higginbottom University of Agriculture, Technology, and Sciences (SHUATS), Allahabad – 211007, India

[2]Department of Pharmaceutics, School of Pharmaceutical Education and Research, Jamia Hamdard (Hamdard University), New Delhi – 110062, India

ABSTRACT

According to the American College of Rheumatology, conventional medicines have limited effectiveness and are highly toxic. Therefore, 60%–90% concentrate on complementary and alternative medicine and people are dissatisfied with the available therapies. Herbs have enormous potential that are not often seen in synthetic drugs of large structural complexity. Different plant constituents, including terpenoids, flavonoids, fatty acids, steroids, have investigated the anti-rheumatic action. These all target different inflammatory mediators such as nitric oxide (NO), cytokines, chemical substances, conformity molecules, NF-kβ, LLOX, and arachidonic acid (AA). They often target various inflammatory mediators. The text presented details on the phytoconstituents based on targeted action on inflammatory biomarkers.

2.1 INTRODUCTION

Rheumatoid arthritis (RA) is an immune-based joint inflammatory disorder that starts when the immune system attacks its own body tissue or bone, which affects almost 1% of the world population. The most evince pathogenesis is T-cell activation which associated with the increase of different inflammatory bio-marks and a bunch of variation (CD) in the T-cells. These involve cytokines, NF-Kβ, arachidonic, nitric oxide (NO), chemokines, lipoxygenase (LOX), adhesion molecules, and matrix metalloproteinase (MMP) (Anderson et al., 1985). Finally, these all damage bone and cartilage by degeneration and alteration. On the basis of this interaction of bioactive such as thymoquinone, curcumin, hesperidin, gambogic acid (GA), polyphenols, celastrol, and resveratrol display high anti-arthritic activity against RA which is dependent on the concentration of dose via targeting inflammatory bio-marks.

RA is affiliated with synovial tissue polyarticular inflammation, which leads to damage the articular cartilage and bones (Anderson et al., 1985). Factors that influence the progression of RA are the change in the shape of an immunological phenomenon, environmental, and genetic and can change the shape of the immunological phenomenon (Scrivo et al., 2007). RA may appear due to abnormal immune response leads to synovial inflammation and joint destructions, but still, its etiology is not clear (Rahman et al., 2015). T cell activation causes CD and simultaneously enhances the secretion of cytokines including TNF-a, IL-1, IL-3, IL-6, inhibitory factors, and macrophage migration (Ismail et al., 2015). These inflammatory biomarkers are involving in the proliferation, secretion of PGs, chemokines, and adhesion molecules (Rahman et al., 2015; Ismail et al., 2015). Whereas adhesion molecule expression causes T-cells excessive binding to synovial type B cells, results to produce a large quantity of MMP (Araki et al., 2016). For angiogenesis in aggravation of RA, there are many factors involving such as cyclooxygenase, neutral proteases, NO synthase, and group of antibodies including IgG, IgM, and IgA respectively (Firestein, 2003; Araki et al., 2016). These all play a role in fixing complements, screen macrophages, cytokines, lymphocytes by ligating the macrophages Fc-c receptors which abnormally lead to inflammation in RA (Smolen et al., 2016; Rahman et al., 2016). Furthermore, the IgA immune complex also involving in the production of higher intraarticular tissue growth factor-β secretion as well as bone erosion, results to RA symptoms (Song et al., 2014). Overall, the pathogenesis of RA involves angiogenesis, synovial cell proliferation, cellular immune system activation by B and T-cells, macrophages, and pannus formation, all these results to produces cartilage deformation and bone erosion. Thus, all these factors are actively involving in the pathogenesis of RA (Song et al., 2014). For the management of RA, there are several drug molecules such as glucocorticoids (GCs), non-steroidal anti-inflammatory drugs (NSAIDs), disease-modifying anti-rheumatic drugs (DMARDs), and biological agents including IL-1 receptor antagonist (IL-1Ra) and TNF-a blockers, reduce inflammation and pain in RA (Smolen et al., 2016). However, there is a need to develop to improve the antirheumatic drugs with the safety and efficacy in the management of RA with fewer side effects. In the current treatment approaches, many of the drugs are withdrawn from the market due to cardiotoxicity associated with cyclooxygenase-2 inhibitors and DMARDs associated with fungal infections, tuberculosis, liver injury, lymphomas, and myelosuppression with long term use (Cannon et al., 2004). Biologic agents act by inhibiting IL-6, IL-1ß, and TNF-a immune mediators. Despite their availability and the high cost of injectables, patients are often unable to continue biological therapy or they discontinue their medication after short-term use (Cannon et al., 2004).

2.2 HERBAL PHARMACOTHERAPY IN RA

According to the American College of Rheumatology, conventional medica-tion has limited efficacy and high toxicity. Nowadays people are dissatis-fied with the available conventional therapies and 60–90% of people are dependent on complementary and alternative medicines (Tamhane et al., 2014). But herbs have great potential and no side effects with wide structural diversity which is not commonly seen with synthetic drug molecules. The various phytoconstituents such as flavonoids, terpenoids, steroids, and fatty acids have anti-RA action which has been explored (Kumar et al., 2015). These all phytoconstituents act on inflammatory mediators such as cytokines, chemokines, NO, NF-κB, adhesion molecules, LOX, and arachidonic acid (AA) (Kumar et al., 2015). It is also illustrated in Figure 2.1.

Pomegranate extracts (PE) are obtained from the fruit of *Punica granatum*, which contains polyphenols, ellagitannins, quercetin, gallic, and ellagic acid. The oral administration of PE prevents cartilage destruction in the arthritic rat models (Rasheed et al., 2010).

Thymoquinone (TQ) is a major bioflavonoid isolated from *Nigella sativa* seeds. In Far and middle-Eastern Countries, it is extensively used as an alter-native medicine to treat several diseases. Various literature surveys indicate the benefits of TQ in inflammation such as osteoarthritis. RA and inflam-matory bowel disease (Umar et al., 2015). In a study on adjuvant-induced arthritis (AIA) conducted by Tekeoglu and Colleagues explored when TQ is administered by injection into the intraperitoneal (I.P) cavity it exhibits the same therapeutic value as MTX (Tekeoglu et al., 2007). Another study confirmed that TQ on oral administration at 5 mg/Kg/day leads to inhibition of the serum TNF-a and IL-1β level in RA (Ahmed et al., 2013).

Resveratrol is a polyphenolic compound present in the epidermis of grapes (*Vitis vinifera*). In various literatures, the medicinal use of resveratrol has been reported (Elmali et al., 2007). In Japan and China grape epidermis along with polygonum, cuspidatum roots which are rich in resveratrol are used as indigenous medicine. In rat models, resveratrol on intra-articular injection is effective against RA by retarding the level of ROS, IL-1, PGE2, tumor protein (p53), induced apoptosis, MPPs, and LTB-4 (Baur and Sinclair, 2006).

Citrus flavonoid hesperidin is known for its pharmacological activity and for its therapeutic effect. It has been extensively investigated in arthritis rat models. Studies showed that hesperidin suppresses the proliferation of synoviocytes in the model of rat adjuvant arthritis (Umar et al., 2013). When hesperidin is given an intragastric dose of 80 mg and 160 mg/kg successfully reduced secondary paw-swelling and decreased the production of TNF-a, IL-6, and IL-1 in RA (Umar et al., 2013).

Curcumin is a tetraterpenoid isolated from rhizomes of *Curcuma longa*. It has a broad range of pharmacological activities such as anticancer, anti-inflammatory, and antioxidant effects (Funk et al., 2006). Due to its lipid solubility, its bioavailability is low and clinically not administrated orally. Currently, curcumin is under study for its action against RA. it suppresses the catabolic and inflammatory mediators such as stimulated NO, MMP-3, MMP-9, IL-b, IL-8, COX-2, PGE2, when given intra-peritoneal in a dose of 23 mg total curcuminoids per kg, per day. Furthermore, it also inhibits mediators like JAK/STAT pathways, NF-κB, and JNK in human chondrocytes (Zheng et al., 2015).

Camellia (family Theaceae) is a species of evergreen shrub or small tree whose leaves and leaf buds are used to produce tea. Extract of green tea shows anti-arthritic potential when given orally at 200 mg/kg. Extract of green tea contains epigallocatechin-3-gallate (EGCG) as active constituents. Whereas its administration into the arthritic rats' results to retards the release of IL-1 induced glycosaminoglycan via blocking the activity of NF-κB in chondrocytes. Furthermore, it also inhibits NO synthase (iNOS) which stimulated by IL-1, JNK action, and NO. These three inflammatory biomarkers induce the destruction of cartilage (Ahmed, 2010; Datta et al., 2012). Whereas the RA synovial fibroblasts contain TNF-a-induced ERK (extracellular signal-regulated kinase), MMP-3, MMP-1, JNK, p38, and AP-1 are promptly inhibited by EGCG and also TNF-a-induced ERK (extracellular signal-regulated kinase), MMP-3, MMP-1, JNK, p38, and

AP-1 and inhibits the expression of oncostatin M stimulated CCL2 chemokines in human osteoblasts and significantly lowers the severity of arthritis induced by collagen (CIA). Therefore, *in vitro* and *in vivo* evaluation concluded that EGCG reduces cartilage degradation, synovial hyperplasia, and bone resorption through different targets in the affected joints (Min et al., 2015).

Trypterigium wilfordii contains pentacyclic triterpene called celastrol. It shows anti-inflammatory and anti-tumor activity (Salminen et al., 2010). In China, *T. wilfordii* has traditionally been used as a treatment of RA. Salminen et al. reported the I.P administration of fixed-dose of celastrol at every day to AIA rats, which exhibits an anti-inflammatory potential via inhibition of NF-κB activation and downregulation of caspase 1 (Salminen et al., 2010; Astry et al., 2015). Furthermore, it also down-regulated the TNF and IL-1β secretion in a rat model of AIA. Now, this study reached to clinical trial phase 1 (Astry et al., 2015).

Sinomenine is an alkaloid isolated from the *Sinomenium acutum* plant, which is traditionally used in herbal medicine in Japan and China for RA. Other compounds isolated from the plant include madecassoside, asiaticoside, Asiatic acid, and centelloside. Sinomenine I.P administration of sinomenine suppressing MMP-2, MMP-9, and IL-6 in the animal model of arthritis. A recent study reported that asiaticoside successfully exhibits anti-inflammatory potential by CIA mice. After oral administration of madecassoside at 10, 20, and 40 mg/kg body weight (BW) dose in CIA mice, the histopathology revealed that inflammatory cells infiltration and synovial hyperplasia helps in providing protection against joint destruction (Tong et al., 2015).

The seeds of *Vitex negundo* (Nirgundi) have been widely used as a traditional Ayurvedic and Chinese herbal medicine which is rich in lignans metabolites and used in the treatment of rheumatism and joint inflammation. The entire lignans of *Vitex negundo* (Nirgundi) seeds (TOV) were offered to play an important role in the treatment of arthritis (Rui et al., 2019).

TOV significantly inhibited the paw edema and decreased the arthritis index, with no influence on the BW and the indices of thymus and spleen of CIA rats. Meanwhile, TOV dose-dependently reduced the infiltration of inflammatory cells, synovial hyperplasia, and attenuated cartilage damage (Rui et al., 2019). Additionally, the serum levels of IL-1β, IL-6, IL-8, IL-17A, TNF-α, MMP-3, and MMP-9 were markedly decreased, while the level of serum IL-10 was increased in TOV-treated rats. The significant reduction of the expression of COX-2, iNOS, and p-IκB and the notable increase of IκB in synovial tissues were also observed in TOV-treated animals (Rui et al., 2019). TOV also significantly inhibited acetic acid-induced writhing and decreased xylene-induced ear edema in mice. Furthermore, due to its high efficacy and safety, TOV can be regarded as a promising drug candidate for RA treatment (Rui et al., 2019).

The whole dried *M. pentaphylla* plants were reflux with 70% ethanol for its extracts. The anti-osteoarthritic effect of MPE was checked in a Sprague-Dawley rat model of MIA-induced OA and anti-inflammatory in *in-vitro* lipopolysaccharide (LPS)-treated RAW264.7 cells (Lee et al., 2019). MPE exhibited anti-inflammatory activity via inhibition of the production of NO (57.8%), PGE2 (97.1%), and IL-6 (93.2%) in LPS-treated RAW264.7 cells at 200 µg/m L. In addition, MPE suppressed IL-1β (60.9%), TNF-α (37.9%), and IL-6 (40.9%) production and suppressed the synthesis of MMP-2, MMP-9, and COX-2 in the MIA-induced OA rat model. Furthermore, the results suggest that MPE has significant anti-inflammatory activity and protects cartilage in an OA in the rat model (Lee et al., 2019).

Anoectochilus roxburghii, with rich in the polysaccharide, has been widely used as Chinese herbal medicine for the treatment of RA, liver disease, and diabetes. Pharmacological results displayed that ARP significantly ameliorated the inflammatory cell infiltration, decrease the arthritis index, and the synovial tissue destruction in CIA rats (Guo et al., 2019). It also shows that ARP possessed antioxidant activity and inhibit NO production. Further investigation showed that the anti-inflammatory mechanism of ARP significantly inhibited the activation of nuclear factor-Kβ (NF-Kβ) by suppressing the phosphorylation of I_B and P65, which subsequently down-regulate the mRNA expression of IL-1β and IL-6 in LPS stimulated RAW 264.7 cells. Result suggested that ARP has great potential for the treatment of type II collagen-induced arthritis (CIA) (Guo et al., 2019).

Apigenin (API) is a natural potent compound found in the flavone which is an aglycone part of the glycoside that was suggested as the suppressor of dendritic cell maturation and migration and protects against CIA. In a study found that CIA mice, API suppress arthritis development through the modulation of dendritic cell functions (Chang et al., 2015). Bone marrow-derived dendritic cells (BMDCs) were stimulated *in vitro* with LPS and treated with API for 24 hrs; DC functions, including phenotype expressions, cytokine secretion, phagocytosis, and chemotaxis, were then investigated (Chang et al., 2015). The effects of API on CIA were examined *in vivo*, and purified DCs from the lymph nodes (LNs) of API-treated CIA mice were analyzed for phenotypes and subsets. In *in-vitro*, API efficiently restrained the phenotypic and functional maturation of LPS-stimulated BMDCs while maintaining phagocytotic capabilities. Moreover, API inhibited the chemotactic responses of LPS-stimulated BMDCs, which may be related to the depressive effect on chemokine receptor 4 (CXCR4). In *in-vivo*, API treatment delayed the onset and reduced the severity of arthritis in CIA mice, and diminished secretion of pro-inflammatory cytokines in the serum and supernatants from the LN cells of the CIA mice (Chang et al., 2015). Similar to the *in vitro* findings, the API-treated mice exhibited reduced expression of co-stimulatory molecules and major histocompatibility complex II on DCs. Furthermore, API treatment strongly down-regulated the number of Langerhans cells, but not plasmacy-toid DCs (pDCs) in LNs, which may be related to the depressive effect of API on the expression of CXCR4 on DCs of peripheral blood. These data provide new insight into the mechanism of action of API on arthritis and indicate that the inhibition of maturation and migration of DCs by API may contribute to its immunosuppressive effects (Chang et al., 2015). Therefore, all the above bioactive has also summarized in Table 2.1.

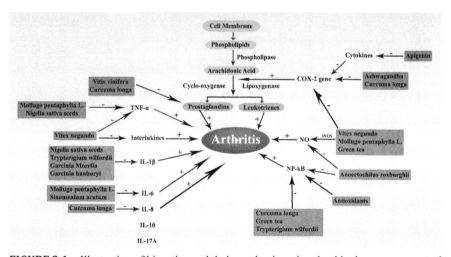

FIGURE 2.1   Illustration of bioactive and their mechanisms involved in the management of rheumatoid arthritis.

2.2.1   ANTIOXIDANT AND ARTHRITIS

In RA patient's administration of high doses of vitamin E were effective in reducing pain symptoms. However, in the *in-vitro* studies show that foods rich in antioxidants have anti-inflammatory effects to be linked to the down-regulation of NF-κB (Sukkar and Rossi, 2004).

TABLE 2.1 Therapeutic Applications of Bioactive in Arthritis

Sl. No.	Phytoconstituents	Sources	MOA and Significance	Challenges	References
1.	Thymoquinone (TQ)	TQ is obtained from the black Caraway seed (*Nigella sativa* Ranunculaceae family)	It exerts antiarthritic action against carrageenan-induced paw edema in rats by inhibiting the inflammatory mediators	It is safe and may cause allergic rashes	Ahmed et al., 2013
2.	Resveratrol	It is obtained from grapes and red wine	It mediated antiarthritic action by targeting NF-Kb and simultaneously decreases AGEs-stimulated expression and prevented AGEs mediated destruction of CIA	Poor oral bioavailability	Baur and Sinclair, 2006
3.	Hesperidin	It is obtained from the fruit of *Citrus aurantium*	It suppresses the T lymphocyte proliferation and IL-2 production in AA rats too.	Limited bioavailability	Umar et al., 2013
4.	Tumeric/Curcumin (*Curcuma longa*)	Curcumin	It acts by inhibition of COX, 5-LOX, and glutathione S Transferase	Higher dose and long-term administration cause nausea and diarrhea	Zheng et al., 2015
5.	Epigallocatechin-3-gallate (EGCG)	Camellia	It acts by blocking the activity of NF-κB. And inhibits nitric oxide synthase (iNOS)	–	Ahmed, 2010; Datta et al., 2012
6.	Celastrol	*Tripterygium wilfordii* (lei gong teng; Thunder of God Vine), which belongs to the Celastraceae family	Celastrol has beneficial antiarthritic effects by suppression of proinflammatory cytokines such as IL-17A, NF-jB mediated MMP-9 expression and lipopolysaccharides	Diarrhea, headache, nausea, and infertility, especially at a high dose.	Salminen et al., 2010; Astry et al., 2015

Sl. No.	Phytoconstituents	Sources	MOA and Significance	Challenges	References
7.	Sinomenine	*Sinomenium acutum*	Sinomenine suppressing MMP-2, MMP-9, and IL-6	Not founds	Tong et al., 2015
8.	Lignans	Seeds of *Vitex negundo*	Reduction of the expression of COX-2, iNOS, and p-IκB and the notable increase of IκB in synovial tissues	—	Rui et al., 2019
9.	*M. pentaphylla*	Dried whole plant used suppressed the NO, PGE2, MMP-2, MMP-9, and COX-2		—	Lee et al., 2019
10.	Polysaccharide	*Anoectochilus roxburghii*	Antioxidant activity and inhibit NO production significantly inhibited the activation of nuclear factor KB	—	Guo et al., 2019
11.	*Boswellia Serrate* (Indian frankincense) Salai/*Salai guggul*	The resin of Boswellia species	Acts via 5-LOX inhibition	Stomach pain, nausea, diarrhea, and allergic rashes reported	Anthoni et al., 2003

— Not founds.

In the experiments on animals, strongly suggest the anti-inflammatory role of an antioxidant such as superoxide dismutase (SOD) and vitamin E in experimentally induced arthritis. Vitamin E seems to withdraw joint destruction and joint inflammation in the transgenic KRN/NOD mouse model of RA, on joint destruction. An antioxidant combination or dose of vitamin E adding high therapeutic value to the treatment for the rheumatoid disease, which can better control the symptoms of arthritis from the first month, and by the second month it controls the rheumatoid disease (Sukkar and Rossi, 2004). Cerhan et al. recommended that intake of certain antioxidants, micronutrients, including of β-cryptoxanthin and supplement zinc and possibly diet rich in fruits and cruciferous vegetables, which has dominant effect in protective role against the development of RA (Cerhan et al., 2003).

2.2.2   TRADITIONAL MEDICINE AND HERBS

Many herbs are still unknown to us and their potential for the treatment of arthritis. But the scientific research has uncovered some of them which have synergistically work to reduce chronic joint inflammation in osteoarthritis, RA, and other types of arthritis (Patwardhan et al., 2010).

2.2.2.1   ASHWAGANDHA

In animal studies, Ashwagandha was found more potent than the phenylbutazone in controlling inflammation. The studies show that animal groups treated with Ashwagandha decrease inflammation proteins, whereas animals treated with phenylbutazone, as well as the control group, had increased inflammatory proteins (Begum et al., 1988). When Ashwagandha extract is compared with hydrocortisone to decrease inflammation, Ashwagandha is far potent. One of the studies shows Ashwagandha had a remarkable effect in decreasing swelling of an arthritic paw, which may have due to COX-2 inhibition (Begum et al., 1988). In another study, 46 patients with RA were given Ashwagandha root powder, in a dose of 4, 6, or 9 grams for 3–4 weeks, which remarkably relieved the pain and swelling in 14 patients, and showed considerable improvement in 10 patients and mild improvement in 11 patients. In one double-blind, placebo-controlled study, the combination of Ashwagandha with zinc and turmeric showed positive effects in osteoarthritis patients with significant improvement in pain severity and disability score (Sharma et al., 2001).

2.2.2.2   WITHANIA

Withania root extract in 1000 mg/kg given orally daily for 15 days to Freund's AIA in rats which shows a significant reduction in both paw swelling and bony degenerative changes as observed by radiologic examination (Begum et al., 1988).

2.2.2.3   BOSWELLIA SERRATA (BS)

The bark of Boswellia (family Burseraceae) having sweet, cooling, and tonic effect and contain boswellic acid resin as the main chemical constituent and it's β-form has anti-inflammatory and anti-arthritic activities. Commonly Boswellia is useful in fever, cough, asthma, urethrorrhea, diaphoresis, convulsion, chronic laryngitis, and jaundice and is analgesic, antihyperlipidemic, and anti-atherosclerotic (James et al., 1991). In both adults and children with RA experienced effective relief from the symptoms when treated with Boswellia, despite having responded poorly in the past to standard therapies such as (NSAIDs) (Kimmatkar et al., 2003). In an animal study, Boswellic acid show significantly reduced in the infiltration of leukocytes in the knee joint and in turn, significantly reduced inflammation (Kimmatkar et al., 2003). A clinical study was conducted to assess the efficacy, safety, and tolerability of *Boswellia serrata* (BS). BS extract was given to the 30 patients of arthritis, 15 each receiving active drug or placebo for 8 weeks founds decrease in knee pain, increase knee flexion, and a decrease in the frequency of swelling in the knee joint (Anthoni et al., 2003).

Aujaie is one of the herbal products prepared by Hamdard Laboratories (Waqf) Pakistan, is believed to have the potential for providing relief from joint pain in (arthritis with or without swelling of joints), gout, lumbago, sciatica, and stiffening of joints and it helps in the excretion of uric acid. Aujaie is prepared from nine different plants; most of these plants have been used in traditional medicines for treating rheumatism and gout-such as *Balsamodendron mukul*, which is very potent in various type of joint problems such as RA, osteoarthritis, gout, inflammatory joints, swelling, and tenderness in inflammatory joints (Akhtar et al., 2003). In order to understand the anti-inflammatory mechanism and antinociceptive activity of the Aujaie. The animal experimental studies in carrageenan induce mice has been carried and founds significant anti-inflammatory results with the dose-dependent manner via inhibition of kinins, cyclooxygenase, histamine, and prostaglandins (Akhtar et al., 2003). Further, the antino-ciceptive activity of Aujaie was evaluated using of the writhing test in mice. Algesia produces by the administration of acetic acid which liberates endogenous substance leads to excite the pain nerve endings. Whereas the Aujaie exerted a significant inhibitory activity on the writhing response with a dose range of 60–240 mg/kg of BW. Therefore, the studies reported that Aujaie a significant anti-inflammatory action and up to the dose of 300 mg/kg/p.o. in mice and 6000 mg/kg/p.o. in rats, did not report any toxic effects (Akhtar et al., 2003).

2.3   CONCLUSION

Treatments for RA have several demerits that hinder their efficacy. Based on inflammatory biomarkers, herbal pharmacotherapy has wide structural diversity and great potential against RA treatment, which is not commonly seen with synthetic treatments. Administration of phyto molecules such as polyphenols, thymoquinone, resveratrol, hesperidin, curcumin, celastrol, and GA, in a dose-dependent manner, gives high efficacy against RA. The benefits are attributed to their targeting action against cytokines, chemokines, adhesion molecules, NF-kβ, NO, etc.

KEYWORDS

- **adjuvant-induced arthritis**
- **arachidonic acid**
- **bone marrow-derived dendritic cells**
- **chemokine receptor 4**
- **collagen-induced arthritis**
- **disease-modifying anti-rheumatic drugs**

REFERENCES

Ahmed, A., Husain, A., Mujeeb, M., et al., (2013). A review on therapeutic potential of *Nigella sativa*: A miracle herb. *Asian Pac. J. Trop. Biomed., 3*, 337–352.

Ahmed, S., (2010). Green tea polyphenol Epigallocatechin 3-gallate in arthritis: Progress and promise. *Arthritis Res. Ther., 12*, 208.

Akhtar, M. S., Malik, A., Saleem, M. S., & Murtaza, G., (2013). Comparative analgesic and anti-inflammatory activities of two polyherbal tablet formulations (Aujaie and Surangeen) in rats. *Tropical Journal of Pharmaceutical Research, 12*(4), 603–607.

Anderson, K. O., Bradley, L. A., Young, L. D., et al., (1985). Rheumatoid arthritis: Review of psychological factors related to etiology, effects, and treatment. *Psychol. Bull., 98*, 358–387.

Anthoni, C., Laukoetter, M. G., & Rijcken, E., (2003). Mechanisms underlying the anti-inflammatory actions of boswellic acid derivatives in experimental colitis. *Indian J. Exp. Biol., 41*(12), 1460–1462.

Araki, Y., Tsuzuki, W. T., Aizaki, Y., et al., (2016). Histone methylation and STAT3 differentially regulate IL-6-induced MMP gene activation in rheumatoid arthritis synovial fibroblasts. *Arthritis Rheumatol., 68*, 1111–1123.

Astry, B., Venkatesha, S. H., Laurence, A., et al., (2015). Celastrol, a Chinese herbal compound, controls autoimmune inflammation by altering the balance of pathogenic and regulatory T-cells in the target organ. *Clin. Immunol., 157*, 228–238.

Baur, J. A., & Sinclair, D. A., (2006). Therapeutic potential of resveratrol: The *in vivo* evidence. *Nat. Rev. Drug Discov., 5*, 493–506.

Begum, V. H., & Sadique, J., (1988). Long term effect of herbal drug *Withaniasomnifera* on adjuvant induced arthritis in rats. *Indian J. Exp. Biol.,26*(11), 877–882.

Cannon, G. W., Holden, W. L., Juhaeri, J., Dai, W., et al., (2004). Adverse events with disease modifying antirheumatic drugs (DMARD): A cohort study of leflunomide compared with other DMARD. *J. Rheumatol., 31*, 1906–1911.

Cerhan, J. R., Saag, K. G., Merlino, L. A., Mikuls, T. R., & Criswell, L. A., (2003). Antioxidant micronutrients and risk of rheumatoid arthritis in a cohort of older women. *Am. J. Epidemiol., 157*(4), 345–354.

Chang, X., He, H., Zhu, L., et al., (2015). Protective effect of apigenin on Freund's complete adjuvant-induced arthritis in rats via inhibiting P2X7/NF-κB pathway. *Chem. Biol. Interact., 236*, 41–46.

Datta, P., Sarkar, A., Biswas, A. K., et al., (2012). Antiarthritic activity of aqueous extract of Indian black tea in experimental and clinical study. *Orient Pharm. Exp. Med., 12*, 265–271.

Elmali, N., Baysal, O., Harma, A., et al., (2007). Effects of resveratrol in inflammatory arthritis. *Inflammation, 30*, 1–6.

Firestein, G. S., (2003). Evolving concepts of rheumatoid arthritis. *Nature, 423*, 356–361.

Funk, J. L.,Oyarzo, J. N., Frye, J. B., et al., (2006). Turmeric extracts containing curcuminoids prevent experimental rheumatoid arthritis. *J. Nat. Prod., 69*, 351–355.

Guo, Y., Ye, Q., Yang, S., et al., (2019). Therapeutic effects of polysaccharides from *Anoectochilus roxburghii* on type II collagen-induced arthritis in rats. *Int. J. Biol. Macromol., 122*, 882–892.

Ismail, H. M., Yamamoto, K., Vincent, T. L., Nagase, H., et al., (2015). Interleukin-1 acts via the JNK-2 signaling pathway to induce aggrecan degradation by human chondrocytes. *Arthritis Rheumatol., 67*, 1826–1836.

James, J., Gormley, H. P., & Ammon, (1991). *Boswellia serrata*: An ancient herb for arthritis, cholesterol, and more better nutrition. *Planta Med., 57*(3), 203–207.

Kimmatkar, N., Thawani, V., Hingorani, L., et al., (2003). Efficacy and tolerability of *Boswellia serrata* extract in treatment of osteoarthritis of knee-a randomized double blind placebo controlled trial. *Phytomed., 10*(1), 3–7.

Kumar, V., Al-Abbasi, F. A.,Verma, A., et al., (2015). Umbelliferone b-Dgalactopyranoside exerts an anti-inflammatory effect by attenuating COX-1 and COX-2. *Toxicol. Res., 4,* 1072–1084.

Lee, Y. M., Son, E., Kim, S. H., et al., (2019). Anti-inflammatory and anti-osteoarthritis effect of *Mollugo pentaphylla* extract. *Pharmaceutical Biology, 57,* 74–81.

Min, S. Y., Yan, M., Kim, S. B., et al., (2015). Green tea epigallocatechin-3-gallate suppresses autoimmune arthritis through indoleamine 2, 3-dioxygenase expressing dendritic cells and the nuclear factor, erythroid 2- like 2 antioxidant pathways. *J. Inflamm (Lond)., 15,* 53.

Patwardhan, K. K., Kaumudee, S. B., & Sameer, S. G., (2010). Coping with arthritis using safer herbal options. *Int. J. Pharm. Sci., 2*(1), 1–8.

Rahman, M., Beg, S., Sharma, G., et al., (2015). Emergence of lipid based vesicular carriers as nanoscale pharmacotherapy in rheumatoid arthritis. *Recent Pat. Nanomed., 5,* 111–121.

Rahman, M., Beg, S., Sharma, G., et al., (2016). Lipid-based vesicular nanocargoes as nanotherapeutic targets for the effective management of rheumatoid arthritis. *Recent Pat. Antiinfect Drug Discov., 11,* 3–15.

Rasheed, Z., Akhter, N. H. T., Haqqi, T. M., et al., (2010). Pomegranate extract inhibits the interleukins-1b-induced activation of MKK-3, p38 a-MAPK and transcription factor RUNX-2 in human osteoarthritis chondrocytes. *Arthritis Res. Ther., 12,* R195.

Rui, J.,Yanfei, B.,Weiheng, X., et al., (2019). Therapeutic effects of the total lignans from *Vitex negundo* seeds on collagen-induced arthritis in rats. *Phytomedicine., 58,* 152825.

Salminen, A., Lehtonen, M., Paimela, T., et al., (2010). Celastrol: Molecular targets of thunder god vine. *Biochem. Biophys Res. Commun., 394,* 439–442.

Scrivo, R., Di Franco, M., Spadaro, A., et al., (2007). The immunology of rheumatoid arthritis. *Ann. N.Y. Acad. Sci., 1108,* 312–322.

Sharma, P. C., Yelne, M. B., & Dennis, T. J., (2001). *Database on Medicinal Plants Used in Ayurveda* (Vol. 1, p. 120). New Delhi: Central Council for Research in Ayurveda and Siddha.

Smolen, J. S., Breedveld, F. C., Burmester, G. R., Bykerk, V., et al., (2016). Treating rheumatoid arthritis to target, 2014 update of the recommendations of an international task force. *Ann. Rheum. Dis., 75,* 3–15.

Song, F., Tang, J., Geng, R., et al., (2014). Comparison of the efficacy of bone marrow mononuclear cells and bone mesenchymal stem cells in the treatment of osteoarthritis in a sheep model. *Int. J. Clin. Exp. Pathol., 7,* 1415–1426.

Sukkar, S. G., & Rossi, E., (2004). Oxidative stress and nutritional prevention in autoimmune rheumatic diseases. *Autoimmun. Rev., 3,* 199–206.

Tamhane, A., Gerald, M. J. R.,David, T. R., et al., (2014). Complementary and alternative medicine use in African Americans with rheumatoid arthritis. *Arthritis Care Res. (Hoboken), 66,* 180–189.

Tekeoglu, I., Dogan, A., Ediz, L., et al., (2007). Effects of thymoquinone (volatile oil of black cumin) on rheumatoid arthritis in rat models. *Phytother. Res., 21,* 895–897.

Tong, B., Yu, J., Wang, T., et al., (2015). Sinomenine suppresses collagen-induced arthritis by reciprocal modulation of regulatory T cells and Th17 cells in gut-associated lymphoid tissues. *Mol. Immunol., 65,* 94–103.

Umar, S., Hedaya, O., Singh, A. K., et al., (2015). Thymoquinone inhibits TNF-alpha-induced inflammation and cell adhesion in rheumatoid arthritis synovial fibroblasts by ASK1 regulation. *Toxicol. Appl. Pharmacol., 287,* 299–305.

Umar, S., Kumar, A., Sajad, M., et al., (2013). Hespiridininhibits collagen induced arthritis possibly through suppression of free radical load and reduction in neutrophil activation and infiltration. *Rheumatol. Int., 33*, 657–663.

Zheng, Z., Sun, Y., Liu, Z., et al., (2015). The effect of curcumin and its nanoformulation on adjuvant induced 21 arthritis in rats. *Drug Des. Devel. Ther., 9*, 4931–4942.

CHAPTER 3

Curcumin Nanomedicine and Their Application in the Management of Disease

SADAF JAMAL GILANI,[1] SYED SARIM IMAM,[2] MOHAMMED JAFAR,[3] SULTAN ALSHEHRI,[2] MOHAMAD TALEUZZAMAN,[4] and MOHAMMED ASADULLAH JAHANGIR[5]

[1] College of Basic Health Sciences, Princess Nourah bint Abdulrahman University, Riyadh 11671, Saudi Arabia

[2] College of Pharmacy, King Saud University, Riyadh, Saudi Arabia

[3] College of Clinical Pharmacy, Imam Abdulrahman Bin Faisal University, Dammam, Saudi Arabia

[4] Faculty of Pharmacy, Maulana Azad University, Jodhpur, Rajasthan, India

[5] Nibha Institute of Pharmaceutical Sciences, Rajgir, Nalanda, Bihar, India

ABSTRACT

Curcumin is a naturally occurring bioactive compound obtained from the rhizomes of *Curcuma longa* Linn. The therapeutic application of curcumin has shown a wide range of biological actions in various diseases. It has shown excellent therapeutic benefits in various diseases (cancer, inflammation, cardiac disease, skin disease, Alzheimer's disease (AD), etc.). Despite having great therapeutic application their clinical use is limited due to low solubility, physicochemical instability, poor bioavailability, rapid metabolism, and poor pharmacokinetics (PKs). These problems can be overcome by delivering an efficient nanodelivery system. The curcumin's PKs, systemic bioavailability, and biological activity have been established by loading curcumin into nanoformulations. By developing a nanoformulations of curcumin their bioavailability can be enhanced due to the nanosize the greater surface area available for the absorption. The current chapter provides an overview of an efficient curcumin nanoformulation administered by different routes for various human diseases.

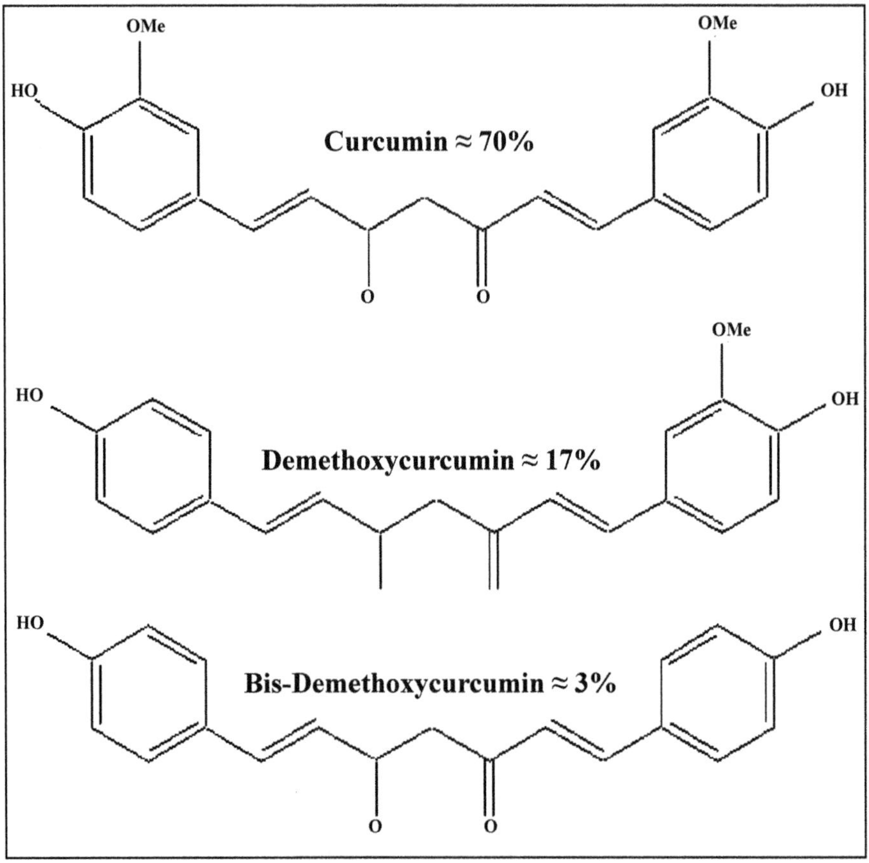

FIGURE 3.1 Three major constituents of curcumin.

3.1 INTRODUCTION

The use of *Curcuma longa* (Linn.), i.e., turmeric as a medicine for treating different local and systemic diseases is not new; it was since antediluvian time of Ayurveda. This herb is widely cultivated in tropical, sub-tropical, and southeast areas for wide use as an ingredient spice (Figure 3.1). Curcumin

(CUR) is a naturally occurring polyphenolic herbal compound isolated from the rhizomes of *Curcuma longa* Linn (Zingiberaceae). The chemical formula of CUR is (1,7-bis[4-hydroxy-3-methoxyphenyl]-1,6-heptadiene-3,5-dione). The structure of curcumin is first identified by Lampe and Milobedeska in 1910 and curcumin is also known as diferuloylmethane (Milobedeska et al., 1910). It contains heptadiene-dione moiety with a molecular mass of 368.37 g/mole and a melting temperature of 183°C. The two para hydroxyl groups, keto groups, methoxy groups, an active methylene group. However, the solution of curcumin has an enol group while it is more stable in keto form (Meeta et al., 2017). The reported solubility of CUR was only approximately 11 ng/mL in plain aqueous buffer (pH = 5.0) (Tonnesen et al., 2002). There are different chemical constituents have been isolated from turmeric, and curcumin was found to be the most important polyphenol constituents cited in the number of literature (Tyagi et al., 2015). The three different major chemical constituents available in turmeric include curcumin I (~75%), dimethoxy curcumin (~20%), and bisdemethoxycurcumin (~5%) (Figure 3.1). It is unstable in neutral or alkaline conditions owing to rapid hydrolytic degradation but found stable in an acidic environment (pH~ 3) (Wang et al., 1997). Curcumin has reported poor oral absorption due to its low solubility in acidic or neutral conditions and poor stability in gastrointestinal fluids (Min, 2012). The poor solubility of curcumin in water leads to poor absorption and low bioavailability upon oral administration. The concentration of curcumin in human plasma is consistently in the nanomolar range even after high oral doses (i.e., 10–12 g/day) (Vareed et al., 2008). There are about major amount curcumin (60–70%) undergoes fast clearance and is eliminated mostly in the feces. However, it is soluble in lipid, which could still induce changes in biomarkers with oral doses as little as 50 mg. Moreover, it can easily bind to different proteins in the body, including a plasma protein albumin; these proteins can act as a carrier for curcumin (Gupta et al., 2012). The rapid elimination could also be an important factor leading to low systemic bioavailability of curcumin (Ireson et al., 2002). It is metabolized in the liver and intestine to form different metabolites such as glucuronide and sulfate conjugates (Lee, 2014). Recently curcumin is gaining popularity among the researchers due to their wide range of therapeutic efficacy and is nicknamed as next-generation multipurpose drug' owing to its multifaceted roles (Figure 3.2). There is a wide range of therapeutic efficacy like anti-cancer, anti-diabetic, antioxidant, antiangiogenic, anti-inflammatory, and antimicrobial activities (Gupta et al., 2012; Lee et al., 2013, 2014). There are different nanoformulation based delivery systems such as nanoparticles

(NPs), liposomes, and nanoemulsions have been designed for curcumin to enhance its poor aqueous solubility (Nair et al., 2012; Gosangari et al., 2012). Moreover, recent reports are emphasizing the role of novel curcumin formulations in ameliorating clinical response and alleviating the toxic effects of curcumin that appeared in the scientific literature (Lee et al., 2014). Although several nanosized delivery systems have been developed, high importance is given on discussing nanoparticles, liposomes, micelles, nanoemulsions, and cyclodextrin due to their significant role in the safe and effective delivery of curcumin in the required site. Both invasive and noninvasive application routes have been studied for effective local, circulatory, affinity, or active targeting of curcumin (Gupta et al., 2013). The improved bioavailability has been reported by these delivery systems, but the application of novel formulations pays attention to efficient targeting of curcumin at the diseased area with the aid of antibody, aptamer, and peptide mediation (Yallapu et al., 2013). The effective nanoformulation loaded with curcumin enhances solubility and stability and prevent rapid drug metabolism and degradation.

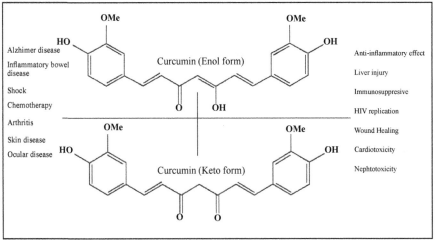

FIGURE 3.2   Curcumin form (Keto and Enol) with their wide range application in various disease.

3.2   CURCUMIN NANOFORMULATIONS

In this chapter, the main emphasis is given on the latest developments in curcumin nanoformulation for improved therapeutic outcomes. There was significant progress that took place in the development of curcumin nanoformulations like liposome, polymeric nanoparticles, solid lipid nanoparticles (SLN), micelles, NLCs since the past few years. Curcumin exhibits poor physicochemical stability, limited aqueous solubility, and undergoes acidic/alkaline degradation, susceptible oxidation, and photo-degradation. There are many research reports published of curcumin nanoformulations that proved the enhancement in the physicochemical stability after loading in nanosized particles (Table 3.1).

3.2.1   APPLICATION OF CURCUMIN NANOFORMULATION IN CANCER

There are numerous studies reported the anticancer activity of curcumin at concentrations between 5 and 50 M (Lee et al., 2015). The formulations loaded with curcumin significantly internalize in cancer cells through endocytosis in the existence of endocytosis inhibitors and active form of curcumin releases to produce the therapeutic effects (Yallapu et al., 2014; Nagahama et al., 2015). Research group Mangalathillam et al. reported about curcumin chitin nano gel formulation and evaluation for *in vitro* anticancer activity on breast cancer cell line and reported the amelioration in bioavailability and anticancer effects (Mangalathillam et al., 2012). The cationic liposome-encapsulated with curcumin was developed and evaluated for antitumor effects were reported by researchers Sun et al. (2010). The result of the study revealed an enhanced anti-tumor effect on colon/melanoma tumor growth in mice. The curcumin/LPPC formulations showed a greater anti-proliferative effect by a rapid burst of the tumor cells (Sun et al., 2010). The major development takes place by the development of curcumin nanoparticles (nano-curcumin) by researchers from Johns Hopkins University School of Medicine and the University of Delhi and dispersed the nano curcumin into aqueous media. The prepared coated nanoparticle enhances the water solubility and rapidly absorbed into the bloodstream. The formulation of nano curcumin evaluated on human cancer cells, such as inhibition of NF-kB and down-regulation of interleukin-6 (IL-6). The result of the depicted better therapeutic effects than pure curcumin. (Bisht et al., 2007). In another research study, curcumin-loaded nanoemulsion (CUR-NEM) prepared and showed particles of 200 nm (PDI 0.2) with negative zeta potential (–30 mV) and a high curcumin yield (95%).

The formulation CUR-NEM further evaluated for *in vitro* assays and showed that CUR-NEM is safe in non-cancerous human cells (HEK-293T) and cytotoxic in gastric (AGS), colon (HT29-ATCC, HT29-US), breast

TABLE 3.1 Curcumin Loaded Nanoformulation with Their Expected Benefits in Different Disease

Formulation	Disease	Findings	References
Nano-micelle	Diabetes	Significant decrease was found in HbA1C, FBG, TG, and BMI comparing results of each subject before and after the treatment (p<0.05).	Rahimi et al., 2016
PLGA microspheres	Diabetes	In type 2 diabetic rats, the Cur-loaded scaffold also showed a greater bone formation capability compared to the pure scaffold.	Li et al., 2018
Nanoparticles	Diabetes	Nano-curcumin and AGE suspension have shown therapeutic potential in the treatment of Diabetic cardiomyopathy, by attenuating cardiac inflammation, myocardial fibrosis, and programmed myocardial cell deaths through inhibiting OS and AGEPs accumulation in diabetic heart tissue.	Abdel-Mageid et al., 2018
Nano–particulate	Cancer	A ten-fold increase in solubility, a three-fold increase in anti-cancer activity, and a significant reduction in the levels of cellular HIF-1α and nuclear p65 (Rel A) were observed for cur-PLGA-NP, when compared to free curcumin.	Khan et al., 2018
Nanoemulsion	Toxoplasmosis	Decrease of cyst numbers was verified by the downregulation of BAG1 in treatment groups compared with a negative control group with a minimum relative expression in CR-NE (1.12 ± 0.28), CR-S (11.76 ± 0.87), and NE-no CR (14.67 ± 0.77), respectively (P<0.001).	Azami et al., 2018
Niosomes	Cervical cancer	The niosomes exhibited higher antitumor efficiency than free Cur. Cur-loaded niosomes induced HeLa229 cells to apoptosis by destroying mitochondrion of cervical tumor cells, simultaneously changing nuclear morphology, and blocking tumor cell proliferation.	You et al., 2019
Polymeric nanoparticles	CNS disorder	Pharmacokinetic analysis after oral delivery of nano-curcumin in mice demonstrated an approximately 20-fold reduction in dose requirement when compared to unformulated curcumin to achieve comparable plasma and central nervous system (CNS) tissue concentrations.	Szymusiak et al., 2016

Formulation	Disease	Findings	References
Nanoparticle	Antimicrobial	*In vitro* antibacterial activity of Nanocurcu was evaluated against *Escherichia coli*, *Staphylococcus aureus*, and *Pseudomonas aeruginosa*. The cream containing Nanocurcu was found to be effective against human bacterial pathogens and hence can be used for the treatment of bacterial diseases.	Pandit et al., 2015
Nanoparticle	Anti-bacterial, Anti-oxidant, Anti-cancer	The Minimum inhibitory concentration of CMNPs against *S. aureus* (~250 µg/mL) was lower than CM-DMSO (~500 µg/mL). Meanwhile, CM NPs showed effective antioxidant ability at a concentration ranging from 125–2000 µg/m L. CM NPs showed time-dependent intracellular internalization ability, resulting in an enhanced anti-cancer effect on colorectal cancer cells.	Xie et al., 2015
Nanoparticle	Alzheimer disease	The results from the Morris water maze proved that PLGA-PEG-B6/Cur improves the spatial learning and memory capability of APP/PS1 mice. The *ex vivo* assays including Bielschowsky silver staining, immunostaining, and western blotting demonstrated that PLGA-PEG-B6/Cur could reduce hippocampal β-amyloid formation and deposit and tau hyperphosphorylation.	Fan et al., 2018
Nanoemulsion gel	Arthritis	A 28-day anti-arthritic evaluation (body weight, paw edema, tibiotarsal joint thickness, TNF-α, and IL-1β levels, and histopathology) on Freund's complete adjuvant-induced arthritic rat model after topical application of CR-NE gel in Wistar rats demonstrated substantial reversal of arthritic symptoms.	Naz and Ahmad, 2015

(MDA-MB-231) and melanoma (B16F10) cells. Further, *in vivo* studies, results revealed that the single dose-treated C57BL/6 mice demonstrated sufficient to completely prevent re incidence tumor growth and spontaneous lung metastasis. The untreated animals showed the incidence and metastasis in about 70% of animals (Guerrero et al., 2018). The research group Martey et al. (2017) used second-generation curcumin derivative in the formulation of styrene-maleic acid (SMA) micelles. The study result showed the formulation of treated group animals enhance biodistribution and drug accumulation about 16-folds in the tumor treated group as compared to control. It also significantly suppressed tumor growth compared to control in a xenograft model of triple-negative breast cancer. The curcumin encapsulated micelle treated mice showed a decrease in angiogenesis and an increase in apoptosis. Another research group developed curcumin SLN and evaluated for human breast adenocarcinoma cells. The optimized formulation showed nanoparticle size, PDI, and encapsulation of 226.8 ± 3.92 nm, 0.24 ± 0.02, and $67.88 \pm 2.08\%$, respectively. The cellular uptake study was evaluated on human breast adenocarcinoma cells at 1 h and 4 h time points. The developed formulation showed enhanced cellular uptake compared to free CUR. The cell viability study performed at 50 µg/mL after 24 h treatments and the study result revealed reduced cell viability ($43.97 \pm 1.53\%$) compared to free CUR ($59.33 \pm 0.95\%$) (Bhatt et al., 2018).

In another study, the *in vitro* efficacy on DU145 prostate cancer cells were evaluated for the curcumin and resveratrol-loaded calcium alginate nanoparticles. The developed formulation showed the particle size (12.53 ± 1.06 nm) with the entrapment efficiency for curcumin ($49.3 \pm 4.3\%$) and resveratrol ($70.99 \pm 6.1\%$). The cytotoxic effects on DU145 cells were observed from the drug-loaded nanoparticles (Saralkar and Dash, 2017). Anitha et al. developed and evaluated curcumin-loaded N, O-CMC nanoparticles, and the formulation showed the nanoparticle size (150 ± 30 nm) with high entrapment efficiency. Further, the developed formulation evaluated for the cytotoxicity studies using MTT assay. The result of the study revealed that curcumin-N, O-CMC nanoparticles found specific toxicity towards cancer cells and non-toxic to the normal cells (Anitha et al., 2012). Thadakapally et al. formulated serum stable long-circulating curcumin polymeric nanoparticles with modification with albumin-bound technology. The polyethylene glycol-albumin-curcumin nanoparticles were evaluated for tissue uptake and kupffer cell uptake study in rats after i.v. administration and further the cell viability assay was performed using a breast cancer cell line MD-MB-231. The comparative antiproliferative activity of polyethylene glycol-albumin-curcumin nanoparticle and neat curcumin was performed and nanoparticle formulation was found more effective. So from the result of the study, it has been concluded that the curcumin nanoparticles can be easily used in breast cancer with enhanced efficacy compared to conventional treatment therapies (Thadakapally et al., 2016).

In another study, the nanoformulation loaded with curcumin was developed by ionotropic pre-gelation followed by polycationic cross-linking using alginate (ALG), chitosan (CS), and pluronic (Das et al., 2010). The developed formulation was evaluated for cytotoxicity assay and the result of the study showed that composite NPs at a concentration of 500 mcg/mL were nontoxic to HeLa cells. The green fluorescence inside the HeLa cells was used to confirm the cellular internalization of curcumin-loaded composite NPs. The half-maximal inhibitory concentrations for free curcumin and encapsulated curcumin were found to be 13.28 and 14.34 muM, respectively.

3.2.2 APPLICATION OF CURCUMIN NANOFORMULATION IN INFLAMMATION

In one of the investigations, the research group prepared curcumin nano-emulsion by titration method and further converted to Carbopol 934 gel. The developed formulation was evaluated for the anti-inflammatory effect by using the carrageenan-induced paw edema method in rats using Diclofenac as a reference. The anti-inflammatory study results were found comparable with standard Diclofenac. The histology of the formulation-treated skin showed insignificant changes in skin integrity (Al-Rohaimi, 2015). In another research study, curcumin nanoemulsion was prepared and disclosed in the results that significant enhancement in the plasma concentrations achieved in mice after oral administration (Youg et al., 2014). The *in-vivo* immuno-suppressive effect of curcumin nanoemulsion was further examined to better understand the therapeutic potential. The oral administration of curcumin nanoemulsion resulted in a reduction of blood monocytes, decreased levels of both TLR4 and RAGE expression, and inhibited secretion of MCP-1. The result of the study demonstrated that curcumin can suppress inflammation by inhibiting macrophage migration via NFB and MCP-1 inhibition. In another study, Kakker et al. reported about tetrahydrocurcumin (THC) as a stable colorless hydrogenated product of curcumin with superior antioxidant and anti-inflammatory properties. In the present study, topical bioavailability of THC was enhanced by formulating into a nano-carrier system based hydrogel. The formulation THC-SLNs gel showed higher skin permeation (about 17 folds) as compared to free THC gel. The pharmacodynamic anti-inflammatory activity was assessed in an excision wound mice model and the result revealed the enhanced biological activity of THC-SLNs gel (Kakker et al., 2018).

Other research groups developed curcumin in CD44-targeting hyaluronate-polylactide (HA-PLA) nanoparticles (NPs) for the modulation of macrophage polarity from the pro-inflammatory M1 to the anti-inflammatory M2 pheno-type. The results of the study revealed that the curcumin nanoparticle found with an average diameter of 102.5 nm and also showed greater cellular uptake. The results suggested that the curcumin CD44-targeting HA-PLA NPs formu-lation showed a promising result for the treatment of inflammatory diseases (Farajzadeh et al., 2018). The curcumin nano-formulation was prepared with embryonic stem cell exosomes (MESC-occur), restored neurovascular loss following ischemia-reperfusion (IR) injury in mice. The MESC curcumin-treated animals decreased the astrocytic GFAP expression and alleviated the expression of NeuN positive neurons in IR-injured mice (Kalani et al., 2016).

The research group formulated curcumin nanoemulsion to assess the *in-vivo* anti-inflammatory activity and arthritic activity using carrageenan-induced paw edema and FCA induced arthritic rat model. The optimized curcumin nanoemulsion with emu oil was converted into carbopol gel and their biological activities were measured. The curcumin formulation in combination with emu oil showed significant improvement in anti-inflammatory activity and arthritic scoring, paw volume, biochemical, molecular, radiological, and histological examinations (Jeengar et al., 2016). The formulation of curcumin loaded self-nano emulsifying drug delivery system (SNEDDS) has been prepared and evaluated. The optimized formu-lation comprised of ethyl oleate:tween 80:PEG 600 (50:40:10% w/w) with 11.2-nm uniform droplets showed a significant increment of 3.95 times in Cmax, and the curcumin bioavailability was enhanced by 194.2%, compared to the curcumin suspension in water (Nazari et al., 2017).

3.2.3   APPLICATION OF CURCUMIN NANOFORMULATION IN MICROBIAL INFECTIONS

There are many antimicrobial activities that have been reported about curcumin to get insight into the aspect of controlling pathogens. It has shown a wide range of activity against different microorganisms such as

B. subtilis, S. aureus, P. aeruginosa, E. coli, A. niger, P. notatum, S. para-typhi, M. tuberculosis, and certain different pathogenic fungi (Meeta et al., 2017). The formulation of silver-curcumin nanoconjugates (Ag-CurNCs) were prepared and evaluated for cytotoxicity study on different skin cell lines and antibacterial activity. The developed formulation was evaluated for antibacterial activity and results showed significant antibacterial activity against *E. coli* with minimal toxicity to skin cells (Abdellah et al., 2018). Curcumin solubility and dispersing ability has been improved by preparing the nanoformulation and lead to enhanced antibacterial activity. In 2015, Gera et al. prepared a nano-curcumin formulation and the result of the study concluded that the developed formulation showed controlled drug release efficacy and also greater bioactivity against different pathogenic and non-pathogenic microbial strains (Meeta et al., 2015). In another research, Vimala et al. reported the entrapment of curcumin with CS-PVA-silver nano-composite films and evaluated for the anti-microbial wound/burn dressings. The result showed that there is significant inhibition in the growth of *E. coli* in comparison with native curcumin or CS-PVA-silver nanoparticles film discretely (Vimala et al., 2010).

Another research group Madan et al. developed liposomal gel formulation of curcumin and their efficacy compared with azithromycin for treatment of Acne. The curcumin liposomal dispersion depicted greater stability and was further converted into carbopol gel. The pharmacokinetics (PKs) study results revealed curcumin liposomal gel achieved quick Tmax for curcumin within 1 h due to quick penetration of nano-sized liposomes. The stratum corneum Cmax was found to be 688.3 ng/mL and AUC0-t of 5857.5 h×ng/mL, while the skin samples displayed Cmax of 203.3 ng/gm and AUC0-t of 2938.1 h×ng/gm. The antibacterial activity was performed using agar diffusion assay method and their co-application (1:1) displayed significantly greater antibacterial effect against both macrolide-sensitive (1.81 versus 1.25 folds) and resistant strains of P. acnes (2.93 versus 1.22 folds). The *in vivo* study revealed that co-application of curcumin and lauric acid liposomal gel in rat ear model displayed a 2 fold reduction in comedones count and cytokines (TNF- and IL-1) in compare to placebo-treated group (Madan et al., 2018).

Another antibacterial study reported by research group Ghaffari et al. by formulating curcumin and ampicillin SLNs. The prepared nanoparticles were found spherical in shape and particle size (112–121 nm), with low zeta potential. The developed formulations were evaluated for antibacterial assessment and showed reasonable anti-bacterial effects with an increase in the rate of wound healing (Ghaffari et al., 2018). In another study, curcumin nanoparticles were developed by wet-milling techniques to enhance its aqueous-phase solubility and antimicrobial properties. The nano-curcumin was found with a narrow particle size range of 2–40 nm. The developed formulation was further evaluated for minimum inhibitory concentration for a variety of bacterial and fungal strains. The result showed that the aqueous dispersion of nano-curcumin was much more effective than neat curcumin against different microorganisms like *S. aureus, B. subtilis, E. coli, P. aeruginosa, P. notatum,* and *A. niger.* The mechanism involved in the antibacterial action of curcumin nanoparticles revealed that these particles entered inside the bacterial cell by completely breaking the cell wall, leading to cell death. There was a marked enhancement in the water solubility and antimicrobial activity of developed nanoparticle due to the reduction in particle size up to the nano range. The activity was more effective against Gram-positive bacteria than Gram-negative bacteria (Bhawana et al., 2011). In this study, it reports the antimicrobial assessment of poly (–caprolactone)/curcumin/grape leaf extract-Ag hybrid nanoparticles (PCL/Cur/GLE-Ag NPs) were evaluated. The antimicrobial characteristics were evaluated against gram-positive and gram-negative bacteria in addition to two fungal strains. The study revealed hybrid NPs have potent antimicrobial activity against pathogenic bacteria species and could be considered as an alternative antibacterial agent (El-Sherbiny et al., 2016).

3.2.4 APPLICATION OF CURCUMIN NANOFORMULATION IN CARDIAC DISEASES

One of the studies was designed to evaluate the cardioprotective effect of curcumin and nisin loaded polylactic acid (PLA) nanoparticle (CurNisNp) on isoproterenol (ISO) induced MI in guinea pigs. The different parameters like electrocardiogram (ECG), blood samples, and tissue biopsies were collected for analyses. The formulation CurNisNp showed LC$_{50}$ of 3258.2 g/mL and MI induction caused atrial fibrillation was prevented by pretreatment of CurNisNp. The increased expressions of cardiac troponin I (CTnI) and kidney injury molecule-1 (KIM-1) were significantly decreased in guinea pigs pretreated with metoprolol or CurNisNp (P<0.05). This study result revealed the formulated nanoparticle confers a significant level of cardioprotection in the guinea pig (Nabofa et al., 2018). The curcumin nanoparticles were prepared for the treatment of monocrotaline (MCT)-induced pulmonary arterial hypertension (HTN) in Sprague Dawley rat. The curcumin nanoparticles administration was associated with reduced right ventricular (RV) wall thickness and a decreased right ventricle weight/body weight (BW) ratio (Rice et al., 2016).

3.2.5   APPLICATION OF CURCUMIN NANOFORMULATION IN CNS DISORDERS

Curcumin was encapsulated in the NPs to develop a delivery platform to treat diseases involving oxidative stress affecting the CNS. The curcumin loaded nanoparticles able to avoid the oxidative stress and linked to polymer architecture (Rabanel et al., 2015). The study reported by researchers Huo et al. about the development of curcumin nanoformulation and their therapeutic potential in Alzheimer's disease. The curcumin loaded selenium-PLGA nanospheres (NSs) able to decrease the amyloid-load in the brain samples. The specific binding of curcumin selenium PLGA NSs with A plaques was observed by fluorescence microscopic technique. The curcumin loaded Se-PLGA nanoformulation has shown the delivery system able to target the disease and effective way to treat Alzheimer's disease (Huo et al., 2019). In another research, curcumin-encapsulated PLGA nanoparticles (Cur-PLGA-NPs) was prepared and evaluated to induce *in vitro* neuronal differentiation in the hippocampus and subventricular zone of adult rats. The developed formulation significantly increases the gene expression involved in cell proliferation and neuronal differentiation. The nanoparticles reverse learning and memory impairments in an amyloid beta-induced rat model by inducing neurogenesis. These findings of the study revealed that curcumin nanoparticles may offer a healing approach to treat neurodegenerative diseases such as Alzheimer's disease, by increasing brain self-repair mechanism (Tiwari et al., 2014).

The curcumin loaded nanoliposomes designed to maintain the planar structure required for interaction with Amyloid. The curcumin loaded liposomes had shown the size in the nano range (131–207 nm) with slightly negative-potential values. They explained that the developed formulation with a very high affinity for A1–42 fibrils, to be exploited as vectors for the targeted delivery of new diagnostic and therapeutic molecules for Alzheimer's disease (Mourtas et al., 2011). The curcumin nanoformulation was prepared by Ramalingam et al. (2015) using N-trimethyl CS administered by the oral route. The developed formulation was surface-modified with solid lipids for successful brain distribution. The formulation poly (N-isopropyl acrylamide) curcumin nanoformulation has depicted greater neurobehavioral activity and reduced cytokine levels in middle cerebral artery occlusion induced cerebral ischemic rats (Ahmad et al., 2014). In another study curcumin, SLN formulation prepared and evaluated for the behavioral, oxidative, nitrosative stress, and physiological parameters in cerebral ischemic-reperfusion injury in rats. The study result revealed curcumin SLN formulation showed a protective role to the treated group (Kakkar et al., 2013).

3.2.6   APPLICATION OF CURCUMIN NANOFORMULATION IN SKIN DISEASE

The hydrogel loaded curcumin nanoparticle (Cur-NP/HG) formulation as topical delivery was developed by Kamar et al. for skin disease. The application Cur-NP/HG treated rats showed marked improvement in the healing process with complete re-epithelization. The developed formulation showed effective improved the healing process in diabetic skin wound with substantial differences in the wound healing kinetics (Kamar et al., 2018). In another study cationic solid lipid nanoparticles (CSLN) were prepared and evaluated for the skin disorder. The formulation showed a monodispersed particle size of 218.4–238.6 nm with a polydispersity index of 0.15–0.35. The formulations had shown the drug release of 14.74–21.23% and suggest the potential of this CSLN as a controlled CUM delivery system for the treatment of skin disorder (Gonçalez et al., 2017).

The topical curcumin (CUR) SLNs were developed by probe ultrasonication method. The formulation was prepared using the Precirol ATO5 as lipid and Tween-80 as a surfactant. The developed formulation was converted into the gel and their biological activity was evaluated against hyperpigmentation through the inhibition of tyrosinase enzyme. The optimized formulation showed skin permeation in a controlled manner. The formulation can suppress the ear swelling and also reduced the skin water content in the BALB/c mouse (Shrotriya et al., 2018). In another research, the curcumin poly (lactic-co-glycolic acid) (PLGA) nanoparticles (NPs) were formulated and assessed for imiquimod (IMQ)-induced psoriasis-like mouse model by topical route. The results demonstrated that higher drugs penetrated in the skin compared to the drug suspension loaded hydrogel. The IMQ-induced psoriasis-like mouse model results revealed that the developed NPs performance was superior to Cur-NPs hydrogel. The formulation showed sustained drug release, greater drug accumulation, skin penetration, and reached to the blood circulation, which significantly enhanced the anti-psoriasis activity in mice (Sun et al., 2017). The anti-inflammatory, antimicrobial, and wound-healing activity have been evaluated by preparing curcumin nanoparticle by topical route. The developed nanoparticles were of 193.1 ± 8.9 nm with a zeta potential of 20.6 ± 2.4 mV. The animal study result revealed that CS/poly-glutamic acid/pluronic/curcumin nanoparticles promoted neo-collagen regeneration and tissue reconstruction (Lin et al., 2017). The curcumin loaded nanoparticles prepared using ethylcellulose and/or methylcellulose (MC). The administration of curcumin nanoparticles to the skin and subsequent UVB-irradiation resulted in less radical formation compared to curcumin lotion (Suwannateep et al., 2012). A cream-based curcumin solid-lipid-based nanoformulation formulated and the result showed nano size (440 nm) with high drug load (70%) and found stable for six months (Tiyaboonchai et al., 2007).

3.2.7   APPLICATION OF CURCUMIN NANOFORMULATION IN OTHER DISEASES

Sankar et al. (2013) prepared curcumin nanoformulation and reported a significant reduction in the lipid peroxidation (LPO) and also showed improved enzymatic and nonenzymatic antioxidants in the treated brain. In another study, Gandapu et al. (2011) developed apo transferrin tagged curcumin nanoparticles for improved uptake in T-cells through transferrin-mediated endocytosis. The result of the study disclosed a higher anti-HIV activity of nano curcumin (IC (50) <1.75 M) compared to sol curcumin (IC (50) = 5.1 M).

The curcumin loaded CS nanoformulation suggested its antimalarial activity (AMA) by inhibiting hemozoin synthesis. The lethal strain-infected mice survived for five more days upon treatment with this nanoformulation (Akhtar et al., 2012). The anti-malarial activity of curcumin lipid nanopar-ticles was evaluated by parenteral administration. The *in-vivo* evaluation results showed a 2-fold increase in anti-malarial activity over free curcumin (Nayak et al., 2010). In another reported study, the AMA of curcumin was evaluated by formulating curcumin loaded PEGylated liposome showed the marked and statistically significant therapeutic *in-vivo* effect against *Plasmodium berghei* infected (murine model of malaria) mice (Isacchi et al., 2012).

The ocular use of curcumin nanoparticles was reported by evaluating the retention of curcumin in the corneal region (Pradhan et al., 2015). The therapeutic efficacy of curcumin nanoparticles was evaluated by delivering through local inhalation in an orthotopic mouse model of human lung cancer. The result of the study revealed the accumulation and retention of most of the nanoparticles in the mice lungs for at least 24 h for inducing its effects (Garbuzenko et al., 2014). The curcumin nanoemulsion and micro-suspension were prepared for lung delivery and administered by nebulization. The curcuminoid nanoemulsion formulations average fine particle fraction (FPF) and mass median aerodynamic diameter (MMAD) ranged from 46% and 4.9 μm to 44% and 5.6 μm, respectively. The aerosol performance of nanoemulsion did not dependent on the curcuminoids concentration and their genotoxicity results suggest the suitability for studies in animals (Al Ayoub et al., 2018).

3.3   CONCLUSION

Curcumin is a polyphenol compound extracted from *Curcuma longa* and has shown a wide range of pharmacological actions. The pure curcumin is widely consumed by humans, and there is not any major limitation by USFDA. There are numbers of *in vitro*, and *in vivo* studies have revealed the use of the bioactive role of curcumin in the treatment of various human diseases. Solubility is the major problem associated with curcumin and to overcome this development of nanoformulations efficiently tackle the solubility and bioavailability problem. The curcumin encapsulated by adding ingredients or excipients that help to enhance the curcumin's overall stability. The curcumin nanoformulations are likely to be approved as a choice for the treatment in the near future. There are pre-clinical animal study has been done and reported in the literature so the major shortcoming is our lack of understanding of curcumin nanoformulations risks in humans. The clinical trials of nanoformulations on humans show their bioavailability and safety.

KEYWORDS

- **cancer**
- **chitosan**
- **curcumin**

- **nanoformulation**
- **silver-curcumin nanoconjugates**
- **skin disease**

REFERENCES

Abdellah, A. M., et al., (2018). Green synthesis and biological activity of silver-curcumin nanoconjugates. *Future Med Chem. 10*(22),2577–2588.

Abdel-Mageid, A. D., et al., (2018). The potential effect of garlic extract and curcumin nanoparticles against complication accompanied with experimentally induced diabetes in rats. *Phytomedicine. 43*,126–134.

Ahmad, N., et al., (2014). PNIPAM nanoparticles for targeted and enhanced nose-to-brain delivery of curcuminoids: UPLC/ESI-Q-ToF-MS/MS-basedpharmacokinetics and pharmacodynamic evaluation in cerebral ischemia model. *Drug Deliv.* 1–20.

Akhtar, F., Rizvi, M. M., & Kar, S. K., (2012). Oral delivery of curcumin bound to chitosan nanoparticles cured Plasmodium yoelii infected mice. *Biotechnol Adv., 30*(1),310–20.

Al Ayoub, Y., et al., (2018). Development and evaluation of nanoemulsion and microsuspension formulations of curcuminoids for lung delivery with a novel approach to understanding the aerosol performance of nanoparticles. *Int. J. Pharm.,557,* 254–263.

Al-Rohaimi, A. H., (2015). Comparative anti-inflammatory potential of crystalline and amorphous nano curcumin in topical drug delivery. *J. Oleo Sci., 64*(1),27–40.

Anitha, A., et al., (2012). Curcumin-loaded N,O-carboxymethyl chitosan nanoparticles for cancer drug delivery. *J. Biomater. Sci. Polym. Ed., 23*(11),1381–400.

Azami, S. J., et al., (2018). Curcumin nanoemulsion as a novel chemical for the treatment of acute and chronic toxoplasmosis in mice. *Int. J. Nanomedicine.,13,*7363–7374.

Bhatt, H., et al., (2018). Development of curcumin loaded solid lipid nanoparticles utilizing glyceryl monostearate as single lipid using QbD approach: Characterization and evaluation of anticancer activity against human breast cancer cell line. *Curr. Drug Deliv.,15*(9),1271–1283.

Bhawana., et al., (2011). Curcumin nanoparticles: preparation, characterization, and antimicrobial study. *J. Agric. Food Chem., 59*(5), 2056–61.

Bisht, S., et al., (2007). Polymeric nanoparticle-encapsulated curcumin ("nanocurcumin"): a novel strategy for human cancer therapy. *J. Nanobiotechnol., 5*, 3.

Das, R. K., Kasoju, N., & Bora, U., (2010). Encapsulation of curcumin in alginate-chitosan-pluronic composite nanoparticles for delivery to cancer cells. *Nanomedicine., 6*(1), 153–60.

El-Sherbiny, I. M., El-Shibiny, A., & Salih, E., (2016). Photo-induced green synthesis and antimicrobial efficacy of poly (ε-caprolactone)/curcumin/grape leaf extract-silver hybrid nanoparticles. *J. Photochem. Photobiol. B., 160*, 355–63.

Fan, S., et al., (2018). Curcumin-loaded PLGA-PEG nanoparticles conjugated with B6 peptide for potential use in Alzheimer﹥s disease. *Drug. Deliv., 25*(1), 1091–1102.

Farajzadeh, R., et al., (2018). Macrophage repolarization using CD44-targeting hyaluronic acid-polylactide nanoparticles containing curcumin. *Artif Cells Nanomed Biotechnol., 46*(8), 2013–2021.

Meeta, G., et al., (2015). Preparation of a novel nanocurcumin loaded drug releasing medicated patch with enhanced bioactivity against microbes. *Adv. Sci. Eng. Med.*, 7, 485–91.

Ghaffari, S., et al., (2018). Nanotechnology in wound healing; Semisolid dosage forms containing curcumin-ampicillin solid lipid nanoparticles, *in-vitro*, *Ex-vivo* and *in-vivo* characteristics. *Adv. Pharm. Bull.* 8(3), 395–400.

Guerrero, S., et al., (2018). Curcumin-loaded nanoemulsion: a new safe and effective formulation to prevent tumor reincidence and metastasis. *Nanoscale.*, 10(47), 22612–22622.

Gonçalez, M. L., et al., (2017). Curcumin-loaded cationic solid lipid nanoparticles as a potential platform for the treatment of skin disorders. *Pharmazie.*,72(12), 721–727.

Gosangari, S. L., & Watkin, K. L., (2012) Effect of preparation techniques on the properties of curcumin liposomes: characterization of size, release and cytotoxicity on a squamous oral carcinoma cell line. *Pharm. Dev. Technol.*, 17, 103–9.

Gupta, S. C., et al., (2012). Discovery of curcumin, a component of golden spice, and its miraculous biological activities. *Clin Exp Pharmacol Physiol.*, 39, 283–99.

Gupta, S. C., et al., (2013). Multitargeting by turmeric, the golden spice: from kitchen to clinic. *Mol. Nutr. Food Res.*, 57(9), 1510–28.

Heo, D. N., et al., (2014). Inhibition of osteoclast differentiation by gold nanoparticles functionalized with cyclodextrin curcumin complexes. *ACS Nano.*, 8(12), 12049–62.

Huo, X., et al., (2019). A novel synthesis of selenium nanoparticles encapsulated PLGA nanospheres with curcuminmolecules for the inhibition of amyloid β aggregation in Alzheimer's disease. *J. Photochem. Photobiol. B.*, 190, 98–102.

Ireson, C. R., et al., (2002). Metabolism of the cancer chemopreventive agent curcumin in human and rat intestine. *Cancer Epidemiol. Biomarkers Prev.*, 11(1), 105–111.

Isacchi, B., et al., (2012). Artemisinin and artemisinin plus curcumin liposomal formulations: enhanced antimalarial efficacy against Plasmodium berghei-infected mice. *Eur. J. Pharm. Biopharm.*, 80(3), 528–34.

Jeengar, M. K., et al., (2016). Emu oil based nano-emulgel for topical delivery of curcumin. *Int. J. Pharm.*, 506(1–2), 222–36.

Kakkar, V., et al., (2013). Curcumin loaded solid lipid nanoparticles: an efficient formulation approach for cerebral ischemic reperfusion injury in rats. *Eur. J. Pharm. Biopharm.*, 85(3Pt A), 339–45.

Kakkar, V., et al., (2018). Topical delivery of tetrahydrocurcumin lipid nanoparticles effectively inhibits skin inflammation: in vitro and in vivo study. *Drug Dev Ind Pharm.*, 44(10), 1701–1712.

Kalani, A., et al., (2016). Curcumin-loaded embryonic stem cell exosomes restored neurovascular unit following ischemia-reperfusion injury. *Int. J. Biochem. Cell Biol.*, 79, 360–369.

Kamar, S. S., Abdel-Kader, D. H., & Rashed, L. A., (2018). Beneficial effect of Curcumin Nanoparticles-Hydrogel on excisional skin wound healing in type-I diabetic rat: Histological and immunohistochemical studies. *Ann Anat.*, 222, 94–102.

Khan, M. N., et al., (2018). Polymeric Nano-Encapsulation of Curcumin Enhances its Anti-Cancer Activity in Breast (MDA-MB231) and Lung (A549) Cancer Cells Through Reduction in Expression of HIF-1α and Nuclear p65 (Rel A). *Curr. Drug Deliv.*, 15(2), 286–295.

Lee, W. H., et al., (2013). Curcumin and its derivatives: their application in neuropharmacology and neuroscience in the 21st century. *Curr. Neuropharmacol.*, 11, 338–78.

Lee, W. H., et al., (2014). Recent advances in curcumin nanoformulation for cancer therapy. *Expert Opin. Drug Deliv.*, 11(8), 1–19.

Li, Y., & Zhang, Z. Z., (2018). Sustained curcumin release from PLGA microspheres improves bone formation under diabetic conditions by inhibiting the reactive oxygen species production. *Drug Des. Devel. Ther., 12,* 1453–1466.

Lin, Y. H., Lin, J. H., & Hong, Y. S., (2017). Development of chitosan/poly-γ-glutamic acid/ pluronic/ curcumin nanoparticles in chitosan dressings for wound regeneration. *J. Biomed. Mater. Res. B. Appl. Biomater., 105*(1), 81–90.

Madan, S., et al., (2018). Design, preparation, and evaluation of liposomal gel formulations for treatment of acne: in vitro and in vivo studies. *Drug Dev. Ind. Pharm.,16,* 1–10.

Mangalathillam, S., et al., (2012). Curcumin loaded chitin nanogels for skin cancer treatment via the transdermal route. *Nanoscale., 4,* 239–50.

Martey, O., et al., (2017). Styrene maleic acid-encapsulated RL71 micelles suppress tumor growth in a murine xenograft model of triple negative breast cancer. *Int. J. Nanomedicine., 12,* 7225–7237.

Meeta., G., et al., (2017). Nanoformulations of curcumin: an emerging paradigm for improved remedial application. *Oncotarget., 8*(39) 66680–66698.

Milobedeska, J., Kostanecki, V., & Lampe, V., (1910). Structure of curcumin. *Ber. Dtsch. Chem. Ges., 43,* 2163–2170.

Min, S., (2012). Advances in nanotechnology-based delivery systems for curcumin. *Nanomedicine, 7*(7), 1085–1100.

Mourtas, S., et al., (2011). Curcumin-decorated nanoliposomes with very high affinity for amyloid-β1-42 peptide. *Biomaterials., 32*(6),1635–45.

Mulik, R., Mahadik, K., & Paradkar, A., (2009). Development of curcuminoids loaded poly(butyl) cyanoacrylate nanoparticles: physicochemical characterization and stability study. *Eur. J. Pharm. Sci., 37*(3–4), 395–404.

Nabofa, W. E. E., et al., (2018). Cardioprotective Effects of Curcumin-Nisin Based Poly Lactic Acid Nanoparticle on Myocardial Infarction in Guinea Pigs. *Sci. Rep., 8*(1), 16649.

Nagahama, K., Sano, Y., & Kumano, T., (2015). Anticancer drug-based multifunctional nanogels through self-assembly of dextrancurcumin conjugates toward cancer theranostics. *Bioorg. Med. Chem. Lett., 25*(12), 2519–22.

Nair, K. L., et al., (2012). Purely aqueous PLGA nanoparticulate formulations of curcumin exhibit enhanced anticancer activity with dependence on the combination of the carrier. *Int J Pharm., 425,* 44–52.

Nayak, A. P., et al., (2010). Curcuminoids-loaded lipid nanoparticles: novel approach towards malaria treatment. *Colloids Surf B: Biointerfaces., 81*(1), 263–73 .

Naz, Z., & Ahmad, F. J., (2015). Curcumin-loaded colloidal carrier system: formulation optimization, mechanistic insight, ex vivo and in vivo evaluation. *Int. J. Nanomedicine., 10,* 4293–307.

Nazari-Vanani, R., Moezi, L., & Heli, H., (2017). In vivo evaluation of a self-nanoemulsifying drug delivery system for curcumin. *Biomed. Pharmacother., 88,* 715–720.

Pandit, R. S., et al., (2015). Curcumin nanoparticles: physico-chemical fabrication and its in vitro efficacy against human pathogens. *3 Biotech., 5*(6), 991–997.

Pradhan, N., et al., (2015). Curcumin nanoparticles inhibit corneal neovascularization. *J. Mol. Med., 93*(10), 1095–106.

Rabanel, J. M., et al., (2015)., Effect of polymer architecture on curcumin encapsulation and release from PEGylated polymer nanoparticles: Toward a drug delivery nano-platform to the CNS. *Eur. J. Pharm. Biopharm., 96,* 409–20.

Rahimi, H. R., et al., (2016). The effect of nano-curcumin on HbA1c, fasting blood glucose, and lipid profile in diabetic subjects: a randomized clinical trial. *Avicenna J Phytomed., 6*(5), 567–577.

Ramalingam, P., & Ko, Y. T., (2015). Enhanced oral delivery of curcumin from N-trimethyl chitosan surface-modified solid lipid nanoparticles: pharmacokinetic and brain distribution evaluations. *Pharm. Res., 32*(2), 389–402.

Rice, K. M., et al., (2016). Curcumin nanoparticles attenuate cardiac remodeling due to pulmonary arterial hypertension. *Artif Cells Nanomed Biotechnol., 44*(8), 1909–1916.

Sankar, P., et al., (2016). Oral nanoparticulate curcumin combating arsenicinduced oxidative damage in kidney and brain of rats. *Toxicol. Ind. Health., 32*(3), 410–21.

Saralkar, P., & Dash, A. K., (2017). Alginate Nanoparticles Containing Curcumin and Resveratrol: Preparation, characterization, and *In-vitro* evaluation against DU145 prostate cancer cell line. *AAPS Pharm. Sci. Tech., 18*(7), 2814–2823.

Shrotriya, S., et al., (2018). Skin targeting of curcumin solid lipid nanoparticles-engrossed topical gel for the treatment of pigmentation and irritant contact dermatitis. *Artif Cells Nanomed Biotechnol., 46*(7), 1471–1482.

Sun, L., et al., (2017). Enhanced topical penetration, system exposure and anti-psoriasis activity of two particle-sized, curcumin-loaded PLGA nanoparticles in hydrogel. *J. Control Rel., 254*, 44–54.

Sun, M., et al., (2010). Enhancement of transport of curcumin to brain in mice by poly (n-butylcyanoacrylate) nanoparticle. *Nanopart. Res., 12.,* 3111–22.

Suwannateep, N., et al., (2012). Encapsulated curcumin results in prolonged curcumin activity in vitro and radical scavenging activity ex vivo on skin after UVB-irradiation. *Eur. J. Pharm. Biopharm., 82*(3), 485–90.

Szymusiak, M., et al., (2016). Bioavailability of curcumin **and** curcumin glucuronide in the central nervous system of mice after oral delivery of nano-curcumin. *Int. J. Pharm., 511*(1), 415–423.

Thadakapally, R., et. al., (2016). Preparation and Characterization of PEG-albumin-curcumin nanoparticles intended to treat breast cancer. *Indian J. Pharm. Sci., 78*(1), 65–72.

Tiwari, S. K., et al., (2014). Curcumin-loaded nanoparticles potently induce adult neurogenesis and reverse cognitive deficits in Alzheimer's disease model via canonical Wnt/β-catenin pathway. *ACS Nano., 8*(1), 76–103.

Tiyaboonchai, W., Tungpradit, W., & Plianbangchang, P., (2007). Formulation and characterization of curcuminoids loaded solid lipid nanoparticles. *Int. J. Pharm., 337*(1–2), 299–306.

Tonnesen, H. H., Másson, M., & Loftsson, T., (2002). Studies of curcumin and curcuminoids. XXVII. Cyclodextrin complexation: solubility, chemical and photochemical stability. *Int. J. Pharm., 244*(1–2), 127–135.

Tyagi, A. K., et al., (2015). Identification of a novel compound (β-sesquiphellandrene) from turmeric (Curcuma longa) with anticancer potential: comparison with curcumin. *Invest New Drugs., 33*, 1175–86.

Vareed, S. K., et al., (2008). Pharmacokinetics of curcumin conjugate metabolites in healthy human subjects. *Cancer Epidemiol Biomarkers., 17*, 1411–17.

Vimala, K., et al., (2010). Fabrication of porous chitosan films impregnated with silver nanoparticles: a facile approach for superior antibacterial application. *Colloids Surf B Biointerfaces., 76*, 248–58.

Wang, Y. J., et al., (1997). Stability of curcumin in buffer solutions and characterization of its degradation products. *J. Pharm. Biomed. Anal., 15*(12), 1867–1876.

Xie, M., et al., (2015). Nano-curcumin prepared via supercritical: Improved anti-bacterial, anti-oxidant and anti-cancer efficacy. *Int. J. Pharm., 496*(2),732–40.

Yallapu, M. M., et al., (2014). Anti-cancer activity of curcumin loaded nanoparticles in prostate cancer. *Biomaterials., 35*(30), 8635–48.

Yallapu, M. M., Jaggi, M., & Chauhan, S. C., (2013). Curcumin nanomedicine: a road to cancer therapeutics. *Curr. Pharm. Des., 19*(11), 1994–2010.

You, L., et al., (2019). Synthesis of multifunctional Fe_3O_4@PLGA-PEG nano-niosomes as a targeting carrier for treatment of cervical cancer. *Mater. Sci. Eng. C. Mater. Biol. Appl., 94,* 291–302.

Young, N. A., et al., (2014). Oral administration of nano-emulsion curcumin in mice suppresses inflammatory-induced NFκB signaling and macrophage migration. *PLoS One.,* (11),111559.

Garbuzenko, O. B., et al., (2014). Biodegradable Janus nanoparticles for local pulmonary delivery of hydrophilic and hydrophobic molecules to the lungs. *Langmuir: ACS J. Surf. Colloids., 30*(43), 12941–9.

CHAPTER 4

Ursolic Acid: A Pentacyclic Triterpene from Plants in Nanomedicine

MONALISHA SEN GUPTA,[1] MD. ADIL SHAHARYAR,[1]
MAHFOOZUR RAHMAN,[2] KUMAR ANAND,[1] IMRAN KAZMI,[3]
MUHAMMAD AFZAL,[4] and SANMOY KARMAKAR[1]

[1]Department of Pharmaceutical Technology, Jadavpur University, Kolkata, West Bengal, India

[2]Department of Pharmaceutical Sciences, SIHAS, SHUATS, Allahabad, Uttar Pradesh, India

[3]Glocal University, Near Mirzapur Pole, Saharanpur, Uttar Pradesh, India

[4]Departmnt of Pharmacology, College of Pharmacy, Jouf University, Sakaka, Kingdom of Saudi Arabia

ABSTRACT

Ursolic acid (UA) is the most promising member of the triterpenoid groups, is a naturally derived pentacyclic triterpenoid. The basic structure is composed of ursane, lupane, and oleanane, which is leading to different pharmacological activities of UA. Though having numerous physiological properties like anti-inflammatory, anticancerous, bone regeneration, antifungal, hepatoprotective, antioxidant, it possesses one major drawback is less solubility in water, followed by poor bioavailability in the drug delivery system. Another drawback of UA is the off-target drug delivery system which results in less use in the medical world. Having these major side-effects, the use of UA is not restricted and overcome with the help of nanotechnology, by developing different formulations like liposomes, nanoemulsions, micelles, solid lipid nanoparticles (SLNs), and nanostructured lipid carriers (NLCs), etc.

4.1   INTRODUCTION

Ursolic acid (UA) is a naturally derived pentacyclic triterpenoid, an important bioactive phytochemical. Ursolic acid is the most promising member of the triterpenoid groups. Depending upon the quantities of different structural isoprene units, families of triterpenoids are classified. By squalene cyclization, these triterpenoids are synthesized which generally found in natural sources like many plants and fruits (Jäger et al., 2009). Roots of *Catharanthus trichophyllus*, leaves of *Plumeria obtuse*, *Eriobotrya japonica*, and *Rosmarinus officinalis*, etc., are some source of UA (Shanmugam et al., 2013). Pentacyclic triterpenes, exhibit numerous biological functions due to the presence of different functional groups. It also possesses activity like cytotoxicity on different cancer cell lines. Having many potential benefits, some physical limitations restrict the oral and systemic delivery of UA (Jeong et al., 2007; Jäger et al., 2008; Yin et al., 2012). To increase the solubility and to improve the bioactivity of UA, formulations like liposomes, nanoemulsions, nanoparticles (polymeric, solid, and metallic, among others) and cyclodextrin drug complexes, among other systems try to develop successfully (Jäger et al., 2015; Xie et al., 2016; Li et al., 2015). The main focus of this chapter will be different evaluation techniques (*in-vitro* and *in-vivo*) regarding the antitumor effects of pentacyclic triterpene, i.e., UA. Not only that, but the contribution of nanotechnology to facilitate the effective delivery of UA will be also concerned.

4.2   CHEMICAL PROPERTY

Ursolic acid (UA) (3-3-hydroxy-urs-12-ene-28-oic-acid) is a naturally derived pentacyclic triterpenoid and a hydroxy monocarboxylic acid which derived by substituting a beta-hydroxy group in urs-12-en-28-oic acid at position 3, from a hydride of a ursane (Figure 4.1). It is an isomer of oleanolic acid (OA). It has been isolated as an isomeric mixture of OA (Liu, 1995; Vasconcelos et al., 2006).

The basic framework of pentacyclic triterpenoids molecules is composed of ursane, lupane, and oleanane. The presence of these functional groups is leading to different pharmacological activities of UA.

4.3   PHYSICAL PROPERTIES

UA a pentacyclic triterpenoid is widely distributed in plant kingdom like fruits, medicinal herbs, and other plants. It exerts many major physiological activities, among which chemopreventive and chemotherapeutic actions are most important. Large, lustrous prisms shaped crystals of UA are obtained from the absolute alcohol extract, whereas extract with dilute alcohol provides fine hair-like needle-shaped crystals (O'Neil, 2006). A higher melting point (284°C) of UA makes it more preferable among other phytochemicals (Lide, 2008). It is soluble in alcoholic NaOH solution as well as hot glacial acetic acid but insoluble in petroleum ether (O'Neil, 2006). The toxicity of UA is very low which also contributes to the more use in therapeutics. The solubility of UA in water is very poor. Due to less solubility in water, UA becomes poorly bioavailable in the drug delivery system. Another drawback of UA is the off-target drug delivery system which results in less use in the medical world. Having these major side-effects, the use of UA is not restricted. By using the knowledge of nanotechnology, different formulations are developed to overcome the limitations related to targeting and solubility of UA.

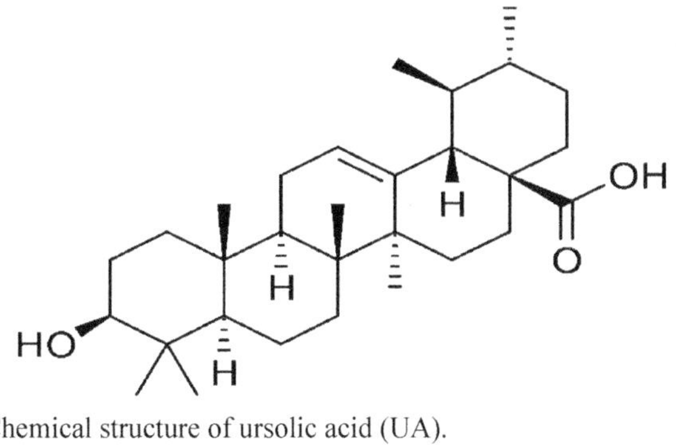

FIGURE 4.1 Chemical structure of ursolic acid (UA).

4.4 PHARMACOKINETICS (PKS)

Different analytical methodologies have been developed for triterpenes, with high selectivity, sensitivity, accuracy, and precision. Pharmacokinetic studies constitute an important stage during the development of new medicines. Discerning the disposition process (i.e., absorption, distribution, and elimination) of new drug candidates facilitates selecting the most appropriate administration route and best dose regimen. The pharmacokinetic parameters of UA in rats after an oral administration suggested rapid absorption, but plasmatic concentrations were extremely low (Liao et al., 2005). Additionally, a lower dose like 10 mg/kg of UA presented rapid absorption with distribution primarily through blood-supplied tissues, such as the lungs, spleen, and liver.

The half-life of UA in the plasma was less than 1 h, indicating rapid elimination (Chen et al., 2011). The study of safety and pharmacokinetic parameters after administering an ascending oral dose of UA shows low and variable UA bioavailability due to the poor water solubility of this compound. This trait led to decreased intestinal absorption and rapid elimination through gut wall/ liver metabolism (Hirsh et al., 2014).

There is limited data to demonstrate the mechanism of pharmacokinetics (PKs) especially absorption of UA which indicated the involved mechanism of absorption was passive diffusion and P-glycoprotein transporter-mediated active transport. It is established by conducting a study with the Caco-2 cell monolayer model. A previous PK study of UA in rats showed the rapid absorption of UA at 1st hour along with the peak concentration after oral administration though the concentrations were extremely low in plasma (Liao et al., 2005). Recently, another PK study among rats demonstrated the time of peak plasma concentration of UA was about half an hour, which ultimately indicating the rapid absorption of UA. Rapid elimination of UA was determined by the lower half-life, i.e., less than 1 hour (Chen et al., 2011). As a result, by enhancing the solubility of UA making it more bioavailable for therapeutic development becomes really challenging. Table 4.1 summarizes the pharmacokinetic properties of UA by using different animal models.

TABLE 4.1   Pharmacokinetic Parameters in Different Animal Models

Animal	Route	Dose	C_{max}	t_{max}	$T_{1/2}$	AUC	References
Rats	Oral	40 g extract/ kg	294.8 ng/mL	1.0 h	4.3 h	1175.3 ng h/mL	Liao et al., 2005
Rats	Oral	10 mg/ kg	1.10 ± 0.3 µg/ mL	0.42 ± 0.11 h	0.71 ± 0.09 h	1.45 ± 0.21 µg h/mL	Chen et al., 2011
Albino rabbits	Oral	1 g extract/ kg	306.8 µg/mL	2.5 h	3.2 h	2245.4 µg h/mL	Shetty et al., 2007

4.5   PHARMACOLOGICAL ACTIVITIES

UA posses numerous physiological properties in which anti-inflammatory, anti-cancerous, bone regeneration, antifungal, hepatoprotective, antioxidant, antimicrobial, antiallergic, antiviral activity, cytotoxic activities are most common and are of great importance among others. It also works as a plant metabolite.

4.6 ANTI-INFLAMMATORY ACTIVITY

In immunity, like innate and adaptive, the inflammation is critical for both due to the quick and spontaneous response against infection or injury by our body. The response can be reviewed as a segment of the complex biological reaction of vascular tissues to detrimental stimuli alike infective agents, blemished or dead cells, and irritants. The exploring of natural compounds and phytochemicals will be able to intrude into the mechanisms which can be useful for the health of human by arresting the prolonged inflammation.

4.6.1 OCULAR INFLAMMATION

Ocular inflammation prevalent complications after eye surgery. Due to the complex structure of the eye, the major challenge in ocular medication is the ability to maintain a therapeutic level of the medicament at the site of action for an extended duration (Agnihotri andVavia, 2009) Generally ocular efficacy is closely associated with the bioavailability of ocular drugs, which may be increased by increasing corneal drug penetration (Gupta et al., 2010). Ocular delivery of drugs is f the most challenging and fascinating venture faced by the pharmaceutical scientist because the development of novel delivery systems for ocular instillation is currently a demand (Araújo et al., 2009; Holden et al., 2012; Karalezli et al., 2008). Several approaches have been proposed but nanoparticles (NPs) represent itself as promising drug transporter for ophthalmic use, by delivering ease of execution just like eye drop having a lesser frequency of administration and extended the duration on the extraocular part (Nagarwal et al., 2009).

UA acts by inhibiting enzymes like cyclooxygenase and phospholipase A2 which involved in the production of eicosanoids. It also helps to avoid the release of cytokines, histamine, serotonin. Not only that, the interaction between serine/threonine kinases and ursolic acid is also avoided (Kwon et al., 2009).

4.7 ANTICANCER ACTIVITY

Cancer is a sort of illness presuming unnatural cell growth with the possibilities to occupy or spread to other portions of the body. Growing cancer incidence and increased mortality trends implied that more efforts should be made to overcome the challenges in the treatment of cancer.

As adjuvant therapy, chemotherapeutic agents have been used independently or integrated with other or integrated with other treatments. Ursolic acid shows a promising inhibitory effect in different cell lines. UA has recently attracted great attraction for its potential as a chemotherapeutic as well as chemopreventive factor. UA kills the fastly growing and dividing cancerous cells as a solitary chemotherapeutic agent, and also destroys the growing regular cells. It may cause adverse effects like congestive heart failure (CHF) during clinical treatment. Limitations of solubility and bioavailability can be solved by incorporating the convenient and safe delivery system, which also helps to maximize the therapeutic activity and minimize the side effects.

UA has its tasks at various phases of tumor enlargement. Still, the exact mechanism of action of its anticancer activity is yet to uncover. But several studies show the inhibitory activities of UA to proliferate and influence apoptosis of numerous tumor cell lines (Sultana, 2011).

Studies also show that apoptosis induced by UA happens due to the involvement of multiple pathways like:

1. The inhibition of DNA replication (Kim et al., 2000).
2. Induction of Ca^{2+} release (Baek et al., 1997).
3. Activation of caspases (Choi et al., 2000; Harmand et al., 2005).
4. C-Jun N-terminal kinase (Xavier et al., 2012; Zhang et al., 2010).
5. Phosphorylation of glycogen synthase kinase 3-, down-regulation of antiapoptotic genes (Kassi et al., 2009).
6. Inhibition of cyclooxygenase-2 and inducible nitric oxide (NO) synthase (Subbaramaiah et al., 2000; Suh et al., 1998).
7. Suppression of matrix metallopeptidase (Cha et al., 1998; Hollosy et al., 2000).
8. The suppression of protein tyrosine kinase (Wu et al., 2012).
9. Phosphatidylinositol-3-kinase (Pathak et al., 2007).
10. Single transducer and activator of transcription (Kim et al., 2000; Zheng et al., 2012).
11. Adenosine 5-monophosphate-activated protein kinase (Shishodia et al., 2003).
12. Nuclear factor-light-chain-enhancer of activated B cell pathways (Kanjoormana et al., 2010).

The abilities of UA to inhibit the different major activities like angiogenesis, invasion, differentiation, and metastasis of tumor cells has been demonstrated by different studies. Functions of numerous enzymes, responsible for DNA synthesis and repair are also interfered by UA (Kim et al., 2000; Novotny et al., 2001; Ovesna et al., 2004) (Table 4.2).

TABLE 4.2 *In Vivo* Potential Antitumor Effects of Ursolic Acid

Animal Model	Mouse Xenograft Model	Treatment	Route of Admini–stration	No. of Animals Per Group	Effects	References
NOD/ SCID mice	U937 (2 × 106 cells/ animal), SC	50 mg/kg for 20 days	IP	10	Induces tumor cell apoptosis	Zheng et al., 2013
Kunming mice, male, and female	H22 cells of exponential growth phase, SC	2.53 mg/ mouse for 10 days	O	10	Induces tumor cell apoptosis	Wang et al., 2011
Athymic nude mice	GBC-SD (2 × 106 cells/ animal), SC	16 mg/kg and 32 mg/ kg	IP	15	Antitumoral effects by suppressing cell proliferation	Weng et al., 2014
Swiss female albino mice	Ehrlich ascites carcinoma (15 × 106 cells/ animal), IP	25, 50 and 100 mg/ kg/d/bw for 14 day	IP	10	Inhibits tumor angiogenesis and induces apoptosis	Saraswati et al., 2013
Balb/c nude female mice	HCT15 (1 × 106 cells/ mice), SC	75 mg/kg bw for 14 days	O	10	Cell death induction and autophagy modulation	Xavier et al., 2013

GBC-SD: Cell line human; IP: Intraperitoneal; bw: Bodyweight; O: Oral; NOD/SCID: Non-obese diabetic/spontaneous mutant model; SC: Subcutaneous.

4.8 HEPATOCELLULAR CARCINOMA (HCC) ACTIVITY

Hepatocellular cancer still remains one of the most threatening cancers, accounts for almost 90% of major liver cancer cases worldwide (Siegel et al., 2013; Parkin et al., 2001). Regardless of the advancement of recent treatments, the resistance to standard chemotherapy has led to less response rates and poor overall survival. Due to the high frequency of recurrence along with poor diagnosis, an immediate need to overcome the recent limitations of chemotherapeutics is arise to improve the therapeutic efficacy. Existing studies have already exhibited the restraining power of ursolic acid (UA), on the progression of a series of cancer cells (Parkin et al., 2001; Shanmugam et al., 2013). Recent works have also demonstrated the antitumor activity of UA through the induction of apoptosis and retardation of angiogenesis (Gao et al., 2012; Shanmugam et al., 2012). However, the restriction of UA is accredited clinically mainly to the low solubility and deficiency of the ability to target tumor areas. In one another study, the *in vivo* utilization of UA was remarkably impaired by its poor solubility, which in consequence leads to poor PKs (Limami et al., 2011). As a result, UA counts a serious and unavoidable side effect, i.e., disability to the target tumor.

4.9   ANTI-BREAST CANCER THERAPY

Ursolic acid (UA) has demonstrated having broad-spectrum anti-tumor activities, but its limitations restrict its clinical application and efficiency. As an *in vitro* model of using MCF-7 cells for anti-cancer mechanistic studies, it is found that the internalization of UA by cancer cells through a folate receptor-mediated endocytic pathway may become easy when it incorporated in a suitable matrix. A lysosomal product of UA shows a great activity by destructing the permeability of the lysosomal membrane, and then got released from lysosomes and localized into mitochondria but not nuclei. The extended retention of UA from the suitable matrix in mitochondria induced excess generation of ROS and demolition of mitochondrial membrane potential which ultimately results in the unrepairable apoptosis in carcinogenic cells. *In vivo* experiments demonstrated that UA in the suitable matrix could significantly reduce the burden of breast cancer particularly in the MCF-7 xenograft mouse model. These outcomes suggested that incorporated UA in a suitable matrix, can be a future prospect as an anti-cancer drug candidate against breast cancer and an upcoming perspective can provide a platform to create a novel anti-drug delivery system against cancer.

4.10   ANTI-CERVICAL CANCER THERAPY

Cervical cancer is f the most common cancers amongst the women which can be concluded from the estimation of 528,000 new cases per year (Bast et al.,

2009), and the mortalities caused by cervical cancer in the world is approximately 266,000, which counts for almost 7.5% of all mortalities related to women cancer (Phongsavan et al., 2010). Approximately 87% of the death caused by cervical cancer, mainly in undeveloped nations and regions. Generally, the women, of 30 to 50 ages, are more prone to this cancer due to factors like environment, gene mutation, job stress, and emotion (Agarwal et al., 2011). Important novel strategies to diminish the cancer progression in therapeutically along with invasion of cervical tumor, metastasis were disclosed through research works regarding molecular mechanisms (Kawase et al., 2010, p. 59).

Among the members of pentacyclic triterpenoids, the imberbic acid, betulinic acid, zeylasteral, and ursolic acid have been reported to show the anticancer activities. Ursolic acid is also familiar to increase apoptotic response in different human cancer cell lines (Gong et al., 2014). However, there are finite numbers of documents which reported the key role of ursolic acid in the ruling of cervical cancer progression. ELISA, western blotting, flow cytometry, and immunohistochemistry assays of ursolic acids were done to investigate the molecular mechanism of modulating cervical cancer progression by ursolic acid nanoparticles. Data indicated that cervical cancer cell proliferation can be suppressed significantly, invasion, and migration compared to the control group, and also apoptosis was induced by ursolic acid nanoparticles through activating caspases, p53, and inhibiting anti-apoptosis-related signals. Furthermore, in the *in-vivo* experiments, the size of the tumor was reduced by the treatment of ursolic acid nanoparticles. In conclusion, ursolic acid can suppress cell proliferation of cervical cancer via apoptosis induction, which can be a potential approach in the future for clinical therapeutic strategy (Table 4.3).

4.11 BONE REGENERATION ACTIVITY

Trauma, infectious, tumor resection, and other diseases cause bone defects. These are the most challenging factors in orthopedics (Tansik et al., 2016; Xie et al., 2017; Nabiyouni et al., 2018). The bone defects make bring unhappiness and economic burden to the patient. Over the past several decades, a number of bone grafts have been used in the sector of bone tissue regeneration like autografts, allografts, and xenografts, which can significantly make a decent result for the patients. An autologous graft is believed as a gold standard (Kim et al., 2017), but it has some negative actions such as donor-site morbidity, lack of availability (Lin et al., 2017). Allografts and xenografts have also their disadvantages including disease transmission and immunogenicity (Duan et al., 2017; Chen et al., 2017). Therefore, it is crucial to originate novel bone

TABLE 4.3 *In Vitro* Potential Anticancer Effects of Ursolic Acid

Cell Line	Cytotoxicity Evaluation Method (Dose and Incubation Time)	Effects	References
HepG2, Hep3B, Huh7, and HA22T cell lines, L-02 cell (human normal liver cell line)	MTT assay (2, 4 and 8 μmol/l UA for 48 h) DNA fragmentation (2, 4 and 8 μmol/l UA for 48 h)	Induces apoptosis	Yan et al., 2010
BGC-803 cell and hepatocellular carcinoma cell line H22	MTT assay (10–60 μM for 12, 24, 36 and 48 h)	Inhibits proliferation, Induces apoptosis	Wang et al., 2013
SW480 and LoVo Human colon cancer cell lines	MTT assay (20 and 40 μM for 48 h) FITC-annexin V/PI (20 and 40 μM for 48 h)	Inhibits proliferation, Induces apoptosis	Weng et al., 2014
GBC-SD and SGC-996 (human cell lines)	MTT assay (40–70 μmol/l for 24, 48 or 72 h) FITC-annexin V (40–70 μmol/l for 36 h)	Antitumoral effects	Nam and Kim, 2013
SW480 (human-colon adenocarcinoma cells)	MTT assay (1–32 μM for 24 h) DNA fragmentation (1–8 μM for 24 h)	Induces apoptosis	Lin et al., 2014
U937 (human leukemia cells)	NBT reduction assay (30 μmol/l for 4 days)	Differentiation-inducing agent for leukemia therapy	Park et al., 2013
PC-3, DU145, LNCaP (prostate cancer cells), Raw 264.7 (leukemic monocyte-macrophage cells) HEK293 (human embryonic kidney 293)	MTT assay (5–80 μM for 24 h) DAPI (30 μM for 24 h)	Induces apoptosis	Kim et al., 2011
MDA-MB-231, human breast cancer cell line	MTT assay (5–100 μM for 24 or 48 h) FACS (40 μM for 24 or 48 h)	Induces apoptosis	Shin and Park, 2013
LNCaP, PC3, DU145, A549, MCF7, HCT116 and HeLa cells	MTT assay (30 μM for 24 h)	Induces apoptosis	Zheng et al., 2013
T24 and BIU-87 lines (human bladder cancer cell)	MTT assay (219 μM for 72 h) FACS/PI (219 μM for 48 h)	Induces apoptosis	Zheng et al., 2012

TABLE 4.3 *(Continued)*

Cell Line	Cytotoxicity Evaluation Method (Dose and Incubation Time)	Effects	References
T24 (human bladder cancer cell)	MTT assay (6.25–400 µg/mL for 24 h; 50, 100 and 200 µg/mL for 24 and 48 h)	Contributes to growth inhibition and apoptosis	Xavier et al., 2013
	FACS/PI (50, 100 and 200 µg/mL for 24 h)		
HCT15 and CO115 (human colon carcinoma-derived cells)	TUNEL assay (4 µM for 48 h)	Induces apoptosis, Autophagy modulation	Limami et al., 2012
	PI (4 µM for 48 h)		
HT-29 (human colorectal) DU145 (human prostate carcinoma cells)	DNA fragmentation (25 µM for 48 h)	Induces apoptosis	Shin et al., 2012
PC3 and DU145 cells	MTT assay (10–40 µM for 24 h) DNA fragmentation (30 and 40 µM for 24 h)	Induces apoptosis	Huang et al., 2011
	PI (30 and 40 µM for 24 h)		
HNBE (human normal lung cells) A549, H3255, and Calu-6 (lung cancer cells)	MTT assay (2, 4, 8 and 16 µmol/l for 48 h)	Inhibition of cell proliferation, invasion, and migration	Limami et al., 2011
	LDH assay (2, 4, 8 and 16 µmol/l for 48 h)		
	DNA fragmentation (2, 4, 8 and 16 µmol/l for 48 h)		
HT-29 and HCT116 (human colorectal cell line)	DNA fragmentation (20 and 30 µM for 24 and 48 h)	Induces apoptosis	Messner et al., 2011
	DAPI (30 µM for 48 h)		
HUVECs (isolation and culture of human umbilical vein endothelial cells)	XTT assay (3.125–50 µM for 24 and 48 h)	Inhibits endothelial proliferation, Inducer of endothelial cell death	Bari et al., 2017
	Annexin V-FITC/PI (6.25 and 12.5 µM for 6, 12, 18, 24 and 48 h)		

DAPI: 4′,6-Diamidino-2-phenylindole; FACS: Fluorescence-activated cell sorting; FITC: Fluorescein isothiocyanate; GBC-SD: Cell line human; HeLa: Cell line human (epitheloid cervix carcinoma); HNBE: Normal human bronchial epithelial cells; HUVEC: Human umbilical vein endothelial cells; LDH: Lactate dehydrogenase; LoVo: Cells line human colon; MTT: 3-(4,5-dimethylthiazol-2-yl)-2,5-diphenyltetrazolium bromide; NBT: Nitroblue tetrazolium; PI: Propidium iodide; TUNEL: Transferase dUTP nick end labeling; UA: Ursolic acid; XTT: 2,3-bis- (2-methoxy-4-nitro-5-sulfophenyl)-2H-tetrazolium-5-carboxanilida.

repair materials for treating efficaciously bone defects (Rezwan et al., 2006). Excellent biocompatibility, osteoconductivity, and bioactivity should be exhibited by optimal bone repair materials (Kim et al., 2016; Chen et al., 2018).

UA is rarely employed for bone tissue regeneration as the few studies were performed in the field of bone tissue repair. Most importantly, osteoblast differentiation also involves the Smad signaling pathway. The release profile of UA from the suitable incorporated dosage form remarkably increased the alkaline phosphatase (ALP) activity, osteogenic differentiation-related gene type I collagen, runt-related transcription factor 2 expression, and osteoblast-associated protein expression. Moreover, the results of micro-CT images, observations from histomorphological data demonstrated that the UA in a suitable dosage form can improve new bone formation ability. Therefore, the UA can be used as novel bone tissue engineering materials by incorporating into a suitable matrix.

4.12 NANOTECHNOLOGY

Nanotechnology has emerged as an efficient tool to address issues of solubility, stability, and oral bioavailability (Valdes et al., 2014). Indeed, a nanosystem-based delivery of drugs, photosensitizers, biomolecules, phytochemicals, and other compounds of interest presents numerous advantages to traditional delivery methods, including facilitated transport across biological barriers, enhanced bioavailability when water solubility is poor, targeted delivery, protection from biological and/or environmental degradation (particularly for sensitive compounds) and controlled release (Morales et al., 2015; Li et al., 2015). Recent improvements in therapeutic efficiency through the use of nanotechnology have gained attention due to enhanced phytochemical delivery to tumors and cancer cells (Gao et al., 2014; Bertrand et al., 2014; Amiji, 2006; Wang et al., 2014).

In oncology, numerous potential benefits, such as protecting the entrapped therapeutic drug from degradation, reducing toxicity to normal cells, modifying the pharmacokinetics and tissue distribution profile to increase drug distribution in the tumor are offered by targeted drug delivery systems. Preventing the side effects of clinical formulations for improving solubility; and increasing cellular uptake and internalization in cancer cells (Bertrand et al., 2014). Several delivery nanosystems like liposomes, nanoemulsions, micelles, solid lipid nanoparticles (SLNs), and nanostructured lipid carriers (NLCs), etc., have been used to enhance the physicochemical nature of phytochemicals. These are the most commonly used nanosystems and can be administered orally, intravenously, intraperitoneally, or transdermally, among other routes (Pattni et al., 2015).

4.12.1 LIPOSOMES

In vesicles formed by nonionic surfactants (niosomes) and phospholipids (liposomes), the different regions (i.e., aqueous medium, interface, and hydrocarbon chains) allow interactions with a wide variety of substrates (Uchegbuk and Florence, 1995; Sandoval et al., 2015). For example, electrostatically charged species would bind to the interface, whereas hydrophobic substrates would locate inside the bilayer. Specifically, many advantages for drug delivery, include good biocompatibility, biodegradability, low toxicity, and a controlled release of the entrapped drug are represented by liposomes (Han et al., 1997) (Figure 4.2).

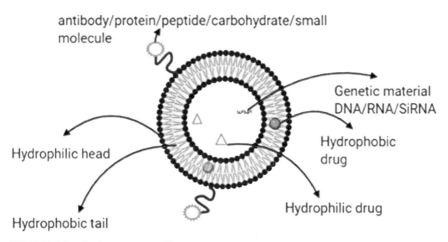

FIGURE 4.2   Basic structure of liposomes.

4.12.1.1 RELATIONSHIP BETWEEN UA AND LIPOSOMES

Regarding UA incorporation into the liposomes Han et al. was the first who studied the effect of triterpenes on membrane fluidity, with 1,2-dipalmitoyl-sn-glycerol-3-phosphocholine (DPPC) liposomes. The study wants to find that UA has a strong condensing effect on the liposomal membrane not only in the liquid-crystalline state but also in the crystalline state. UA displays fewer effects in decreasing the fluidity of the liquid-crystalline liposomal membrane as well as higher membrane-stabilizing effects are comparable with another triterpenes and natural products (Both et al., 2002).

In another study, injection formed liposomes with a low concentration of UA (3 mM) was incorporated into a gel of Carbopol 981. This study reported that UA incorporation into liposomes increased both the ceramide content of cultured normal human epidermal keratinocytes and the collagen content of cultured normal human dermal fibroblasts (Caldeira et al., 2013).

Caldeira et al. proposed the pH-sensitive liposomes containing UA. This was prepared with the lipid hydration method in a total lipid concentration of 20 mM using the same amount of dioleoyl-phosphatidyl-ethanolamine and cholesteryl-hemisuccinate and di-stearoyl-phosphatidyl-ethanolamine-polyethyleneglycol (PEG) 2000 in very low concentration. All materials should be dissolved in chloroform, with a UA equivalent at 0.1% or 0.05% (w/v). Then the whole solution will be added to the lipid solution. Approximately 88% of the vesicles were < 300 nm, had almost neutral surface charges, showed no effects on stability, and had a UA entrapment of 0.77 ± 0.01 mg/mL which proves that UA can be successfully incorporated into it (Yang et al., 2014).

A recent study of Yang et al. reported the antitumor effects of a folate-targeted UA stealth liposome prepared by the thin film dispersed hydration method. The lipid compositions were soybean phosphatidyl-choline/CHOL/monomethoxy polyethylene glycol 2000-distearoyl-phosphatidyl-ethanolamine and soybean phosphatidylcholine/CHOL/ mPEG-DSPE2000/folate-PEG cholesteryl hemisuccinate, with a 1: 20 (w/w) UA to lipid ratio. The lipid suspension was then extruded to produce unilamellar vesicles. Liposome characterizations were similar in both cases, with mean size distributions (150160 nm), potentials (–23.15 and –21.24 mV), and UA entrapment efficiencies (86.7 and 88.9%) (Qian et al., 2015). The result determines that UA can be successfully incorporated into these matrixes.

4.12.1.2   IN-VITRO AND IN-VIVO EFFECTS OF LIPOSOMES

In vitro and *in vivo* models both have been used to assess the anti-inflammatory, anti-proliferative, and pro-apoptotic effects of triterpenoids in relation to potential anticancer activities.

The effect of pH-sensitive liposome-UA on breast and prostate cancer cell line viabilities were also studied by MTT assays, revealing that IC50 values obtained after liposome-UA treatment (48 h) were significantly lower than IC50 values obtained after free-form UA treatment of MDA-MB-231 cancer cells (Yang et al., 2014).

Regarding *in vivo* studies, Yang et al. evaluated PEGylated liposome and folate-receptor-targeted liposome antitumor efficacies using the human KB tumor xenograft model in female Balb/c nude mice. The obtained results demonstrated that free-form UA did not decrease tumor growth, which was in contrast to mice treated with folate-receptor-targeted-liposome-UA, which resulted in a 55% reduction in tumor volume compared with PBS-treated mice (Qian et al., 2015).

Qian et al. recently examined the safety and activity of UA liposomes against tumors in 20 subjects of age 18–75, in whom the presence of advanced solid tumors had already confirmed by cytological or histological data. All subjects received intravenously administered UA liposomes at doses of 56, 74, and 98 mg/m^2 for 14 consecutive days over a 21-day time period. All the subjects were evaluated at the tolerability and toxicity scale. The results demonstrating the safety profile of UA liposome treatment particularly for subjects with advanced solid tumors. Indeed, 60% of patients achieved stable disease status after two treatment cycles (Wang et al., 2013).

Wang et al. evaluated the toxicity and single-dose PKs of intravenous UA liposomes. All subjects received a single-dose of UA liposomes (11, 22, 37, 56, 74, 98, and 130 mg/m^2) administered as a 4 h intravenous infusion. The clinical data reported, for the first time, that the UA liposome had manageable toxicities, with a maximum tolerated a dose of 98 mg/m^2. Dose-limiting toxicity was encountered at 74, 98, and 130 mg/m^2, and consisted of hepatotoxicity and diarrhea. The single-dose pharmacokinetic parameters revealed a linear relationship between Cmax, AUC024 h (Merisko-Liversidge et al., 2003).

4.12.2 NANOLIPOSOMES

For years the use of nanocarrier-mediated drug delivery systems into the improvement of the therapeutic activity and safety of drugs. Formulations for poorly water-soluble drugs like nanoliposome is a promising approach (Zhu et al., 2013). The new technologies for the encapsulation and delivery of bioactive agents are nanoliposome, or submicron bilayer lipid vesicle. The immense list of bioactive material ranging from pharmaceuticals to cosmetics and nutraceuticals can be incorporated into nanoliposomes. Due to the nanosize along with their biocompatibility and biodegradability, their, nanoliposomes have demonstrated their potential applications in numerous fields. By improving the solubility, bioavailability, *in vitro*, and *in vivo* stability, along with the prevention of unwanted interactions with other molecules, nanoliposomes are able to enhance the performance of bioactive agents. Cell-specific targeting is an another advantage of nanoliposomes, which is a prerequisite to attain drug concentrations, required for obtaining maximum therapeutic efficacy in the target site while minimizing adverse effects on healthy cells and tissues. It is used mainly in cosmetics, food technology, and agriculture and also including nano-therapy like diagnosis, cancer therapy and gene delivery (Figure 4.3).

4.12.2.1   RELATIONSHIP BETWEEN UA AND NANOLIPOSOMES

Thus, for the first time development of UA nanoliposomes (UANL) were happening in the People's Republic of China. Because due to bypassing the stomach by nanoparticles the bioavailability of UANL is considered to be improved at intravenous (IV) administration. Till date, a wide range of preclinical studies have been completed in China (Li, unpublished data, 2005). A further unpublished study has demonstrated the induced minimal toxic effects even with the long-term application by UAN L.

4.12.2.2   IN-VITRO AND IN-VIVO EFFECTS OF NANOLIPOSOMES

There are some studies which revealed the inhibition of the growth of various human cancer cells and nude mice xenografts by the nanoliposome-encapsulated UA. That the concept of the first entry of UANL into the stomach and intestines, followed by the rapid declination of its concentrations is suggested by tissue distribution experiments in mice. Conversely, the hepatic concentration of UA increases rapidly and exceeded the concentrations in the stomach and intestines at 4 hours after IV injection. The results demonstrated that UANL delivers UA to the liver, where it accumulates. Consequently, the drug disposition behavior changes *in vivo*, and the toxic and side effects of UA on other tissues is decreased (unpublished data). The antitumor activities and the minimal toxic effects of UA t were observed in preclinical studies and promoted the human clinical trials of UAN L.

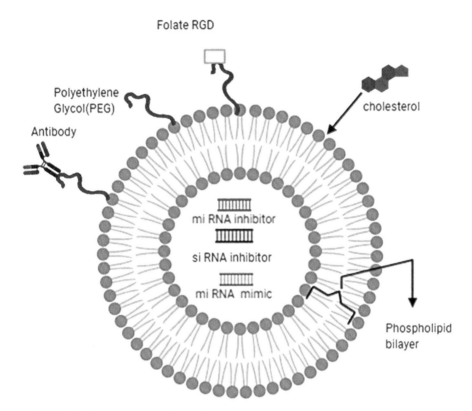

FIGURE 4.3   Basic structure of nanoliposome.

In Phase I, a nanoliposome study by Zhu et al., the UA nanoliposome exhibited a relatively linear pharmacokinetic behavior at dose levels between 37 and 98 mg/m². Furthermore, there was no such evidence of drug accumulation with repeated doses of UANL was observed, and the intravenous infusion in patients with advanced tumors and by healthy volunteers was well tolerated (Alvarado et al., 2015).

4.12.3   *NANOEMULSIONS*

Generally, nanoemulsions ranges from 10 to 1,000 nm are a system of colloidal particles in the submicron size range which enacting as a transporter of drug molecules. The surface of these carriers is amorphous and lipophilic with a negative charge and with the solid spheres. To enhance site-specificity, magnetic nanoparticles can be used. They may enhance the therapeutic effectivity of the drug and customize the adverse effect and toxic reactions as a drug delivery system. The treatment of infection of the reticuloendothelial system (RES), enzyme replacement therapy in the liver, treatment of cancer, and vaccination are included as major applications. An emulsion a biphasic system, is a thermodynamically unstable system, can be stabilized by the addition of an emulsifying agent (emulgent or emulsifier), where one phase is dispersed into the other in the form of minute droplets ranging in diameter from 0.1 to 100 m. The dispersed phase is also known as the internal phase or the discontinuous phase while the outer phase is called dispersion medium, external phase, or continuous phase. The intermediate or interphase is an emulsifying agent. The terminology nanoemulsion' is fine oil/water or water/oil dispersion also refers to a mini-emulsion which stabilized by an interfacial film of surfactant molecule having droplet size range 20,600 nm. Because of small size, of nanoemulsions are responsible for the transparent nature of it. There are three types of nanoemulsion as per their formulation technique:

1. Oil in water nanoemulsion: oil/nonaqueous phase are dispersed in the continuous aqueous phase;
2. Water in oil nanoemulsion: water droplets/aqueous phase are dispersed in the continuous oil phase; and
3. Bicontinuousnanoemulsions (Figure 4.4).

4.12.3.1 RELATIONSHIP BETWEEN UA AND NANOEMULSIONS

Alvarado et al. developed nanoemulsions using natural or synthetic UA mixtures. The nanoemulsion composition was obtained from pseudoternary phase diagrams composed of castor oil (oil phase, 20%), a 4:1 ratio mixture of Labrasol (surfactant), and Transcutol P (co-surfactant), propylene-glycol (aqueous phase, 20%) and OA/UA mixtures (0.2%). The sizes of droplets of nano-emulsions (NE) were 200.95 nm (p.i. 0.25) and 139.70 nm (p.i. 0.18), respectively which formed with a natural or synthetic UA mixture, ultimately shows great activity (Zhou et al., 2009).

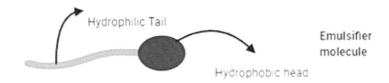

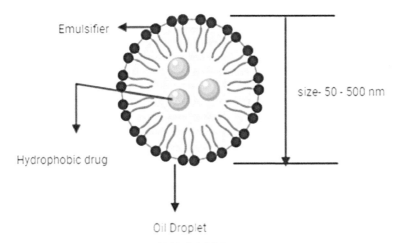

O/W NANOEMULSION

FIGURE 4.4   The basic structure of nanoemulsion droplets.

4.12.4   *NANOPARTICLES*

The existence of nanoparticles is only on the nanometer scale (i.e., below 100 nm in at least one dimension). The physical properties demonstrated by them are uniformity, conductance, or special optical properties. These are the most desirable properties in materials science and biology. Various nanoparticle drug delivery systems have been explored, including nanoparticles, nanospheres (NSs), nanocapsules (NCs), SLNs, and polymeric nanoparticles (Figure 4.5).

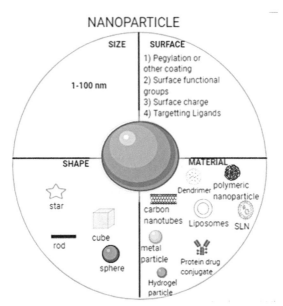

FIGURE 4.5   Basic structure of nanoparticles.

4.12.4.1   RELATIONSHIP BETWEEN UA AND NANOPARTICLES

Zhou et al. prepared powder of UA phospholipid nanoparticles using solvent emulsification evaporation and ultrasonic dispersion. Specifically, soybean phospholipids, UA, and poloxamer 188® were dissolved in an ethanol and ethyl acetate as co-solvent. The UA nanoparticle suspension was added to 5% glucose and mannitol, which serve as cryoprotectants, and samples were freeze-dried. The resulting nanoparticles had an average diameter of 273.8 ± 2.3 nm, a potential of -23.2 ± 1.5 mV, and encapsulation effectivity (EE) of $86.0 \pm 0.4\%$ (Sun et al., 2011).

To improve UA solubility, Sun et al. by using the supercritical antisolvent process developed a nanoparticle, which resulted from 139.4 ± 19.4 nm to 1039.8 ± 65.2 nm. The processed UA dissolution rates were 4.4-fold higher than unprocessed UA (Zhang et al., 2013).

In turn, Zhang et al. proposed a UA delivery system composed of polymeric nanoparticles prepared through a nano-precipitation method. This method used mPEGPCL block copolymers and UA (ratio 2:1), which were dissolved in acetone and then dialyzed in water. The obtained nanoparticles had an average diameter of 144.0 ± 4.0 nm, a potential of -0.99 ± 0.3 mV, and an EE of $87\% \pm 5.3\%$ (Mandelli et al., 2013).

Furthermore, Mandelli et al. developed UA lipid nanoparticles for incorporation into a cosmetic formulation. Nanoparticles were produced through high-pressure homogenization with 1% UA and cetyl-alcohol, methyl soyate, tocopheryl acetate, and sorbitol, among others. Only stability of the UA was evaluated (i.e., a variation of the viscosity and pH), with results revealing that the nano-structured-lipid carrier provided better physical and chemical stability than free-form UA (Singh et al., 2010).

Polymeric nanoparticles were studied by Alvarado et al. to develop an ophthalmic delivery system. The polymeric nanoparticles were prepared using the solvent displacement technique, which employed PLGA, poloxamer 188, and synthetic and natural OA/UA mixtures. The synthetic mixture nanoparticles exhibited a Z-average of 222.75 ± 2.19 nm, a potential of -27.30 ± 1.63 mV, and an EE of $76.55\% \pm 3.92\%$. In turn, natural mixture OA/UA polymeric particles presented a size of 211.80 ± 1.83 nm, a potential of -26.90 ± 0.27 mV, and an EE of $78.45\% \pm 2.40\%$ (Zhou et al., 2009).

4.12.4.2 IN-VITRO AND IN-VIVO EFFECTS OF NANOPARTICLES

In-vitro and *in-vivo* effects related to Zang et al. study who worked on a polymeric delivery UA nanoparticle, had demonstrated that the UA-nanoparticle significantly elicited more cell death by suppressing the expression of COX-2 and activation of caspase 3 with *in-vitro* cytotoxicity and apoptosis tests. Notably, UA-nanoparticle doses were nearly equivalent to free-form UA. These results showing its preference towards the superiority of the UA-nanoparticle over the free-form UA in regard to cell membrane penetration, a requirement for intracellular drug accumulation (Mandelli et al., 2013).

4.12.5 CYCLODEXTRINS INCLUSION COMPLEX

Cyclodextrins inclusion compound is a complex system where designs can be incorporated either in which one component of complex (the host) forms a cavity, or in the case of, spaces of crystal lattice in the shape of long tunnels or channels where second chemical species (the guest) of the molecular entities are located. The guest and host are, attracted by the van der Waals forces, but not by covalent bonding.

The cyclodextrin inclusion complex is one of the most studied pathways in relation to the issue of solubility. For the formation of inclusion compounds, the well-established hosts are cyclodextrins. The illustrative case of ferrocene is insertion under hydrothermal conditions, into the cyclodextrin at

100°C. Cyclodextrin also able to incorporate fragrances into the inclusion compounds, which have reduced vapor pressure, and the stability in exposure to light and air is more. Due to the slow-release action, the fragrance of these molecules lasts much longer when it incorporated into textiles (Cerga et al., 2011), (Figure 4.6).

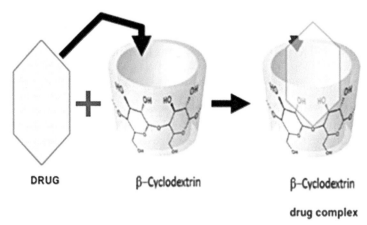

DRUG   β–Cyclodextrin   β–Cyclodextrin

                                                                                    drug complex

FIGURE 4.6   Formation of cyclodextrin-drug inclusion complex.

4.12.5.1   RELATIONSHIP BETWEEN UA AND CYCLODEXTRINS INCLUSION COMPLEX

Cegal et al. evaluated the inclusion of OA and UA in two cyclodextrins (i.e., hydroxyl-propyl-cyclodextrin, and hydroxypropyl cyclodextrin), characterizing the complexation between the acids and cyclodextrins. Differential scanning calorimetry (DSC) and x-ray characterization indicated that the active compounds and cyclodextrin inclusion complexes remained unaltered and could be used as drug delivery systems (Soica et al., 2014).

4.12.5.2   IN-VITRO AND IN-VIVO EFFECTS OF CYCLODEXTRIN COMPLEX

Soica et al. also developed an OA/UA cyclodextrin complex, which was monitored using *in vivo* skin cancer models (SKH1 female mice were exposed to UVB and 7,12-dimethylbenz (a)anthracene). The results showed an increase in antitumor activity for the UA/OA mixture, both alone and in complex with cyclodextrin (Zhang et al., 2015).

4.12.6   BIOGLASS (BGS) SCAFFOLDS

Bioglass (BGs) was originally discovered in 1969 and now commonly used in bone tissue engineering because of its good biocompatibility and osteo-conductivity. After implanted *in vivo*, BGs can bond closely to host bones via the formation of carbonated hydroxyapatite (CHA) layer between them, however, their osteogenic capacity is not enough excellent to effectively heal bone defects especially for the patients with bone diseases (Hench, 2006; Park and Ha, 2018). Fortunately, empty mesoporous microspheres are mainly fit for the restorative scaffolds in which the controlled delivery of osteogenic drugs facilitates *in vivo* bone tissue formation (Kang et al., 2018). The empty interiors in hollow microspheres facilitate drug storage, and the mesoporous features provide the bigger surface areas for bone-like CHA deposition and drug delivery (Kang et al., 2018; Moghaddam et al., 2018; Zhang et al., 2014; Logith et al., 2016). Moreover, chitosan (CS) with 2-acetamido-2-deoxy-d-glucan and 2-amino-2-deoxy-d-glucan units possesses so excellent biocom-patibility, osteoconductivity, and biodegradability that it becomes a fascinating bone repair material (Gupta et al., 2010). The functional groups such as -OH and -NH2 in CS can up-regulate drug loading (DL)-release behaviors via hydrogen-bonding interactions. Hence, it is inferred that hollow mesoporous bioglass (MBG)/CS scaffolds can serve as ideal therapeutic carriers for bone defect healing (Figure 4.7).

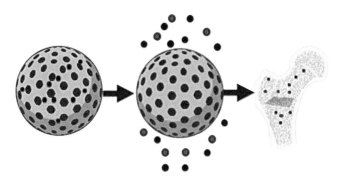

FIGURE 4.7   Basic structure and function of mesoporous bioactive glass scaffolds.

4.12.6.1   RELATIONSHIP BETWEEN UA AND BIOGLASS (BGS) SCAFFOLDS

Generally, it is observed that Ursolic acid (UA) has an *in-vivo* effect on new bone formation and BGs scaffolds have also shown its potential activities in orthopedics. Therefore, Yu-Wei et al. developed the MBG/CS porous scaffolds for the first time, which are loaded with UA (MBG/CS/UA) to increase d bone regeneration. The MBG microspheres were uniformly dispersed on the CS films having particle sizes and pore sizes of ~300 nm and of ~3.9 nm, respectively. The MBG microspheres having mesoporous structure and the hydrogen bonding between the scaffolds and UA drugs, prepared the MBG/CS/UA scaffolds having the controlled drug release activities.

4.12.6.2   IN VITRO AND IN VIVO ACTIVITIES OF BIOGLASS (BGS)

The release of UA drugs from the scaffolds are remarkably increased the activity of ALP, osteogenic differentiation-related gene type I collagen, runt-related transcription factor 2 expression, and osteoblast-associated protein expression. Moreover, the results of micro-CT images, and observations of histomorphological demonstrated that the new bone formation ability can be improved by MBG/CS/UA scaffolds. Therefore, the MBG/CS/UA porous scaffolds can be used as novel bone tissue engineering materials. Hyperlink: "https://www.ncbi.nlm.nih.gov/pmc/articles/PMC3347861/."

4.12.7   POLY LACTIC-CO-GLYCOLIC ACID (PLGA)

Poly lactic-co-glycolic acid (PLGA) is one of the best-known classes of biodegradable polymers for the sustained released drug. PLGA is a biostable polymer, which is degraded into nontoxic oligomers and monomers, lactic acid, and glycolic acid hydrolytically (Araujo et al., 2009). Amongst all these biomaterials, f the biodegradable polymer polylactic-co-glycolic acid (PLGA) has shown immense potential as a carrier and scaffolds for drug delivery and tissue engineering respectively. Amongst the FDA-approved biodegradable polymers PLGA is one which is strong physically and greatly biocompatible and also the use as delivery vehicles for drugs have been extensively studied, proteins, and various other macromolecules like DNA, RNA, and peptides. Due to long clinical experience, favorable degradation properties and possibilities for sustained release drug delivery. Current work has demonstrated that the deterioration of PLGA can be employed for sustained drug release at desirable doses by implantation without surgical procedures. Additionally, it is manageable to tune the overall physical characteristics of the polymer-drug matrix by supervising the relevant criterion of polymer such as molecular weight, ratio of the lactide to glycolide, and drug concentration to execute the desired dosage form and release gap depending upon the drug type (Figure 4.8).

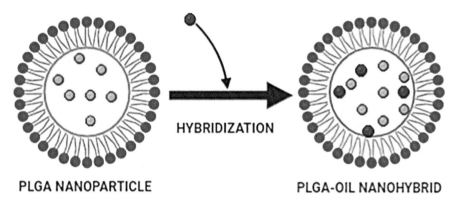

PLGA NANOPARTICLE   **PLGA-OIL NANOHYBRID**

FIGURE 4.8   Basic structure of PLGA nanoparticles.

4.12.7.1   RELATIONSHIP BETWEEN PLGA AND UA

PLGA provides exact particle size and a narrow size range, ensuring less irritation, requisite bioavailability, and stability mainly with ocular tissues (Gonzalez-Mira et al., 2011). The main target of Helen et al. study was to design and optimization of PLGA NPs into vehiculize this natural triterpene compounds in a controlled delivery system for ophthalmic delivery. For this purpose, the response surface methodology (RSM) approach was used to investigate the simple effect and the interaction of different operating conditions, such as amount UA, amount of surfactant and pH of the aqueous phase. Central composite rotatable design (CCRD) was used because requires many few tests and has been shown to be sufficient to describe the majority of the process responses (Uchegbu and Florence, 1995). Since the major drawback of those natural compounds is the limited amount of availability in plants and the secondary objective was the evolution of a synthetic mixture of UA. Moreover, accumulative release operation and penetration capability, as well as, ocular tolerance of the optimized NPs were assessed.

4.12.7.2   DIFFERENT EFFECTS OF PLGA

The evaluation of the ocular tolerability is a mandatory requirement. The study showed that the ocular irritation index (OII) is 0.07 which confirmed that nanoparticles (NPs) did not exert irritation. This was further re-enforced by *in vivo* assay. The application of both types of NPs on the rabbit eyes showed no sign of toxicity or irritation to the external ocular tissues. NPs showed it's best potential to use on damaged or inflamed eyes due to based on biocompatible materials (Araujo et al., 2009). The anti-inflammatory activity in rabbits of NPs exhibited a decrease in the ocular inflammation caused by the installation of sodium arachidonate a solution. In summary, to accomplish the demand for efficient ocular drug delivery systems, this study states that an approach to the use of a CCRD design for the optimization of PLGA NPs of UA elaborated by the solvent displacement method. These formulations exhibited good bioavailability properties due to low Z-ave and PI values, with negative ZP, even upon storage after 6 months at both specified conditions. PLGA NPs exhibited Newtonian behavior and low viscosity allowing sterile filtration and easy administration. Concerning the corneal penetration from NPs, the encapsulated drug was distributed at a constant rate with enhanced accumulation into the ocular tissue creating a reservoir able to prolong the ocular residence time and more powerful effect of the NM. Eye-irritating effects were neither observed *in vitro* nor *in vivo* Draize test. Finally, *in vivo* studies suggested that optimized UA loaded NPs can be expected to gain considerable attention for ocular anti-inflammatory treatment.

4.13   OTHER FORMULATIONS

4.13.1   UA NIOSOMES

Niosomes are non-ionic surfactant vesicles having similar structures and properties to liposomes (Jamal et al., 2015). A recent report on UA encapsulated in pseudo-niosomes prepared vesicles using the film hydration technique which composed of Span 60, cholesterol, and phospholipids, the diameter of the resulted product is 665.45 nm and entrapment efficiency is 92.7%. Vesicles were then incorporated into a standard gel for use as a potential arthritis treatment (Wang et al., 2015), (Figure 4.9).

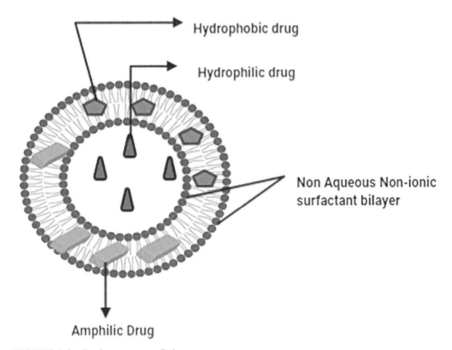

FIGURE 4.9 Basic structure of niosomes.

4.13.2 UA NANOSUSPENSION

In a search of other formulations based on nanotechnology, work by Wang et al. was found. Specifically, this research group tailored the particle size of UA nano-suspensions by using anti-solvent precipitation with a four-stream multi-inlet vortex mixer. It was observed that an increased relative amount of water to ethanol in the final mixture resulted in increased mean particle size. Mean particle sizes of 90 nm (ethanol: water volume ratio of 1:7) and 300 nm (1:15 ratio) were obtained, and the p.i. of all nano-suspensions was <0.3 (Gao et al., 2015).

4.13.3   DENDRIMER-BASED UA PRODRUGS

The use of dendrimers as a targeted drug delivery system is also becoming an attractive alternative due to the small size (115 nm) and high water solubility of these polymers. By applying these properties Gao et al. developed a target for UA on poly-amido-amine (PAMAM; amine-terminated PAMAM [G3-NH2, G5-NH2]), with folic acid used as the targeting agent. Both folic acid and UA were covalently conjugated to the surface of PAMAM through an acid-labile ester bond. The strong hydrophilic properties of PAMAM help the UA to disperse in water very well. The results of particle sizes and potentials of two different formulations (folic acid-G3-UA and folic acid-G5-UA) were suggested that dendrimer-based UA prodrugs have the potential for the targeted delivery of UA into cancer cells (Zhao et al., 2015) (Table 4.4).

4.14   CONCLUSION

Naturally originating pentacyclic triterpenes UA, present significant therapeutic potentials. Notably, more than 30 reports on cancer treatment have assessed the cytotoxic effects of these acids in human cell lines. Despite treatment potential, the poor permeability and water solubility of pentacyclic triterpenes hinder use as galenic agents, an issue starkly evidenced by the limited number of reported clinical studies. Nevertheless, pharmaceutical technologies could vastly improve solubility, stability, and bioavailability, thus favoring the anticancer activities of pentacyclic triterpenes. Many promising *in vitro* work reports have been currently published with the result that the delivery of these compounds through different nanometric systems, such as liposomes, nanoemulsions, nanoparticles, PLGA, BGs, niosomes, and magnetic and polymeric nanoparticles, among others. This is particularly relevant for nanoliposome-UA, which has shown high tolerances and low toxicities in human studies involving healthy and ill individuals. Remaining challenges for the nanopharmaceutical application of these systems include assessing stability, determining elaboration costs, and ultimately, developing the technology required for scaled production. Additionally, obtaining a useful and viable alternative in the near future requires the design of vehicles that employ biocompatible and biodegradable excipients that are approved by regulatory authorities.

TABLE 4.4 *In Vitro* Anticancer Effects of UA Delivered Through Different Nanocarriers

Nanosystem	*In Vitro* (Cell Line)	Cytotoxicity Evaluation Method (Dose and Incubation Time)	Effects	References
Cyclodextrin complex	A2058 and A375 human melanoma cell line	Alarma blue assay (40–100 µM for 48 h)	Cytotoxic	Cerga et al., 2011
PEGylated liposome folate-receptor-targeted liposome	KB cell line (human oral cancer)	MTT assay (6–200 µM for 24 h)	Antitumor	Zhao et al., 2015
Dendrimer	HeLa and HepG2 cells	MTT assay (5–100 µM for 48 h)	Antitumor	Qian et al., 2015
PEG-modified liposomes	EC-304 cancer cells	MTT assay (15.63–500 µg/mL for 24 h)	Antitumor	Zhang et al., 2015
Liposome	LNCaP cell lines (prostate cancer) MDA-MB-231 (breast cancer)	MTT assay (1.2–40 µM for 24 h)	Inhibited proliferation	Yang et al., 2014
Polymeric nanoparticle	SGC7901, gastric cancer cell	MTT assay (20–70 µM for 24, 48 and 48 h)	Apoptotic	Mandelli et al., 2013
		DAPI (20–40 µM for 48 h)		
Nanosuspensions	MCF-7 breast cancer cells	Annexin V-FITC/PI (5 µM for 24 h)	Anticancer	Gao et al., 2015

DAPI: 4′,6-Diamidino-2-phenylindole; FITC: Fluorescein isothiocyanate; UA: Ursolic acid.

KEYWORDS

- **bioglass**
- **central composite rotatable design**
- **encapsulation effectivity**
- **ocular irritation index**
- **pharmacokinetics**
- **response surface methodology**

REFERENCES

Agarwal, S. M., Raghav, D., Singh, H., et al., (2011). CCDB: A curated database of genes involved in cervix cancer. *Nucleic Acids Res., 39(Database),* D975–D979.

Agnihotri, S. M., & Vavia, P. R., (2009). Diclofenac-loaded biopolymeric nanosuspensions for ophthalmic application. *Nanomedicine, 5*(1), 90–95.

Alvarado, H. L., Abrego, G., Souto, E. B., et al., (2015). Nanoemulsions for dermal controlled release of oleanolic and ursolic acids: *In vitro, ex vivo,* and *in vivo* characterization. *Colloids Surf. B. Biointerfaces.,* 130, 40–47.

Amiji, M. M., (2006). *Nanotechnology for Cancer Therapy.* CRC Press, USA.

Araújo, J., Gonzalez, E., Egea, M. A., et al., (2009). Nanomedicines for ocular NSAIDs: Safety on drug delivery. *Nanomedicine, 5*(4), 394–401.

Araujo, J., Vega, E., Lopes, C., et al., (2009). Effect of polymer viscosity on physicochemical properties and ocular tolerance of FB-loaded PLGA nanospheres. *Colloids Surf B Biointerfaces, 72,* 48–56.

Baek, J. H., Lee, Y. S., Kang, C. M., et al., (1997). Intracellular Ca^{2+} release mediates ursolic acid-induced apoptosis in human leukemic HL-60 cells. *Int. J. Cancer, 73*(5), 725–728.

Bari, A., Bloise, N., Fiorilli, S., et al., (2017). Copper-containing mesoporous bioactive glass nanoparticles as multifunctional agent for bone regeneration. *Acta Biomater., 55,* 493–504.

Bast, Jr. R. C., Hennessy, B., & Mills, G. B., (2009). The biology of ovarian cancer: New opportunities for translation. *Nat Rev Cancer, 9*(6), 415–428.

Bertrand, N., Wu, J., Xu, X., et al., (2014). Cancer nanotechnology: The impact of passive and active targeting in the era of modern cancer biology. *Adv. Drug Del. Rev., 66,* 2–25.

Both, D. M., Goodtzova, K., Yarosh, D. B., et al., (2002). Liposome-encapsulated ursolic acid increases ceramides and collagen in human skin cells. *Arch. Dermatol. Res., 293*(11), 569–575.

Caldeira, D. A. L., S., Vinícius, M. N. M., Salviano, T. C., et al., (2013). Preparation, physicochemical characterization, and cell viability evaluation of long-circulating and pH-sensitive liposomes containing ursolic acid. *BioMed. Res. Int.,* 467147.

Cerga, O., Borcan, F., Ambrus, R., et al., (2011). Syntheses of new cyclodextrin complexes with oleanolic and ursolic acids. *J. Agroaliment. Process. Technol., 17,* 405–409.

Cha, H. J., Park, M. T., Chung, H. Y., et al., (1998). Ursolic acid-induced down-regulation of MMP-9 gene is mediated through the nuclear translocation of glucocorticoid receptor in HT1080 human fibro sarcoma cells. *Oncogene., 16*(6), 771–778.

Chen, Q., Luo, S., Zhang, Y., et al., (2011). Development of a liquid chromatography-mass spectrometry method for the determination of ursolic acid in rat plasma and tissue: Application to the pharmacokinetic and tissue distribution study. *Anal. Bioanal. Chem., 399*(8), 2877–2884.

Chen, Y. J., Pao, J. L., Chen, C. S., et al., (2017). Evaluation of new biphasic calcium phosphate bone substitute: Rabbit femur defect model and preliminary clinical results. *J. Med. Biol. Eng., 37*(1), 85–93.

Chen, Y., Kawazoe, N., & Chen, G., (2018). Preparation of dexamethasone-loaded biphasic calcium phosphate nanoparticles/collagen porous composite scaffolds for bone tissue engineering. *Acta Biomater., 67,* 341–353.

Choi, Y. H., Baek, J. H., Yoo, M. A., et al., (2000). Induction of apoptosis by ursolic acid through activation of caspases and down-regulation of c-IAPs in human prostate epithelial cells. *Int. J. Oncol., 17*(3), 565–571.

Duan, X., Liao, H. X., Zou, H. Z., et al., (2017). An injectable, biodegradable calcium phosphate cement containing poly lactic-co-glycolic acid as a bone substitute in *ex vivo* human vertebral compression fracture and rabbit bone defect models. *Connect Tissue Res., 59*(1), 55–65.

Gao, N., Cheng, S., Budhraja, A., et al., (2012). Ursolic acid induces apoptosis in human leukemia cells and exhibits anti-leukemic activity in nude mice through the PKB pathway. *Br. J. Pharmacol., 165*(6), 1813–1826.

Gao, Y., Li, Z., Xie, X., et al., (2015). Dendrimeric anticancer prodrugs for targeted delivery of ursolic acid to folate receptor expressing cancer cells: Synthesis and biological evaluation. *Eur. J. Pharm. Sci., 70*, 55–63.

Gao, Y., Xie, J., Chen, H., et al., (2014). Nanotechnology-based intelligent drug design for cancer metastasis treatment. *Biotechnol. Adv., 32*(4), 761–777.

Gong, Y. Y., Liu, Y. Y., Yu, S., et al., (2014). Ursolic acid suppresses growth and adrenocorticotrophic hormone secretion in AtT20 cells as a potential agent targeting adrenocorticotrophic hormone-producing pituitary adenoma. *Mol. Med. Rep., 9*(6), 2533–2539.

Gonzalez-Mira, E., Egea, M. A., Souto, E. B., et al., (2011). Optimizing flurbiprofen-loaded NLC by central composite factorial design for ocular delivery. *Nanotechnology, 22*(4), 045101.

Gunther, G., Berrios, E., Pizarro, N., et al., (2015). Flavonoids in micro heterogeneous media, relationship between their relative location and their reactivity towards singlet oxygen. *PLoS One, 10*(6), e0129749.

Gupta, H., Aqil, M., Khar, R. K., et al., (2010). Sparfloxacin-loaded PLGA nanoparticles for sustained ocular drug delivery. *Nanomedicine, 6*(2), 324–333.

Han, S. K., Ko, Y. I., Park, S. J., et al., (1997). Oleanolic acid and ursolic acid stabilize liposomal membranes. *Lipids, 32*(7), 769–773.

Harmand, P. O., Duval, R., Delage, C., et al., (2005). Ursolic acid induces apoptosis through mitochondrial intrinsic pathway and caspase-3 activation in M4Beu melanoma cells. *Int. J. Cancer, 114*(1), 1–11.

Hench, L. L., (2006). The story of bioglass. *J. Mater. Sci. Mater. Med., 17*(11), 967–978.

Hirsh, S., Huber, L., Zhang, P., et al., (2014). A single ascending dose, initial clinical pharmacokinetic and safety study of ursolic acid in healthy adult volunteers. *FASEB J., 28*(1), 1044.

Holden, C. A., Tyagi, P., Thakur, A., et al., (2012). Polyamidoamine dendrimer hydrogel for enhanced delivery of antiglaucoma drugs. *Nanomedicine, 8*(5), 776–783.

Hollosy, F., Meszaros, G., Bokonyi, G., et al., (2000). Cytostatic, cytotoxic and protein tyrosine kinase inhibitory activity of ursolic acid in A431 human tumor cells. *Anticancer Res., 20*(6B), 4563–4570.

Hsu, H. Y., Yang, J. J., & Lin, C. C., (1997). Effects of oleanolic acid and ursolic acid on inhibiting tumor growth and enhancing the recovery of hematopoietic system post irradiation in mice. *Cancer Lett., 111*(1, 2), 7–13.

Huang, C. Y., Lin, C. Y., Tsai, C. W., et al., (2011). Inhibition of cell proliferation, invasion, and migration by ursolic acid in human lung cancer cell lines. *Toxicol. In Vitro, 25*(7), 1274–1280.

Jäger, S., Laszczyk, M. N., & Scheffler, A., (2008). A preliminary pharmacokinetic study of betulin, the main pentacyclic triterpene from extract of outer bark of birch (Betulae alba cortex). *Molecules, 13*(12), 3224–3235.

Jäger, S., Trojan, H., Kopp, T., et al., (2009). Pentacyclic triterpene distribution in various plants-rich sources for a new group of multi-potent plant extracts. *Molecules, 14*(6), 2016–2031.

Jamal, M., Imam, S. S., Aqil, M., et al., (2015). Transdermal potential and anti-arthritic efficacy of ursolic acid from niosomal gel systems. *Int. Immunopharmacol., 29*(2), 361–369.

Jeong, D. W., Kim, Y. H., Kim, H. H., et al., (2007). Dose-linear pharmacokinetics of oleanolic acid after intravenous and oral administration in rats. *Biopharm. Drug Dispos, 28*(2), 51–57.

Kang, M. S., Lee, N. H., Singh, R. K., et al., (2018). Nanocements produced from mesoporous bioactive glass nanoparticles. *Biomaterials, 162*, 183–199.

Kanjoormana, M., & Kuttan, G., (2010). Antiangiogenic activity of ursolic acid. *Integr. Cancer Ther., 9*(2), 224–235.

Karalezli, A., Borazan, M., & Akova, Y. A., (2008). Intracameral triamcinolone acetonide to control postoperative inflammation following cataract surgery with pharmacoemulsification. *Acta Ophthalmol., 86*(2), 183–187.

Kassi, E., Sourlingas, T. G., Spiliotaki, M., et al., (2009). Ursolic acid triggers apoptosis and Bcl-2 downregulation in MCF-7 breast cancer cells. *Cancer Invest., 27*(7), 723–733.

Kawase, R., Ishiwata, T., Matsuda, Y., et al., (2010). Expression of fibroblast growth factor receptor 2 IIIc in human uterine cervical intraepithelial neoplasia and cervical cancer. *Int. J. Oncol., 36*(2), 331–340.

Kim, D. K., Baek, J. H., Kang, C. M., et al., (2000). Apoptotic activity of ursolic acid may correlate with the inhibition of initiation of DNA replication. *Int. J. Cancer., 87*(5), 629–636.

Kim, H. D., Amirthalingam, S., Kim, S. L., et al., (2017). Biomimetic materials and fabrication approaches for bone tissue engineering. *Adv. Healthc. Mater., 6*(23), 1700612.

Kim, J. A., Lim, J., Naren, R., et al., (2016). Effect of the biodegradation rate controlled by pore structures in magnesium phosphate ceramic scaffolds on bone tissue regeneration *in vivo. Acta Biomater., 44*, 155–167.

Kim, K. H., Seo, H. S., Choi, H. S., et al., (2011). Induction of apoptotic cell death by ursolic acid through mitochondrial death pathway and extrinsic death receptor pathway in MDA-MB-231 cells. *Arch. Pharmacal. Res., 34*(8), 1363–1372.

Kwon, T., Lee, B., Chung, S. H., et al., (2009). Bull, synthesis and NO production inhibitory activities of ursolic acid and oleanolic acid derivatives. *Korean Chem Soc., 30*(1), 119–123.

Li, C., Zhang, J., ZU, Y. J., et al., (2015). Biocompatible and biodegradable nanoparticles for enhancement of anti-cancer activities of phytochemicals. *Chin. J. Nat. Med., 13*(9), 641–652.

Li, Z., Jiang, H., Xu, C. M., et al., (2015). A review: Using nanoparticles to enhance absorption and bioavailability of phenolic phytochemicals. *Food Hydrocolloid, 43*, 153–164.

Liao, Q., Yang, W., Jia, Y., et al., (2005). LC-MS determination and pharmacokinetic studies of ursolic acid in rat plasma after administration of the traditional Chinese medicinal preparation Lu-Ying extract. *YakugakuZasshi, 125*(6), 509–515.

Lide, D. R., (2007). *CRC Handbook of Chemistry and Physics 88TH Edition 2007–2008* (pp. 3–516). CRC Press, Taylor & Francis, Boca Raton, F L.

Limami, Y., Pinon, A., Leger, D. Y., et al., (2011). HT-29 colorectal cancer cells undergoing apoptosis overexpress COX-2 to delay ursolic acid-induced cell death. *Biochimie., 93*(4), 749–757.

Limami, Y., Pinon, A., Leger, D. Y., et al., (2012). The P2Y 2/Src/p38/COX-2 pathway is involved in the resistance to ursolic acid-induced apoptosis in colorectal and prostate cancer cells. *Biochimie., 94*(8), 1754–1763.

Lin, D., Chai, Y., Ma, Y., et al., (2017). Rapid initiation of guided bone regeneration driven by spatiotemporal delivery of IL-8 and BMP-2 from hierarchical MBG-based scaffold. *Biomaterials, 196*, 122–137.

Lin, D., Zhang, R., Feng, T., et al., (2014). Ursolic acid induces U937 cells differentiation by PI3K/Akt pathway activation. *Chin. J. Nat. Med., 12*(1), 15–19.

Liu, J., (1995). Pharmacology of oleanolic acid and ursolic acid. *J. Ethnopharmacol., 49*(2), 57–68.

Logith, K. R., Keshav, N. A., Dhivya, S., et al., (2016). A review of chitosan and its derivatives in bone tissue engineering, *Carbohyd. Polym., 151*, 172–188.

Mandelli, A. M., Nadia, A., Denise, C. J., et al., (2013). Evaluation of physical and chemical stability of nanostructured lipid carries containing ursolic acid in cosmetic formulation. *J. Appl. Pharm. Sci., 3*(1), 5–8.

Merisko-Liversidge, E., Liversidge, G. G., & Cooper, E. R., (2003). Nanosizing: A formulation approach for poorly-water-soluble compounds. *Eur. J. Pharm. Sci., 18*(2), 113–120.

Messner, B., Zeller, I., Ploner, C., et al., (2011). Ursolic acid causes DNA-damage, p53-mediated, mitochondria-and caspase-dependent human endothelial cell apoptosis, and accelerates atherosclerotic plaque formation *in vivo. Atherosclerosis, 219*(2), 402–408.

Moghaddam, S. P. H., Yazdimamaghani, M., & Ghandehari, H., (2018). Glutathione-sensitive hollow mesoporous silica nanoparticles for controlled drug delivery. *J Control Release, 282*, 62–75.

Morales, J. O., Valdes, K., Morales, J., et al., (2015). Lipid nanoparticles for the topical delivery of retinoids and derivatives. *Nanomedicine, 10*(2), 253–269.

Nabiyouni, M., Bruckner, T., Zhou, H., et al., (2018). Magnesium-based bioceramics in orthopedic applications. *Acta Biomater., 66*, 23–43.

Nagarwal, R. C., Kant, S., Singh, P. N., et al., (2009). Polymeric nanoparticulate system: A potential approach for ocular drug delivery. *J Control Release, 136*(1), 2–13.

Nam, H., & Kim, M. M., (2013). Ursolic acid induces apoptosis of SW480 cells via p53 activation. *Food Chem. Toxicol., 62*, 579–583.

Novotny, L., Vachalkova, A., & Biggs, D., (2001). Ursolic acid: An anti-tumorigenic and chemo preventive activity: Mini review. *Neoplasma., 48*(4), 241–246.

O'Neil, M. J., (2006). *The Merck Index: An Encyclopedia of Chemicals, Drugs, and Biologicals* (p. 1699). Whitehouse Station, NJ: Merck and Co., Inc.

Ovesna, Z., Vachalkova, A., Horvathova, K., et al., (2004). Pentacyclic triterpenoic acids: New chemo protective compounds: Mini review. *Neoplasma., 51*(5), 327–333.

Park, J. H., Kwon, H. Y., Sohn, E. J., et al., (2013). Inhibition of Wnt/β-catenin signaling mediates ursolic acid-induced apoptosis in PC-3 prostate cancer cells. *Pharmacol. Rep., 65*(5), 1366–1374.

Park, S. S., & Ha, C. S., (2018). Hollow mesoporous functional hybrid materials: Fascinating platforms for advanced applications. *Adv. Funct. Mater., 28*, 1703814.

Parkin, D. M., Bray, F., Ferlay, J., et al., (2001). Estimating the world cancer burden: Globocan 2000. *Int.J. Cancer, 94*(2), 153–156.

Pathak, A. K., Bhutani, M., Nair, A. S., et al., (2007). Ursolic acid inhibits STAT3 activation pathway leading to suppression of proliferation and chemo sensitization of human multiple myeloma cells. *Mol. Cancer Res., 5*(9), 943–955.

Pattni, B. S., Chupin, V. V., & Torchilin, V. P., (2015). New developments in liposomal drug delivery. *Chem. Rev., 115*(19), 10938–10966.

Phongsavan, K., Phengsavanh, A., Wahlström, R., et al., (2010). Women's perception of cervical cancer and its prevention in rural Laos. *Int. J. Gynecol Cancer, 20*(5), 821–826.

Qian, Z., Wang, X., Song, Z., et al., (2015). A Phase I trial to evaluate the multiple-dose safety and antitumor activity of ursolic acid liposomes in subjects with advanced solid tumors. *BioMed. Res. Int.,* 809714.

Rezwan, K., Chen, Q. Z., Blaker, J. J., et al., (2006). Biodegradable and bioactive porous polymer/inorganic composite scaffolds for bone tissue engineering. *Biomaterials, 27*(18), 3413–3431.

Sandoval, C., Ortega, A., Sanchez, S. A., et al., (2015). Structuration in the interface of direct and reversed micelles of sucrose esters, studied by fluorescent techniques. *PLoS One., 10*(4), e0123669.

Saraswati, S., Agrawal, S. S., & Alhaider, A. A., (2013). Ursolic acid inhibits tumor angiogenesis and induces apoptosis through mitochondrial-dependent pathway in Ehrlich as cites carcinoma tumor. *Chem. Biol. Interact., 206*(2), 153–165.

Shanmugam, M. K., Dai, X., Kumar, A. P., et al., (2013). Ursolic acid in cancer prevention and treatment: Molecular targets, pharmacokinetics, and clinical studies. *Biochem. Pharmacol., 85*(11), 1579–1587.

Shanmugam, M. K., Ong, T. H., Kumar, A. P., et al., (2012). Ursolic acid inhibits the initiation, progression of prostate cancer and prolongs the survival of TRAMP mice by modulating pro-inflammatory pathways. *PLoS One, 7*(3), e32476.

Shetty, P., Mangaonkar, K., Sane, R., et al., (2007). Pharmacokinetic analysis of ursolic acid in Alstoniascholaris R. Br. by high-performance thin-layer chromatography. *JPC J. Planar. Chromatogr. Modern TLC, 20*(2), 117–120.

Shin, S. W., & Park, J. W., (2013). Ursolic acid sensitizes prostate cancer cells to TRAIL-mediated apoptosis. *Biochim. Biophys. Acta, 1833*(3), 723–730.

Shin, S. W., Kim, S. Y., & Park, J. W., (2012). Autophagy inhibition enhances ursolic acid-induced apoptosis in PC3 cells. *Biochim. Biophys. Acta, 1823*(2), 451–457.

Shishodia, S., Majumdar, S., Banerjee, S., et al., (2003). Ursolic acid inhibits nuclear factor-kappaB activation induced by carcinogenic agents through suppression of IkappaBalpha kinase and p65 phosphorylation: Correlation with down-regulation of cyclooxygenase 2, matrix metalloproteinase 9, and cyclin D1. *Cancer Res., 63*(15), 4375–4383.

Siegel, R., Naishadham, D., & Jemal, A., (2013). Cancer statistics. *CA Cancer J. Clin., 63*(1), 11–30.

Singh, R., Bharti, N., Madan, J., et al., (2010). Characterization of cyclodextrin inclusion complexes: A review. *J. Pharm. Sci. Technol., 2*(3), 171–183.

Soica, C., Oprean, C., Borcan, F., et al., (2014). The synergistic biologic activity of oleanolic and ursolic acids in complex with hydroxypropyl-γ-cyclodextrin. *Molecules, 19*(4), 4924–4940.

Subbaramaiah, K., Michaluart, P., Sporn, M. B., et al., (2000). Ursolic acid inhibits cyclooxygenase-2 transcription in human mammary epithelial cells. *Cancer Res., 60*(9), 2399–2404.

Suh, N., Honda, T., Finlay, H. J., et al., (1998). Novel triterpenoids suppress inducible nitric oxide synthase (iNOS) and inducible cyclooxygenase (COX-2) in mouse macrophages. *Cancer Res., 58*(4), 717–723.

Sultana, N., (2011). Clinically useful anticancer, antitumor, and antiwrinkle agent, ursolic acid and related derivatives as medicinally important natural product. *J. Enzyme Inhib. Med. Chem., 26*(5), 616–642.

Sun, Z., Ma, C. H., Yang, L., et al., (2011). Production of ursolic acid nanoparticles by supercritical antisolvent precipitation. *Adv. Mater. Res., 233–235*, 2210–2214.

Tansik, G., Kilic, E., Beter, M., et al., (2016). A glycosaminoglycan mimetic peptide nanofiber gel as an osteoinductive scaffold. *Biomater. Sci., 4*(9), 1328–1339.

Uchegbu, I. F., & Florence, A. T., (1995). Non-ionic surfactant vesicles (niosomes): Physical and pharmaceutical chemistry. *Adv. Colloid Interface Sci., 58*(1), 1–55.

Valdes, K., Morilla, M. J., Romero, E., et al., (2014). Physicochemical characterization and cytotoxic studies of nonionic surfactant vesicles using sucrose esters as oral delivery systems. *Colloid Surf. B Biointerfaces., 117*, 1–6.

Vasconcelos, M. A., Royo, V. A., Ferreira, D. S., et al., (2006). *In vivo* analgesic and anti-inflammatory activities of ursolic acid and oleanoic acid from *Miconia* albicans (Melastomataceae). *Z Naturforsch C, 61*(7/8), 477–482.

Wang, J., Liu, L., Qiu, H., et al., (2013). Ursolic acid simultaneously targets multiple signaling pathways to suppress proliferation and induce apoptosis in colon cancer cells. *PLoS One, 8*(5), e63872.

Wang, S., Su, R., Nie, S., et al., (2014). Application of nanotechnology in improving bioavailability and bioactivity of diet-derived phytochemicals. *J. Nutr. Biochem., 25*(4), 363–376.

Wang, X. H., Zhou, S. Y., Qian, Z. Z., et al., (2013). Evaluation of toxicity and single-dose pharmacokinetics of intravenous ursolic acid liposomes in healthy adult volunteers and patients with advanced solid tumors. *Expert Opin. Drug Metab. Toxicol., 9*(2), 117–125.

Wang, X., Zhang, F., Yang, L., et al., (2011). Ursolic acid inhibits proliferation and induces apoptosis of cancer cells *in vitro* and *in vivo*. *J. BioMed. Biotechnol.*, 419343.

Wang, Y., Song, J., Chow, S. F., et al., (2015). Particle size tailoring of ursolic acid nanosuspensions for improved anticancer activity by controlled antisolvent precipitation. *Int. J. Pharm., 494*(1), 479–489.

Weng, H., Tan, Z. J., Hu, Y. P., et al., (2014). Ursolic acid induces cell cycle arrest and apoptosis of gallbladder carcinoma cells. *Cancer Cell Int., 14*(96), 1–10.

World Health Organization: International Agency for Research on Cancer. Cervical cancer estimated incidence, mortality and prevalence worldwide in 2012. World Health Organization. 2012.

Wu, B., Wang, X., Chi, Z. F., et al., (2012). Ursolic acid-induced apoptosis in K562 cells involving upregulation of PTEN gene expression and inactivation of the PI3K/Akt pathway. *Arch Pharm. Res., 35*(3), 543–548.

Xavier, C. P. R., Lima, C. F., Pedro, D. F. N., et al., (2012). Ursolic acid induces cell death and modulates autophagy through JNK pathway in apoptosis-resistant colorectal cancer cells. *J. Nutr. Biochem.* [Epub ahead of print].

Xavier, C. P. R., Lima, C. F., Pedro, D. F. N., et al., (2013). Ursolic acid induces cell death and modulates autophagy through JNK pathway in apoptosis-resistant colorectal cancer cells. *J. Nutr. Biochem., 24*(4), 706–712.

Xie, H., Ji, Y., Tian, Q., et al., (2017). Autogenous bone particle/titanium fiber composites for bone regeneration in a rabbit radius critical-size defect model. *Connect Tissue Res., 58*(6), 553–561.

Xie, J., Yang, Z. G., Zhou, C. G., et al., (2016). Nanotechnology for the delivery of phytochemicals in cancer therapy. *Biotechnol. Adv., 34*(4), 343–353.

Yamai, H., Sawada, N., Yoshida, T., et al., (2009). Triterpenes augment the inhibitory effects of anticancer drugs on growth of human esophageal carcinoma cells *in vitro* and suppress experimental metastasis *in vivo*. *Int. J. Cancer, 125*(4), 952–960.

Yan, S. L., Huang, C. Y., Wu, S. T., et al., (2010). Oleanolic acid and ursolic acid induce apoptosis in four human liver cancer cell lines. *Toxicol. In Vitro, 24*(3), 842–848.

Yang, G., Yang, T., Zhang, W., et al., (2014). *In vitro* and *in vivo* antitumor effects of folate-targeted ursolic acid stealth liposome. *J. Agric. Food Chem., 62*(10), 2207–2215.

Yin, M. C., Lin, M. C., Mong, M. C., et al., (2012). Bioavailability, distribution, and antioxidative effects of selected triterpenes in mice. *J. Agric. Food Chem., 60*(31), 7697–7701.

Zhang, H., Li, X., Ding, J., et al., (2013). Delivery of ursolic acid (UA) in polymeric nanoparticles effectively promotes the apoptosis of gastric cancer cells through enhanced inhibition of cyclooxygenase 2(COX-2). *Int. J. Pharm., 441*(1), 261–268.

Zhang, J., Zhao, S., Zhu, Y., et al., (2014). Three-dimensional printing of strontium-containing mesoporous bioactive glass scaffolds for bone regeneration. *Acta Biomater., 10*(5), 2269–2281.

Zhang, Y. L., Xia, L., Zhai, D., et al., (2015). Mesoporous bioactive glass nanolayer-functionalized 3D-printed scaffolds for accelerating osteogenesis and angiogenesis. *Nanoscale, 7*(45), 19207–19221.

Zhang, Y., Kong, C., Zeng, Y., et al., (2010). Ursolic acid induces PC-3 cell apoptosis via activation of JNK and inhibition of Akt pathways *in vitro*. *Mol. Carcinog., 49*(4), 374–385.

Zhao, T., Liu, Y., Gao, Z., et al., (2015). Self-assembly and cytotoxicity study of PEG-modified ursolic acid liposomes. *Mater. Sci. Eng., 53*, 196–203.

Zheng, Q. Y., Jin, F. S., Yao, C., et al., (2012). Ursolic acid-induced AMP-activated protein kinase (AMPK) activation contributes to growth inhibition and apoptosis in human bladder cancer T24 cells. *Biochem. Biophys. Res. Commun., 419*(4), 741–747.

Zheng, Q. Y., Li, P. P., Jin, F. S., et al., (2013). Ursolic acid induces ER stress response to activate ASK1-JNK signaling and induce apoptosis in human bladder cancer T24 cells. *Cell Signal, 25*(1), 206–213.

Zhou, X. J., Hu, X. M., Yi, Y. M., et al., (2009). Preparation and body distribution of freeze-dried powder of ursolic acid phospholipid nanoparticles. *Drug Dev. Ind. Pharm., 35*(3), 305–310.

Zhu, Z., Qian, Z., Yan, Z., et al., (2013). A Phase I pharmacokinetic study of ursolic acid nanoliposomes in healthy volunteers and patients with advanced solid tumors. *Int. J. Nanomed., 8*, 129.

CHAPTER 5

Phytoconstituent-Centered Byproducts and Nanomedicines as Leishmanicidal Scavengers

SABYA SACHI DAS, P. R. P. VERMA, and SANDEEP KUMAR SINGH

Department of Pharmaceutical Sciences and Technology,
Birla Institute of Technology, Mesra – 835215, Ranchi, Jharkhand, India,
E-mail: dr.sandeep_pharmaceutics@yahoo.com (S. K. Singh)

ABSTRACT

Leishmaniasis is considered as clinical expression triggered by the protozoal parasites of the genus *Leishmania*. Almost 1.6 million of new individual cases cutaneous leishmaniasis (CL) and more than half a million of new individual cases of visceral leishmaniasis (VL) ensue every year all over the world. Above half a century, the medical manifestations of this infection have been cured almost entirely with the pentavalent antimonial combinations. The major disadvantage in the management of leishmaniasis includes its advent of resistance to the existing chemotherapeutics. Leishmanicidal agents need to be directed in low doses as the usually procured drugs show severe adverse effects, and henceforth drug resistance can occur promptly. To date, vaccination methods and approaches have been found to be unsuccessful to arrive for clinical trials, chemotherapy centered small molecular ailments are provisionally the exclusive curing strategy. Plants are the innocuous sources of bioactive compounds, which have been reported to be effective primarily, chemically stable, and least harmful as compared with the synthetic molecules. The natural products, chiefly plant-originated phytoconstituents and their byproducts of varied structural groups and classes, displaying the anti-leishmanial activity (ALA), further could be established for their potential efficacy in drug development systems and biomedical research, have been reported in this review. New studies have been emphasized with some biopharmaceutical nano-technologies for designing varied drug delivery approaches, including nanoparticles (NPs), nanocapsules (NCs), liposomes, micelles, cochleate, and nanotubes. Furthermore, the current resistance of anti-leishmanial available drugs and their lethal effects has fetched the drift to measure the ALA of several plant-derived phytoconstituents extracts and their refined compounds further briefed in this review.

5.1   INTRODUCTION

Leishmaniasis is considered as one of the most neglected parasitic disease chiefly caused by *Leishmania* (protozoan parasites) whose transmission and spreading to human beings is assisted through the infected female phlebotomine sandflies bite. The pathology of this disease primarily takes three chief forms: VL (*kala-azar*), CL, and mucocutaneous leishmaniasis (MCL) (*http:// www.who.int/mediacenter/factsheets/fs375/en*, accessed on 18 October, 2017).

World Health Organization (WHO) estimated that almost 1.6 million of fresh leishmaniasis case reports ensue annually, of which half a million cases are related to CL (almost 90% appear in countries like India, Bangladesh, Nepal, Brazil, Sudan, and Ethiopia) and more than half a million cases are related to VL (almost 90% occur in Algeria, Afghanistan, Saudi Arabia, Iran, Brazil, Peru, Syria, and Sudan) (http://whqlibdoc.who.int/publications/2010/9789241564090_eng.pdf). As per the reported data's, Leishmaniasis presently affects an appraised of 12 million individuals and nearly 330 million individuals survive at peril of infection, while a projected count of 500 000 people dies yearly due to VL. Additionally, immunosuppressive disorders like AIDS, add on to the advent of extreme clinical forms of this disease. Till day, the Mediterranean basin has been reported for extreme incidence Leishmania-HIV co-infection (http://www.cdc.gov/parasites/ leishmaniasis/, accessed 20 August, 2013; Columba et al., 2009).

CL, conventionally termed as *Delhi Boil* (Ayub et al., 2003), is frequently prevalent in tropical (humid) and subtropical sections of the world (Alrajhi, 2003). This situation of the disease is not lethal, but the defacement is a disgrace, which primes to communal segregation, mental stress, and minor prospects of fiscal affluence (Rafferty, 2005). The usually reported causative agents for CL are *L. peruviana, Leishmania (L) braziliensis, L. panamensis, L. guyanensis, L. mexicana, L. pifanoi, L. venezuelensis, L. garnhami, L. aethiopica, L. killicki, L. lainsoni, L. major, L. colombiensis, L. amazonensis* and *L. tropica* (Reithinger et al., 2007). Imperfect or no cure of CL may lead to the subsequent expansion of MCL (Goto and Lindoso, 2010).

MCL is predominantly caused by the parasite species, *L. braziliensis*, while additional species (*L. amazonensis* and *L. guyanensis*) have also been reported (Amato et al., 2008). The contamination of mucocutaneous area by these parasites resulted in the extent of contamination at the site of pharyngeal/oronasal mucosa and consequently conquers the soft matters (skin and tissues) as well as cartilages of the nook, which further causes spontaneous erosion. In disparity to CL, these abrasions do not reconcile instinctively. The potency of self-healing of the skin lesions or abrasions primarily depends on the immune response of the individual (Sacks et al., 2002).

If there is a state of immunity failure, the disease tends to be chronic, with infection continuing to the reticuloendothelial system (RES), further causing VL which is systemic and non-curative (Von Stebut and Udey, 2004). Complications caused by VL include episodic or unceasing malaise, cachexia, splenomegaly, limbs, liver megaly, intestinal protruding, trunk devastation, and pancytopenia (Badaro et al., 1996; Neva, 1990). Additionally, about 10% of the patients suffering from the disease, bone marrow are also affected (Feise et al., 2010). VL is commonly caused by *L. donovani*, appears in the Indian subcontinent region, Asia, and East Africa region, while *L. infantum* is liable for contaminations in North Africa, Europe, and Latin America region. Furthermore, if the treatment is not procured properly, VL can also cause death (95% of cases reported). VL is considered lethal because if treatment of the disease is not procured in time then the parasite gets spread systematically (Pearson and Sousa, 1996) (Figure 5.1).

Leishmaniasis (including all forms) has been treated by traditional medications such as extracts of bark, leaves, and other plant parts because of their substantial widespread in underdeveloped and poorest areas of the world. In this context, an effort has been made by us to amass and review the published and infrequent unpublished information's of the naturally occurring phytoconstituents and their purest metabolites, which have been conventionally used for healing leishmaniasis and associated diseases.

5.1.1   LIFE CYCLE OF LEISHMANIA PROTOZOAL PARASITE

Primarily, Knowledge of the *leishmania* (protozoal parasite) life cycle could be implicit by the numerous different phases of diverse species of the sand-fly. The female sand-fly takes a blood meal of humans or terrestrial animals, situation where they require a protein during the period of laying eggs, primes to evolution of leishmanial parasite. The life cycle of the parasite surrogates between two phases, namely promastigote phase and amastigote phase (Figure 5.2a). The promastigote is originated in the midgut of sand-fly and the amastigote mostly exists in humans (macrophages) and other vertebrate congregations (Roy et al., 2010; Ladurner et al., 2000). As the sand-fly slurps the amastigote infested blood from the host, these amastigote gets converted into promastigotes form within 5 hours of incorporation in the inner part of the gut of insect. Within a period of 24–48 hours, the amastigotes wholly get converted into active and motile promastigotes by the procedure of binary separation. In a time period of 7–10 days of consumption of disease-ridden blood the promastigotes get carried to the mid-gut of sand-flies and once this infected sand-fly bites a new host, it gets infected with promastigote. Further, this causes fast penetration of neutrophils and macrophages existing at the site of bite, where the promastigote tends to become immobile and transforms rearer to amastigote form (Figure 5.2b). These amastigotes penetrate and take shelter in the active cells of RES (place where they endure proliferation by binary fusion). Finally, when this developed RES cells get shattered, it primes to deliverance of 40–160 amastigotes and causes interruption of the immunity as the T-helper cell type 1 gets diminished (Kaye and Scott, 2000).

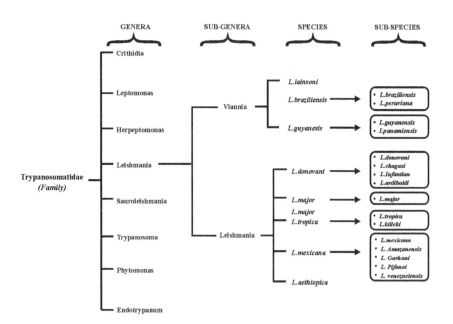

FIGURE 5.1   Taxonomical classification of *Leishmania* parasite.

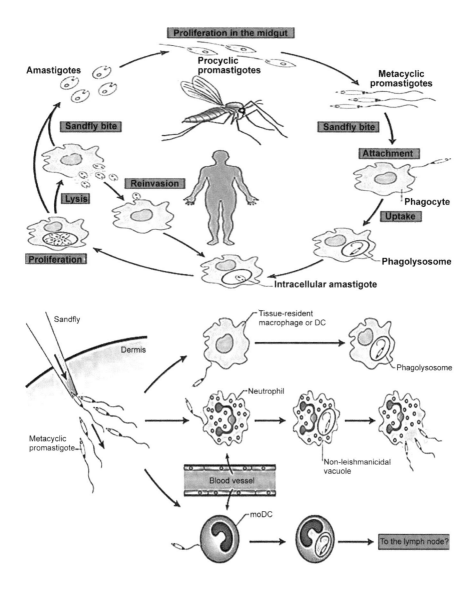

FIGURE 5.2 (a) The life cycle of *Leishmania* parasites and (b) Involvement of multiple cell types in the uptake of *Leishmania* parasites.

Source: Reprinted with permission from Kaye and Scott (2011). © Springer Nature.

5.1.2 PRESENT CHEMOTHERAPY AND RELATED CHALLENGES

The drugs comprising antimony (pentavalent antimonials) as a principal component are primarily the drugs of choice as anti-leishmanial drugs (ALD) for first line cure of Leishmaniasis where confrontation has not been stated (Singh et al., 2006). These comprise of the generic sodium stibogluconate (pentostam, Figure 5.3), the branded meglumine antimoniate, which is been in practice for over five decades. Unfortunately, the Leishmania protozoal parasites have been progressively developed the resistance to these pentavalent antimonial drugs and hence this raised a question for their usage in disease-endemic extents (Maltezou, 2010). Since, these antimonials are directed intravenously (I.V) or intramuscularly (I.M), they are not suitable for patients. They are also concomitant with adverse reactions, which include biochemical pancreatitis, elevation in serum aminotransferases level, and electro-cardiographic oddities (Polonio and Efferth, 2010).

Additionally, second-line ALD consists of amphotericin B (AmP B) (Figure 5.3), particularly used in extents where antimonial resistance is communal (Bern et al., 2006). It displays strong conjugation to ergosterol, the chief sterol of leishmanial and fungal cell membranes. Disappointingly, AmP B is toxic (Hassane et al., 2001; Laborin and Vargas, 2009) despite its high efficacy. Other preparations of AmP B have principally evaded the adverse effects although some are prominently expensive (Singh and Singh, 2012). Other second-line antileishmanial chemotherapeutics contain miltefosine (Figure 5.3), initially established as anticancer molecules. It was the earliest orally administered drug molecule for cure of VL. Having proved its notable efficiency in clinical trials (Sundar, 2006; Bhattacharya et al., 2007), it was reflected as a major discovery in antileishmanial chemotherapy (Jha et al., 1999; Sundar et al., 2006). However, severe apprehensions of its teratogenicity and its long half-life (152 h), which further may boost the appearance of drug resistance, limited its usage (Sundar et al., 2011). Paromomycin (Figure 5.3), alternative second line ALD, cures both VL and CL although its insufficiency has hindered its usage in prevalent regions (Thakur et al., 2000; Thakur, 2003). Sitamaquine (Figure 5.3), the only ALD initially developed to cure VL, provides a benefit for oral administration. Its efficiency and permissibility was confirmed in a phase II clinical experimental in India (Jha et al., 2003). Its potency has also been conveyed in a Kenyan research clinical trial. However, adverse effects like cyanosis, vomiting, dyspepsia, glomerulonephritis, nephritic syndrome, headache, abdominal pain, and kidney dysfunctioning were witnessed in both the clinical trials (Wasunna et al., 2005). Pentamidine (Figure 5.3) is been used to cure antimonial-stubborn VL patients although its deteriorating efficiency has led to its usage (Das et al., 2001).

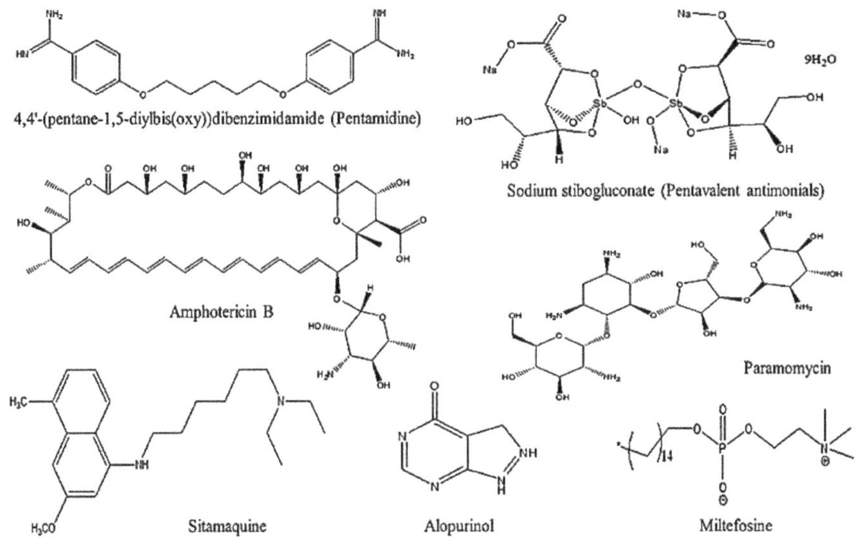

FIGURE 5.3   Presently used anti-leishmanial drugs.

5.1.3   ANTILEISHMANIAL NATURAL COMPOUNDS AND BY-PRODUCTS

The present-day encounters allied with present chemotherapeutic interferences for Leishmaniasis permit rigorous research determinations into unique antileishmanial treatments and therapies. In this segment, we have reviewed for the natural products that have confirmed marked ALA. The ALA of numerous unpolished extracts and parts isolated from plant sources has been accredited to the compounds fitting to varied chemical clusters, which includes terpenoids (monoterpenes, diterpenoids, triterpenes, sesquiterpenes,), phenolic complexes (e.g., flavonols, aurones, chalcones, lignans, quinines, coumarins, tannins), and alkaloidal complex metabolites (indole alkaloids, quinoline alkaloids, isoquinoline alkaloids) (Salem and Werbovetz, 2006).

5.1.3.1   ALKALOIDS

Fournet et al. (1993) demonstrated the actions of some selective quinolone alkaloids isolated from *Galipea longiflora* (Rutaceae) and evaluated their ALA in BALB/c mice diseased with *L. venezuelensis or L. amazonensis*; strains causing CL. The pharmacokinetic *in vitro* and animal model-based *in vivo* studies revealed that: two 3-carbon series quinolones: chimanine D and 2-n-propylquinoline, earlier one was found to be more effective than N-methylglucamine (NMG) antimonate beside *L. amazonensis*. Further, 5 more quinoline alkaloids [2- (3,4-methylenedioxyphenylethyl) quinoline, cusparine, 2- (3,4-dimethoxyphenylethyl) quinoline, chimanine, and skimmianine, were found to be active as that of conventional drug. These active quinolone alkaloids containing derivatives showed no deceptive toxicities throughout the experiment. Bringmann et al. (2000) isolated two new bioactive alkaloids, ancistroealaines A and B and three naphthoic acid derivatives, eleutherolic acid and ancistronaphthoic acids A and B respectively, from *Ancistrocla dusealaensis* (Ancistrocladaceae). Further *in vitro* results showed that ancistroealaines A exhibited IC$_{50}$ (µg/mL) values of 4.1 and 2.35 against *L. donovani* and *T. cruzi*, respectively. Further, Bringmann et al. (2003) isolated a novel naphthylisoquinoline alkaloid, ancistrolikokine D, and likewise 5,80-attached alkaloid ancistroealaine A, further two biosynthetically allied, cis-isoshinanolone, and ancistronaphthoic acid B, from *Ancistrocladus likoko J. Leonard* (Ancistrocladaceae). The compounds showed ALA against *L. donovani*, *T. cruzi*, and *T. brucei* rhodesiense. Muhammad et al. (2003) *Psychotriaklugii* (Rubiaceae) conceded two novel klugine, benzoquino-lizidine alkaloids and 7-O-demethylisocephaeline, collected with earlier known isocephaeline (ICP), cephaeline (CPL) and 7-O-methylipecoside. CPL confirmed effective *in vitro* ALA alongside *L. donovani* (IC$_{50}$ 0.03 µg/mL) and was more effective as compared to pentamidine and AmP B, correspondingly, while klugine (IC$_{50}$ 0.40 µg/mL) and ICP (IC$_{50}$ 0.45 µg/mL) seem to be less potent (<13- and <15-fold) than CPL. Further, emetine (IC$_{50}$ 0.03 µg/mL) was as effective as of CPL, but was >12-fold more toxic than CPL against VERO cells (IC$_{50}$ 0.42 vs. 5.3 µg/mL). Klugine and CPL also displayed strong antimalarial activity (AMA) against *P. falciparum*. Bringmann et al. (2004) isolated three novel naphthylisoquinoline alkaloids; all of the three compounds were S-aligned at position C-3 and endure oxygen at position C-6. Further, *in vitro* studies exhibited their anti-pathogenic activity against leishmaniasis, Chagas' disease, malaria, and African sleeping sickness. Reina et al. (2014) isolated 23 indole alkaloids from various parts of *Aspidosperma desmanthum* and *A. spruceanum*. Further, the antiparasitic activity of these isolated composites experimented against *T. cruzi* and *L. infantum* and their non-précised cytotoxicity on the particular mammalian cells. Larghi et al. (2015) reviewed the present facts about the assortment of the biological actions linked to neocryptolepine (NCL), its correspondents and byproducts. Remarkably, NCL showed weak ALA against *L. donovani*, with IC_{50} 49.5 ± 3.7 µM, nearly two orders of magnitude greater than the standard miltefosine (IC_{50} 0.56 ± 0.07 µM). NCL and other quinoline alkaloids have shown notable docking to LmajMetRS, a protein from *L. major*.

5.1.3.2 TANNINS

Kolodziej et al. (2001) tested the immunomodulatory effect and antiparasitic effect (against intra- and extra-cellular promastigotes) for a series of 27 hydrolyzable tannins and related compounds. Furthermore, of these all compounds, Gallic acid (GAE) and its methyl ester induced murine macrophages. The *in vitro* studies revealed that, tumor necrosis factor-α (TNF-α) inducing potential of examined polyphenols, was found to be highest in oligomeric ellagitannins, and potent interferon (IFN)-like activity was found highest in some ellagitannins and majority of dehydroellegitannins. Furthermore, all polyphenols showed pronounced ALA against *L. donovani*, including possibilities for tempting the release of NO, TNF-α and IFN-like actions in macrophage-like cells. Cortez et al. (2016) evaluated the cytotoxicity, ALA, and curative potential of *Arrabidaea chica*. Further, results stated that the dried extracts confined of flavonoids, tannins metabolites, anthocyanidins complexes, and chalcones. Moreover, the ALA of *A. chica* produced acceptable outcomes in concentrations range of 60–155.9 µg/mL. Cytotoxic assay exposed a 50% decrease in viable cells at an amount of 189.9 µg/mL.

5.1.3.3 TERPENES

Sairafianpour et al. (2001) isolated cryptotanshinone (quinoid diterpene), and 3 novel natural products, 1-oxocryptotanshinone, 1α-hydroxycryptotanshinone and 1-oxomiltirone extracted from the roots of *Perovskia abrotanoides* (Lamiaceae). These composites exhibited ALA *in vitro* (IC_{50} 18–47 mM) which was further used for the management of CL. The isolated terpenes are trained in the development of erudite malarial parasites, drug-sensitive KB-3-1 human carcinoma cell line, multidrug-resilient KB-V1 cell line, and human lymphocytes triggered with phytohaemagglutinin A (IC_{50} 5–45 mM). Tiuman et al. (2005) investigated the *in vitro* ALA of PTL, refined from the hydro-alcoholic extract of varied plant parts of *Tanacetum parthenium*, against *L. amazonensis*. PTL showed substantial activity against the promastigote phases of *L. amazonensis* (IC_{50} 0.37 µg/mL). Foki-alakis et al. (2006) evaluated the ALA of 11 cis-clerodane type diterpenes, 7 labdane oriented diterpene and triterpene, extracted through *Cistus monspeliensis* (Cistaceae), against *L. donovani* promastigotes. The selective isolated compounds exhibited ALA (IC_{50} 3.3 m g/mL, 3.4 m g/mL and 3.5 m g/mL, respectively). Barrera et al. (2008) evaluated the consequence of three plant-derived sesquiterpene complexed lactones, from cultured *L. mexicana* promastigotes. Results displayed that the composites suppressed the *in vitro* development of the selected parasites at moderately lower concentrations, further the effect was fast and irreversible (IC_{50} 2–4 µM). Furthermore, these composites showed lesser cytotoxicity for the mammalian cells. All the three lactones persuaded DNA fragmentation and the aptitude of parasites to attack the Vero cells was reduced by acquaintance to lower concentrations of these composites. Karioti et al. (2009) assessed the ALA of three irregulars, linear sesquiterpene modulated lactones freshly isolated from *Anthemis auriculata*, against *T. brucei rhodesiense* and *T. cruzi*, also for xenic amastigotes of *L. donovani*. The cytotoxic efficiency of these compounds was also evaluated alongside mammalian (rat) skeletal myoblasts (L6 cells). All composites presented strong trypanocidal and ALA. All the three extracts influenced toxicity on mammalian cells; further, this helped to limit their usage as antiprotozoal agents. Maregesi et al. (2010) identified the putative active constituents of *Elaeodendron schlech-teranum* (Celastraceae). Bioassay-directed sequestration managed to empathy of tingenin B; chief antibacterial integrals. Moreover, this compound was found to be vigorous beside *B. cereus*, *S. aureus* and *E. coli* (IC_{50}< 0.25 µg/mL). Furthermore, antiparasitic action was detected against *T. cruzi* (IC_{50}< 0.25 µg/mL), *T. brucei* (<0.25 µg/mL), *L. infantum* (0.51 µg/mL), and *P. falciparum* (0.36 µg/mL). Tingenin B was extremely cytotoxic to MRC-5 cells (CC_{50} 0.45 µg/mL), demonstrating a deprived selectivity. Misra et al. (2010) assessed the *in vitro* activity of terpenoid compounds, isolated from *Polyalthia longifolia*, by means of intracellular transgenic green luminescent protein firmly expressed *L. donovani* parasites. This compound, a clerodane diterpenes, found to be potent as human DNA topoisomerase, introverted recombinant DNA topoisomerase I (TP-1), which eventually persuaded apoptosis. Further, the molecular docking assays specified that five robust hydrogen-bonding interfaces and hydrophobic interfaces of this complex with *L. donovani* DNA-TP-1 was accountable for its ALA. Bharate et al. (2011) carried the quantitative structure-activity relationship (QSAR) study, carrying out a sequence of phloroglucinol-terpene adjuncts showing ALA to invent the essential characteristics which was vital for the bio-chemical action. The QSAR study was conceded out using J. Chem. for Excel and the finest QSAR model was imitated by multiple regression examination. The finest model includes four products shaped correlation coefficient of 0.930 (s = 0.096, F = 65.93, P <0.0001) based on stepwise multiple regression technique. The study concluded, lipophilic oddity (C Log P), Haray index, isoelectric point, and Platt index played a significant role in ALA of these complexes. ALA of numerous architecturally alike naturally arising euglobals was also prophesied using developed QSAR model. Sidana et al. (2012) quarantined the terpenoidal ingredients by isolating the dried extracts using chloroform-methanol mixture of dried leaves of *Eucalyptus loxophleba* for evaluation of ALA against the *L. donovani* promastigotes by means of an Alamar blue assay. Further, results disclosed that 3-acetyl loxanic acid and loxanic acid collectively exhibited ALA (IC_{50} 133–235 µM) in contradiction of the promastigotes of established strain. Moura do Carmo et al. (2012) analyzed the production of essential oils (EOs) gained from the leaves of *Piper demeraranum* and *Piper duckei* by GC-MS technique. The chief constituents found in *P. demeraranum* oil: limonene, β-elemene and in *P. duckei* oil: germacrene D, trans-caryophyllene. *P. duckei* and *P. demeraranum* oils showed potential biological action (IC_{50} 15–76 µg mL^{-1}) against *L. amazonensis*, and hence these EO extracts could be used in the treatment of CL. Tiuman et al. (2014) established the fact that parthenolide (PTN) induced cell death in amastigote forms of *L. amazonensis*. Further, results specified that the ALA of PTN was associated with autophagic vacuole advent, lessening of flexibility, forfeiture of membrane veracity and mitochondrial dysfunction. Rottini et al. (2015) assessed the inhibitory effect of (−) α-bisabolol, in contradiction of promastigotes and amastigotes phases of *L. amazonensis*, caused alterations in cytotoxicity of the treated cells. This compound revealed an important ALA against promastigotes (IC_{50} 4.26–8.07 µg/mL). Approximately around 69% of the promastigotes phases agonized mitochondrial membrane injury after the treatment with this compound, signifying inhibition of the metabolic action of the parasites. Teles et al. (2015) isolated 3β,6β,16β-trihydroxylup-20 (29)-ene from *Combretum leprosum* fruit, assayed for anticancer effects. It showed substantial activity in contradiction to the intracellular amastigotes of *L. (L.) amazonensis*. Results indicated that the metabolite inhibits *L. (L.) amazonensis* amastigote duplication and existence inside the host cells and bioinformatics studies intensely indicated this molecule to be an impending inhibitor of topoisomerase IB. Bufalo et al. (2016) isolated 4 diterpenes from *Salvia deserta* extracted roots. Taxodione was imitated leishmanicidal (IC$_{50}$ 46 μM-0.46 mg/L) against *L. donovani* and showed antifungal and antimicrobial actions. The crude extract section, containing the isolated compounds, exhibited stouter antibacterial activity (1.3 mg/L for *S. aureus* and 1.1 mg/L for methicillin-resilient *S. aureus*). Garcia et al. (2017) evaluated the ALA of *Citrus sinensis* (L.) (Rutaceae) extracts. Further, results of the extracts exhibited ALA (IC$_{50}$ 25.91 ± 4.87). Additionally, 60 μg/mL of sample extract abridged the amount of intracellular amastigotes and the ratio of diseased macrophages in 62% and 37%, respectively. Ulloa et al. (2017) assessed the ALA of enhydrin, uvedalin, and polymatin B, isolated from *Smallanthus sonchifolius*, against *L. Mexicana* and *T. cruzi*. Further, results showed that the three compounds unveiled ALA (IC$_{50}$ 0.42–0. 54 and 0.85–1.64 μg/mL for promastigotes and amastigotes respectively. Want et al. (2017) prepared nanoliposomal artemisinin (ARM), a sesquiterpene lactone, (NLA) using thin-film hydration technique and optimized the formulation by using Box-Behnken design (BBD) with a mean globule size (83 ± 16 nm), PDI (0.2 ± 0.03), zeta potential (–27.4 ± 5.7 mV), and drug loading (DL) (33.2% ± 2.1%). NLA expressively defamed the intracellular infection of *L. donovani* amastigotes and quantity of infected macrophages (IC$_{50}$ 6.1 ± 1.4 μg/mL and 5.2 ± 0.9 μg/mL, respectively). Rodrigues et al. (2018) evaluated the ALA of *Copaifera spp.* oleoresins, the impact of crude dried extracts and parts of oleoresin of samples through *Copaifera paupera* onto parasites: *L. infantum* and *L. amazonensis*. Further, oleoresin comprising of α-copaene (38.8%) showed the best action against *L. amazonensis* (IC$_{50}$ = 62.5 μg/mL) and against *L. infantum* (IC$_{50}$ = 65.9μg/mL). To upsurge the ALA, nano-emulsion encompassing copaiba oleoresin and α-copaene were established and examined against *L. amazonensis* and *L. infantum* promastigotes, which was further showed high ALA. Armah et al. (2018) apprised the ALA of crude plant extract, its portions, and isolated complexes of *E. ivorense* by means of direct totaling assay of promastigotes of *L donovani* using AmP B as positive control. Further, a suggestively active methanol fraction (IC$_{50}$ 2.97 μg/mL) related to AmP B (IC$_{50}$ 2.40 ± 0.67 μg/mL). The unique diterpene complexes extracted showed weak activity. Further, the results presented additional aspect where these composites and their comparative profusions could act as chemotaxonomical bio-markers of the significant genus.

5.1.3.4 LACTONES

Akendengue et al. (2002) isolated klaivanolide (KVL), from the stems of *Uvaria klaineana* (Annonaceae). KVL showed persuasive *in vitro* ALA against both sensitive and AmP B-impervious promastigote forms of *L. donovani* (IC_{50} 1.75 and 3.12 mM, respectively). The molecule also exhibited *in vitro* trypanocidal activity (TPA) contrary to trypomastigote forms of *T. brucei*. Tiuman et al. (2014) investigated the *in vitro* ALA of PTN against *L. amazonensis*. PTN (lactone) refined from the extract of plant parts of *Tanacetum parthenium* exhibited substantial activity against the promastigote form of *L. amazonensis* (IC_{50} 0.37 µg/mL). Barrera et al. (2008) assessed the effects of some selective lactones, using cultured *L. mexicana* promastigotes and further observed that the molecules originated from the plant extracts exhibited strong ALA (IC_{50} of 2–4 µM) as compared pure compound, ketoconazole. Karioti et al. (2009) estimated the *in vitro* ALA as well as TPA activity of extracts, bearing lactones as chief components, against *T. bruceirhodesiense* and *T. cruzi*. Results showed that Compound (2) appeared to be the most active complex against all parasites, predominantly towards *T. bruceirhodesiense* (IC_{50} 0.56 mg/mL). Tiuman et al. (2005) confirmed cell demise in amastigote phases of *L. amazonensis* induced lactone, PTN. Further analysis and results indicated that the ALA of PTN was allied with loss of membrane veracity and mitochondrial dysfunction. Ulloa et al. (2017) estimated the activity of three selective lactones. Enhydrin, uvedalin, and polymatin B, isolated from *Smallanthus sonchifolius*, on *L. Mexicana* and *T. cruzi*. Further, the *in vitro* studies depicted that the three compounds exhibited ALA (IC_{50} 0.42–0. 54 µg/mL).

5.1.3.5 STEROLS

Sartorelli et al. (2007) analyzed the dried extracts and segments from the fruits of *Cassia fistula* used for the treatment of VL. Hexane extract exhibited substantial ALA beside the promastigote stage of *L. chagasi*. The bio-directed degradation ensued in the seclusion of a sterol, clerosterol, further scrutinized in altered models. Promastigotes and intracellular amastigotes established high vulnerability (IC_{50} 10.03 µg/mL and 18.10 µg/mL, respectively).

Mammalian cytotoxicity was also assessed; further results confirmed that clerosterol was less lethal than the conventional drug pentamidine. Radwan et al. (2009) isolated 9 novel cannabinoids from a highly potential variety of *Cannabis sativa*. Some selective compounds exhibited substantial antibacterial and antifungal actions, while some compound displayed strong *in-vitro* ALA. Mazoir et al. (2011) appraised the *in vitro* ALA against *L. infantum* promastigotes and *T. cruzi*e pimastigotes of isolated 25 selective semisynthetic terpenoid metabolites obtained from *Euphorbia resinifera* (α-euphol and α-euphorbol) and *Euphorbia officinarum* (obtusifoliol and 31-norlanosterol). Furthermore, results unveiled that 78% and 62% of the test composites showed antiparasitic actions on *L. infantum* and *T. cruzi*, respectively. Da Silva et al. (2014) examined the *in vitro* ALA against numerous Leishmania species and antibacterial actions against selective bacteria strains isolated from the methanolic extract and segments of *Lacistema pubescens*. Results showed that the hexane fraction of extract showed a resilient activity alongside amastigotes of *L. amazonensis* (IC_{50} = 6.8 μg/mL). Pulivarthi et al. (2015) detected the ALA of *Sassafras albidum* (Lauraceae) bark extract and quoted that this compound has excellent ALA (IC_{50}<12.5 μg/mL) against promastigotes of *L. amazonensis*. Khedr et al. (2016) examined the ALA of two newfangled triterpenoids, ficupanduratin A and ficupanduratin B isolated from the fruits of *Ficus pandurate Hance* (Moraceae). These compounds showed virtuous affinity towards CB2 receptor, with supplanting values of 69.7 and 62.5%, respectively. Rebolledo et al. (2017) estimated the leishmanicidal efficacy of some selected medicinal species (*T. procumbens*, *L. xuul*, and *P. andrieuxii*), *in vivo* against *L. Mexicana*. Results depicted that these selective compounds displayed strong ALA (IC_{50}>30 mg/mL) against *L. Mexicana*. Oghumu et al. (2017) surveyed the immunomodulatory assets of pentalinonsterol (PEN) and assessed its probability as an adjuvant. Further, results confirmed that PEN enhanced the expression of NF-κB and AP1 transcription factors and promoted BMDC-mediated production of IFN-γ by T-cells, henceforth could be castoff as a leishmanicidal agent.

5.1.3.6   TERPENOIDS

Takahashi et al. (2004) inspected the ALA of 46 natural compounds counting several ferns and Betula components. Numerous pterosin and atisene complexes from selective ferns showed great activity. Amongst the triterpenoids, the compounds comprising of carboxyl group seem to be significant for ALA. Moreover, in diarylheptanoids, the linear-type structures and the diphenylether type conjugates exhibited noteworthy activity, and was established that the carbonyl group at C-11 is essential for the ALA of biphenyl-types conjugates. Ibrahim et al. (2016) extracted 3 novel tetracyclic triterpenoids through endophytic fungus *Fusarium* sp. which was sequestered in root part of *Mentha longifolia L.* (Labiatae) and further found that the isolated compounds exhibited high ALA (IC_{50} 6.35 µM). Machumia et al. (2010) synthesized 10 diterpenoid compounds through roots of a Kenyan selective medicinal plant, *Clerodendrumeriophyllum*, these compounds exhibited strong antifungal activity (IC_{50} 0.58 and 0.96 µg/mL, respectively) against *C. neoformans*, additionally, few selective compounds exhibited potent ALA (IC_{50} 0.08 and 0.20 µg/mL, respectively) against *L. donovani*. Das et al. (2017) isolated triterpenoid lupeol from *Sterculia villosa* which was further selected for its ALA *in vitro* and *in vivo*, for the treatment of VL. Lupeol exhibits significant ALA (IC_{50} 65 ± 0.41 µg/mL and 15 ± 0.45 µg/mL beside promastigote and amastigote stages respectively). Further, lupeol executed extreme cytoplasmic membrane impairment of *L. donovani* promastigote. Moreover, lupeol persuades generation of NO in *L. donovani* infected macrophages trailed by up-regulation of pro-inflammatory cytokines and down regulation of anti-inflammatory cytokines.

5.1.3.7 SESQUITERPENE

Tiuman et al. (2005) investigated the *in vitro* ALA of PTN, extracted from several parts of plant *Tanacetum parthenium*, against *L. amazonensis* parasite. Results showed the high potency of these compounds as leishmanicidal agents (IC_{50} 0.37 µg/mL). Karioti et al. (2009) evaluated the *in vitro* antiprotozoal as well as leishmanicidal activity three irregulars, linear sesquiterpene and reported that all compounds exhibited potent trypanocidal and leishmanicidal activity. Moura do Carmo et al. (2012) examined the fabrication of EO found from leaves of *Piper demeraranum* and *Piper duckei* by GC-MS. The main constituents found in *P. demeraranum* oil and *P. duckei* oil showed high potential of ALA (IC_{50} 15–76 µg mL^{-1}) against strains of *L. amazonensis*. Rottini et al. (2015) estimated the inhibitory effect of (–) α-bisabolol, in contradiction of the promastigotes and intracellular amastigotes phases of *L. amazonensis*, and their IC_{50} with effective concentration of 8.07 µg/mL (24 h) and 4.26 µg/mL (48 h) was recorded. Rodrigues et al. (2018) estimated the ALA of Copaifera spp. Oleoresins against *L. amazonensis* and *L. infantum* strains. Further, results showed that these novel compounds exhibited ALA against *L. amazonensis* (IC_{50} = 62.5 *μ*g/mL) and alongside *L. infantum* (IC_{50} = 65.9 *μ*g/mL).

5.1.3.8   QUINONES

Bringmann et al. (2008) isolated a series of novel natural quinones isolated from different parts of plant species *Triphyophyllum peltatum*, Additionally, previously identified quinones plumbagin, droserone, malvone A, and nepenthone A existed in the extract of *A. abbreviatus*. Some compounds exhibited worthy and specific ALA against *L. major*, although they were not vigorous alongside other protozoic parasites. Furthermore, management with certain specific isolated compounds strongly persuaded apoptosis in humanoid tumor cells imitated from two dissimilar cellmalignancies, cell lymphoma, and manifold myeloma, deprived of some noteworthy toxicity concerning normal exterior mononuclear blood cells.

5.1.3.9   CHALCONES

Narender et al. (2004) reported three vigorous metabolites bearing 2′,2′-Dimethyl chromeno dihydrochalcones from the aerial parts of plant *Crotalaria ramosissima* (Leguminosae), rarely found as plant secondary metabolites. Additionally, they also described the plan to expediently manufacture naturally arising chromeno dihydrochalcones through biogenetic kind pyridine or amberlyst-15 metabolized chromenylation of dihydrochalcones and ALA of chromeno dihydrochalcones and associated metabolites. Cortez et al. (2001) examined the cytotoxic, anti-leishmanial, and curative potential of roots of plant species *Arrabidaea chica*. Further, the cytotoxic assessment was conceded out by MTT assay, and the 50% cellular cytotoxicity was firmed. Moreover, the results revealed that the dried isolations contained flavonoids, tannins, anthocyanidins, and chalcones. The ALA *A. chica* produced acceptable outcomes in concentrations of between 62 and 156.9 μg/mL. Cytotoxic assay showed a 50% lessening in viable cells at an amount of 188.9 μg/mL.

5.1.3.10   FLAVONOIDS

García et al. (2010) investigated the ALA of 21 species of hydroalcoholic extracts of plants *Punica granatum L.* (Punicaceae) and *Bidens pilosa L.*

(Asteraceae), were further tested in contradiction of promastigotes and amastigotes stages of *L. amazonensis*. Moreover, level of toxicity was examined beside peritoneal macrophages from BALB/c mice. From the results, it was noticed that the plant extracts introverted the development of intracellular amastigotes (IC_{50} 42.8 and 69.5 μg/mL, respectively). The antiparasitic actions of *B. pilosa* and *P. granatum*was stated alongside other parricidal agents and their actions was due to the presence of flavonoids. Nour et al. (2010) revealed that the extract of dichloromethane synthesized from aerial parts of *Ageratum conyzoides L.* (Asteraceae), showed a protuberant activity (IC_{50} = 0.68 μg/mL) against *T. brucei rhodesiense*, *L. donovani* (IC_{50} = 3.5 μg/mL) as well as *P. falciparum* (IC_{50} = 8.1 μg/mL). Finally, results exhibited that some selective flavonoids pertained ALA against the protozoan pathogens. Gontijo et al. (2012) quarantined some of selective biflavonoids using ethyl acetate isolations of crude and crushed parts of fruit parts of *Garcinia brasiliensis*. All of the composites displayed significant leishmanicidal and antioxidant actions, also exhibited low cytotoxicity. These consequences provided new perceptions on drug development systems for the cure of leishmaniasis and inhibitory enzyme action on *L. mexicana* cysteine proteases and added isoforms. Cortez et al. (2005) evaluated the cytotoxic, ALA, and healing potential of *Arrabidaea chica*. Cytotoxic evaluation was performed through MTT assay. Further, results exhibited that the crude isolations comprise of flavonoids, anthocyanins, tannins, and chalcones. The ALA of *A. chica* produced adequate results in concentrations of 60–155.9 μg/mL. Duarte et al. (2016) examined the ALA of aqueous extract from *Zingiber officinalis* (ginger) was recognized as liable for ALA. The characterization of compound was performed and it was chiefly composed of flavonoids and saponins. The optimized formulation exhibited strong ALA (IC_{50} 125.5 μg/mL). Rahman et al. (2017) isolated bacterial clusters from *Fagonia indica* and screened them for bioactive conjugates and further ALA was examined. Strains of *B. subtilis* exhibited higher phenolic matters, 253 μg/mg of GAE and *S. maltophilia* displayed more flavonoids amount 15.8 μg/mg quercitin (QA), over-all antioxidant capacity (TAC) 37.6 μg/mg of isolation amount, reducing power (RP) 206 μg/mg of extract and (DPPH) free radical scavenging activity (IC_{50} 98.7 μg/mL).

5.1.3.11   ESSENTIAL OILS (EOS) DERIVATIVES

Houel et al. (2015) examined whether the anti-dermatophytic potential of EOs could be utilized as indicator for detection of vigorous natural compounds against parasites of species *L. amazonensis*. In accordance to this, the aerial parts of some selective plant parts were hydrolyzed and to equate the antifungal and antiparasitic effects of significant EOs. Furthermore, utmost fascinating antifungal entrants were the EOs from *Cymbopogon citratus*, *Otacanthus azureus,* and *Protium heptaphyllum.* The *P. hispidum* EO was recognized as the utmost favorable compound in the outcomes from the infected macrophages model (IC$_{50}$: 4.8 µg/mL). Rottini et al. (2015) assessed the inhibitory effect of (–) α-bisabolol, in contradiction of the promastigotes and amastigotes phases of *L. amazonensis*, alterations in cytotoxicity of the treated cells. (–) α-bisabolol composite displayed important ALA against promastigotes (IC$_{50}$ 4.27–8.07 µg/mL). Approximately around 67% of the promastigotes phases agonized mitochondrial membrane injury after the conjugation with this compound, signifying inhibition of the metabolic action of the parasites. Aloui et al. (2016) exemplified the chemical configuration, ALA, and antioxidant activity of *Artemisia campestris* L. and their EOs. Further, effects revealed that selected isolations unveiled diverse antioxidant actions conferring to the used assay. The radical scavenging effects (using DPPH assay) of these extracts considering their IC$_{50}$ = 3.3 mg/mL and IC$_{50}$ = 9.1 mg/mL for *Artemisia campestris* and Artemisia herbal-based EOs, respectively. Andrade et al. (2016) evaluated the ALA of different EOs on *L. amazonensis*, also tested their cytotoxicity on mammalian cells and biochemical configuration. Moreover, EOs from *Cinnamoden drondinisii, Myroxylon peruiferum, Matricaria chamomilla, Salvia sclarea, Ferula galbaniflua, Bulnesia sarmientoi,* and *Siparuna guianensis,* found to be most vigorous against *L. amazonensis* (IC$_{50}$ 54.05–162.25 µg/mL). Investigation of EOs by GC-MS exhibited the occurrence of β-farnesene (52.73%) primarily; the utmost which further persuaded the ALA. Moraes et al. (2018) established nanoemulsions of copaiba and andiroba oils as a drug delivery system and verified their ALA on *L. infantum* and *L. amazonensis*. These nanoemulsions showed an average globule size of 77.1 and 88.1, respectively PDI value of 0.15 to 0.16 and zeta potential ± 2.54 to ± 3.9. The treatment of *L. infantum*-infected BALB/c mice with the optimized nanoemulsion presented favorable consequences reducing the parasitic burden in spleen and liver.

5.1.3.12   PLANT RESINS

Bafghi et al. (2014) evaluated oleo gum resin of *Ferula asafetida* (asafetida) on mortality and morbidity *L. majorin vitro*. Results showed that asafetida reticent the development of parasites in all doses in immobile and logarithmic phases. The ELISA measurement proposed that the feasibility of parasites expressively reduced after 48 h (P < 0.05) and hence these selective oleo gum resins could be moreover used for the cure of leishmaniasis. Regueira-Neto et al. (2018) estimated the antiprotozoan and cytotoxic potentials of red propolis samples and also equated the results with the samples achieved for the extract of plant resins isolated from *Dalbergiae castophyllum* trees. The IC_{50} perceived against the parasitic growths could be utilized without elevating the fibroblast cell damage.

5.1.4 NANOTECHNOLOGICAL STRATEGIES FOR THE TREATMENT OF LEISHMANIASIS

From the past few decades, drug delivery based nanotechnological approaches have been engrossed abundant attention towards its significant usage and drug delivery based application in pharmaceutical arena. The foremost purpose of these nano-based approaches is to overwhelm the key hitches in the orthodox dose and dosage form, including poor bioavailability, unwanted adverse effects, and restricted efficiency, also upsurges the amount of drug at specific notched target sites. Saponins as liposomic formulations and alkaloids as NPs are amongst the chief plant elements used to formulate nanoformulations. Furthermore, these liposomes are mostly arranged by combination of specific lipids such as cholesterol (Chol), phosphatidyl choline (PC) and phosphatidic acid (PA) (Medda et al., 1999; Basu et al., 2005), while NP formulations include polylactide (PLA) specifically as their core ingredient, which provides better constancy, biocompatibility, and effectual delivery systems related to liposomal structures (Lala et al., 2004). Phospholipid-centered liposomic formulations are commonly utilized for the alteration of the pharmacokinetic profile of numerous drugs. Natural yields including dried extracts, segments, or quarantined phytocompounds have been amalgamated into various colloidal transporters, comprising liposomes. Furthermore, as anticipated in the amalgamation of synthetic molecules and their conjugates, lipid-based formulations improve the ability of solubility, efficacy, and bioavailability of the natural isolations and bioactive complexes (Chen et al., 2011; Ajazuddin and Saraf, 2010). The capability of colloidal transporters to increase tissue macrophages circulation may influence the *Leishmania* contamination. Moreover, affinity of systems based on nano-sized structures, specifically liposomes, apprehended through the mononuclear phagocyte system, acted as an extra benefit in the management of leishmaniasis. Moreover, the intraperitoneal (I.P) and I.V administration of liposome formulations ascertained to be a virtuous biodistribution system for ALD in management of VL, since it amplified drug molecule accumulation in the macrophage composed tissue matters such as liver and spleen, thus diminishing the toxicity level (Pierrot et al., 1995). From prehistoric eras, compounds derived from plant and animal sources are being in usage as ancient medicine to combat many humanoid infectious diseases. Presently, the usage of traditional medicine till now has a prodigious influence on well-being of persons having no admittance to current health care practices; an assessed 80% of individuals existing in the emerging countries trust virtually on ancient medicinal apply to encounter their prime treatment desires (Esquenazi et al., 2002; Kim, 2005; Firenzuoli and Gori, 2007). Therefore, the usage of plant-derived compounds as remedies has fascinated the attention of research labs all over the world, looking for novel bioactive molecules. Amongst the utmost studied natural compounds, plant-floras are a valued source of complexes with ALA. Vigorous derivatives originated from plant sources is defined by several labs universally (Braga et al., 2007; Bero et al., 2011). In fact, phytoscience is found to be significant means in the quest for novel ALDs with rarer adverse effects and inferior impending costs. The active secondary metabolites derived from plant extracts could be castoff in numerous approaches for the expansion of medications. Moreover, the nano-centered drug delivery systems seem to be favorable methodology for evolving new ALDs.

Furthermore, flavonoids and affiliates of this class have been termed as bioactive mediators and are amongst the most commonly established phenolic complexes taken as if in the human diet. Quercetin (QCT) loaded nanoformulations was formulated using quality by design (QBD) approach and its biodistribution was studied. Results showed that the optimized formulation could promote the control release, and improves the physical stability of QCT (Kumar et al., 2015) additionally; substantial antiprotozoal actions of the flavonoids have been testified against *Trypanosoma* and *Leishmania* classes. QCT inhibited the parasite arginase activity (Silva et al., 2012; Majolin et al., 2013) and persuades the fabrication of superoxide anion, hydrogen peroxide (H_2O_2), and additional reactive oxygen species (ROS) by the matured infected cells. Consequently, generation of ROS tempted by QCT was found to be vital for the utmost antiparasitic action, since ROS are indeed created by macrophages as an appliance to eradicate intracellular parasites such as *Leishmania* (Fonseca-Silva et al., 2011). Moreover, the liposomal and nanoencapsulated QCT preparations were formulated for estimating finest drug delivery system. Nanoencapsulated QCT was more potent than the non-encapsulated QCT as anti-leishmanial agents; further, its marked activity might be associated to the nanovesicular conformation and globular size (Sarkar et al., 2002).

Noteworthy, the prime advantages of the liposomes over orthodox dosage forms are their globule size, entrapment efficacy, HLB value and their biocompatibility in the human biological system. In current days, experimental works have showed that the liposomes exhibited extreme number of predicted clinical usage of all the specified nanomedicines used for the healing of leishmaniasis in current days. Liposomal formulation of AmP B was found to be a good example for the management of leishmaniasis (Vyas and Gupta, 2006). Perez et al. (2014) examined the *in vitro* ALA of liposomes which showed numerous restorability utilities was loaded with a light sensitizer zinc pthalocyanine (ZnPcAL). Further, the three liposome systems: soyabean PC liposomes, sodium cholate loaded liposomes and an ultra-deformable liposomes (UDL), was compared and it was observed that the photoactive liposomes did not damaged the promastigotes, Fascinatingly, results implicated that liposomes encompassing sodium cholate were merely captivated by macrophages which consecutively led to upsurge in the intracellular distribution (2.5 folds) as compared to UDL. Italia et al. (2011) notified that the formulated doxorubicin (DOX) loaded nanocapsules (NCs) by means of layer by layer (LBL) technique; further layered with specific amount of phosphatidylserine (PS) enhanced the uptake by the cells. Further, the efficiency of DOX-NCs and DOX-NCs covered with PS (DOX-NCs-PS) was targeted to *L. donovani.* Further, when ALA was tested for DOX-NCs and DOX-NCs-PS, the DOX-NCs-PS exhibited an improved uptake by J774A.1 macrophage cell lines when equated to the DOX-NCs specifically in organs including spleen and liver. It was also observed that the ALA with DOX-NCs-PS exhibited highest parasitic reticence of 85.23% as compared to DOX-NCs and the DOX (Gutierrez et al., 2016). Farokhzad et al. (2009) prepared Nanosphere (NS) of PLGA containing AmP B (AmP B-PLGA-NS) which showed a significant ALA. A solo shot injection of PLGA-NS, free AmP B, and AmP B-PLGA-NS was given to the mice infected with the promastigotes. Moreover, results exposed that the AmP B-PLGA-NS was efficient and presented favored accretion in the organs. Further, the cytotoxicity test depicted that the efficiency of AmP B-PLGA-NS was because of the consequences of CD8 t-lymphocytes. Raffie et al. (2014) prepared NPs of andrographolide (AG) which was isolated from the aerial parts and leaves of *Andrographis paniculata,* further exhibited better ALA with minimal toxicity to the macrophage cells. It was observed that the macrophages in Albino mice tested for ALA were found to be significant for NPs synthesis with 4% PVA in around one-fourth of the amount of pure compound AG. Later on, the investigators resolved that AG acts as a chemotherapeutical agent at a reasonably low cost by an unconventional contrivance. Notably, some specific studies were focused to intensify the management of *L. major* infected mice with the ferroportin (Fpn) NPs, which exhibited resistance to the *L. major* but were vulnerable to visceral infections, leading to anemia and lastly death (Want et al., 2015). Further, to get rid of the constancy issues and bioavailability fence, ARMamalgated into PLGA NPs were formulated, categorized, and optimized using BBD. Morphological results revealed the spherical shape of the optimized NPs, exhibited 221 ± 14 nm globule sizes and release was sustained over specific period of time. It was found that reduction in amastigotes/macrophage and % infested macrophages *ex vivo*; after associated to that of blank ARM and were non-toxic in divergence to free compound (Allahverdiyev et al., 2013). In fact, ROS is well recognized for displaying anti-microbial activity. Moreover, different scientific reports have concluded that TiAg-NPs could act via accelerating of ROS formation which basically gets tested for ALA against L. *tropica*and L. *infantum* para-sites (Lopes et al., 2014). Further, mixture of TiAg-NPs with light assists as a favorable substitute against VL management. Cury et al. (2015) premeditated cinnamic acid loaded nanoliposomes and established them against protozoal cultures encompassing mixture of *Leishmania amazonensis* stain and DMSO (dimethylsulfoxide) solution. Further, evident interfaces of byproducts with lipid bilayer during assessment and acquiescent system for eliminating of leishmaniasis were concluded. In fact, dinitroanilines are exclusive chemical moieties with established *in vivo* ALA, but was found to be less aqueous soluble and accrues less at diseased sites were the chief complications in formulations. Despite of issues, Carvalheiro et al. (2015) resolved that nano healing method with addition of novel synthesized particles would be a healthier strategy for effective and enhanced controlling of V L. Observing this scenario, Falcao et al. (2013) established solid lipid nanoparticles (SLNs) and liposomes of oryzalin (OZ), associated there *in vitro* and *in vivo* clinical prospective. OZ loaded liposomes resulted in improved biodistribu-tion profiling with fewer hemolytic activity and cytotoxicity as compared to free drug. Further, scientists also established liposomal clusters of trifluralin byproducts to improve the ALA. The *in vitro* and *in vivo* assessment was performed by means of promastigotes of *L. infantum* parasite and amastigotes on a zoonotic VL murine model respectively. Further, formulated clusters exhibited reduced cytotoxicity and hemolytic activity with petite amastigote quantity in mice spleen. Handman (2001) shaped a nanotube conjugated drug delivery system which comprised of nanotubes, further used to solve out the issue of drug tempted toxicity of ALDs. This system established by the functionalized carbon nanotubes (f-CNTs) were bonded with AmP B and its yields AmP B-f-CNTs. This drug delivery system enhanced the drug efficacy to stop growth of *L. donovani* species. Furthermore, *in vitro* and *in vivo* studies showed reduced noxiousness to liver and kidney in mice.

5.2 FUTURE PROSPECTS

Notwithstanding, the progresses in the parasitological and biological investigations by means of numerous species of *Leishmania* parasites, the management choices available against leishmaniasis are found to be distant from pleasing. In the present situation, the improvement of novel drugs to contest leishmaniasis entail intensification input from the disciplines of chemistry, pharmacology, toxicology, and pharmaceutical technology to accompaniment the improvements in molecular biology. Natural products and their by-products are found to be the potential foundations of novel and discriminating agents used for management of vital tropical diseases instigated by protozoans and varied classes of parasites. The incredible chemical miscellany presented in the phytoconstituents and the favorable leads have already been established substantial implications against parasitic infections are required to be observed and discussed beside leishmania parasites. The development of natural products derived ALDs or their referents as per the concerns sketched above can be a strong positive inspiration on the management of leishmaniasis. Whenever conceivable, the macrophage assay with the significant intracellular amastigote phases should be castoff by rodent models. It must be specified for the tactics of utilizing extracts and parts of floras can serve two purposes: (i) authorization of the ethno-pharmacological usages of the medicinal and therapeutic plants, and (ii) preliminary fact for drug discovery by means of the exemplified results to find novel leads. But as per the reports, utmost studies have been conceded out on the promastigote phase of the parasites using plant isolates. Captivatingly, the promastigote phase is found to be the infectious form of the parasite in mammalian hosts, and supreme assessments conceded out with this type is the merely possible ALA of the plant-derived metabolites. Therefore, there is necessity to transmit out such accomplishments *in vivo*. Further, such varied methodologies will comfort us taking our natural composites or plant-derived metabolites to the next stage of drug discovery or novel drug delivery systems, focused for clinical trials. Additionally, the number of reports engaged towards the recognition of plant isolated metabolites with the aptitude to constrain the vital enzymes of *Leishmania* parasites is also limited. Hence, there is a necessity to perform such studies related to the mechanism of action of these selective plant-based metabolites. A harmless, shorter, and inexpensive treatment, the empathy of the most cost operative scrutiny system and control approaches, appropriate vector control method are some of the most significant characteristics for the control and complete abolition of this lethal disease.

KEYWORDS

- **anti-leishmanial agents**
- **antimalarial activity**
- **leishmaniasis**
- **nanomedicine**
- **nanotechnology**
- **phytoconstituents**

REFERENCES

Ajazuddin, & Saraf, S., (2010). Applications of novel drug delivery system for herbal formulations. *Fitoterapia*, *81*(7), 680–689.

Akendenguea, B. R. F., Loiseauc, P. M., Boriesc, C., Milamaa, E. G., Laurensb, A., & Hocquemiller, R., (2002). Klaivanolide, an antiprotozoal lactone from *Uvaria klaineana*. *Phytochemistry*, *59*, 885–888.

Allahverdiyev, A. M., Abamor, E. S., Bagirova, M., Baydar, S. Y., Ates, S. C., Kaya, F., Kaya, C., & Rafailovich, M., (2013). Investigation of antileishmanial activities of Tio2@Ag nanoparticles on biological properties of *L. tropica* and *L. infantum* parasites, *in vitro*. *Exp. Par.*, *135*(1), 55–63.

Aloui, Z., Messaoud, C., Haoues, M., Neffati, N., Bassoumi, J. I., Essafi-Benkhadir, K., Boussaid, M., et al., (2016). Asteraceae *Artemisia campestris* and *Artemisia herba-alba* essential oils trigger apoptosis and cell cycle arrest in *Leishmania infantum* promastigotes. *Evid. Based Complement Alternat. Med.*, 9147096.

Alrajhi, A. A., (2003). Cutaneous leishmaniasis of the old world. *Skin Ther. Lett.*, 1–7.

Amato, V. S., Tuon, F. F., Bacha, H. A., Neto, V. A., & Nicodemo, A. C., (2008). Mucosal leishmaniasis. Current scenario and prospects for treatment. *Acta. Trop.*, *105*(1), 1–9.

Andrade, M. A., Azevedo, C. D., Motta, F. N., Santos, M. L., Silva, C. L., Santana, J. M., & Bastos, I. M., (2016). Essential oils: *In vitro* activity against *Leishmania amazonensis*, cytotoxicity, and chemical composition. *BMC Complement Altern. Med.*, *16*(1), 444.

Armah, F. A., Amponsah, I. K., Mensah, A. Y., Dickson, R. A., Steenkamp, P. A., Madala, N. E., & Adokoh, C. K., (2018). Leishmanicidal activity of the root bark of *Erythrophleum Ivorense* (Fabaceae) and identification of some of its compounds by ultra-performance liquid chromatography quadrupole time of flight mass spectrometry (UPLC-QTOF-MS/ MS). *J. Ethnopharmacol.*, *211*, 207–216.

Ayub, S. G. M., Khalid, M., Mujtaba, G., & Bhutta, R. A., (2003). Cutaneous leishmaniasis in Multan: Species identification. *J. Pak. Med. Ass.*, *53*(10), 445.

Badaro, R., Benson, D., Euhilio, M. C., Freire, M., Cunha, S., Netto, E. M., Pedral-Sampaio, D., et al., (1996). rK39: A Cloned Antigen of *Leishmania chagasi* that predicts active visceral leishmaniasis. *J. Inf. Dis.*, *173*, 758–761.

Bafghi, A. F., Bagheri, S. M., & Hejazian, S. H., (2014). Antileishmanial activity of Ferulaassa-foetida oleo gum resin against *Leishmania major*: An *in vitro* study. *J. Ayurveda Integr. Med.*, *5*(4), 223–226.

Barrera, P. A., Jimenez-Ortiz, V., Tonn, C., Giordano, O., Galanti, N., & Sosa, M. A., (2008). Natural sesquiterpene lactones are active against *Leishmania mexicana*. *J. Parasitol.*, *94*(5), 1143–1149.

Basu, M. K., (2005). Liposomal delivery of antileishmanial agents. *J. App. Res.*, *5*(1), 221–236.

Bern, C., Moore, J. A., Berenguer, J., Boelaert, M., Boer, M. D., Davidson, R. D., Gradoni, L., et al., (2006). Liposomal amphotericin B for the treatment of visceral leishmaniasis. *Clin. Inf. Dis.*, *43*, 917–924.

Bero, J., Hannaert, V., Chataigne, G., Herent, M. F., & Quetin-Leclercq, J., (2011). *In vitro* antitrypanosomal and antileishmanial activity of plants used in Benin in traditional medicine and bio-guided fractionation of the most active extract. *J. Ethnopharmacol.*, *137*(2), 998–1002.

Bharate, S. B., & Singh, I. P., (2011). Quantitative structure-activity relationship study of phloroglucinol-terpene adducts as anti-leishmanial agents. *Bioorg. Med. Chem. Lett.*, *21*(14), 4310–4315.

Bhattacharya, S. K., Sinha, P. K., Sundar, S., Thakur, C. P., Jha, T. K., Pandey, K., Das, V. R., et al., (2007). Phase 4 trial of miltefosine for the treatment of Indian visceral leishmaniasis. *J. Inf. Dis.*, *196*, 591–598.

Braga, F. G., Bouzada, M. L., Fabri, R. L., De, O. M. M., Moreira, F. O., Scio, E., & Coimbra, E. S., (2007). Antileishmanial and antifungal activity of plants used in traditional medicine in Brazil. *J. Ethnopharmacol.*, *111*(2), 396–402.

Bringmann, G., Dreyer, M., Faber, J. H., Dalsgaard, P. W., Staerk, D., Jaroszewski, J. W., Ndangalasi, H., et al., (2004). Ancistrotanzanine C and related 5,1'-and 7,3'-coupled naphthylisoquinoline alkaloids from *Ancistrocla dustanzaniensis*. *J. Nat. Prod.*, *67*(5), 743–748.

Bringmann, G., Hamm, A., Gunther, C., Michel, M., Brun, R., & Mudogo, V., (2000). Ancistroealaines A and B two new bioactive naphthylisoquinolines, and related naphthoic acids from *Ancistrocla dusealaensis*. *J. Nat. Prod.*, *63*, 1465–1470.

Bringmann, G., Rudenauer, S., Irmer, A., Bruhn, T., Brun, R., Heimberger, T., Stuhmer, T., et al., (2008). Antitumoral and antileishmanial dioncoquinones and ancistroquinones from cell cultures of *Triphyophyllum peltatum* (Dioncophyllaceae) and *Ancistrocladus abbreviatus* (Ancistrocla daceae). *Phytochemistry, 69*(13), 2501–2509.

Bringmann, G., Saeba, W., Ruckerta, M., Miesa, J., Michela, M., Mudogob, V., & Brunc, R., (2003). Ancistrolikokine D a 5,80-coupled naphthylisoquinoline alkaloid, and related natural products from *Ancistrocladus likoko*. *Phytochemistry, 62*, 631–636.

Bufalo, J., Cantrell, C. L., Jacob, M. R., Schrader, K. K., Tekwani, B. L., Kustova, T. S., Ali, A., & Boaro, C. S., (2016). Antimicrobial and antileishmanial activities of diterpenoids isolated from the roots of *Salvia deserta*. *Planta. Med., 82*(1/2), 131–137.

Carvalheiro, M., Esteves, M. A., Santos-Mateus, D., Lopes, R. M., Rodrigues, M. A., Eleuterio, C. V., Scoulica, E., et al., (2015). Hemisynthetic trifluraline analogues incorporated in liposomes for the treatment of leishmanial infections. European journal of pharmaceutics and biopharmaceutics: *Eur. J. Pharm. Biopharm., 93*, 346–352.

Centers for Disease Control and Prevention (2020). http://www.cdc.gov/parasites/leishmaniasis/ (accessed on 25 June 2020).

Chen, M., Wang, S., Tan, M., & Wang, Y., (2011). Applications of nanoparticles in herbal medicine: Zedoary turmeric oil and its active compound beta-element. *Am. J. Chin. Med., 39*(6), 1093–1102.

Colomba, C., Saporito, L., Vitale, F., Reale, S., Vitale, G., Casuccio, A., Tolomeo, M., et al., (2009). Cryptic *Leishmania infantum* infection in Italian HIV infected patients. *BMC Inf. Dis., 9*, 199.

Cortez, D. S. J., Almeida-Souza, F., Mondego-Oliveira, R., Oliveira, I. S., Lamarck, L., Magalhaes, I. F., Ataides-Lima, A. F., et al., (2016). Leishmanicidal, cytotoxicity and wound healing potential of *Arrabidaea chicaVerlot*. *BMC Complement. Altern. Med., 16*, 1.

Cury, T. A., Yoneda, J. S., Zuliani, J. P., Soares, A. M., Stabeli, R. G., Calderon, L. A., & Ciancaglini, P., (2015). Cinnamic acid derived compounds loaded into liposomes: Antileishmanial activity, production standardization, and characterization. *J. Microencapsul., 32*(5), 467–477.

Da Silva, J. M., Antinarelli, L. M., Pinto, N. C., Coimbra, E. S., De Souza-Fagundes, E. M., Ribeiro, A., & Scio, E., (2014). HPLC-DAD analysis, antileishmanial, antiproliferative, and antibacterial activities of *Lacistemapubescens*: An Amazonian medicinal plant. *Biomed. Res. Int.*, 545038.

Das, A., Jawed, J. J., Das, M. C., Sandhu, P., De, U. C., Dinda, B., Akhter, Y., & Bhattacharjee, S., (2017). Antileishmanial and immunomodulatory activities of lupeol, a triterpene compound isolated from *Sterculia villosa*. *Int. J. Antimicrob. Agents,50*(4), 512–522.

Das, V. N. A., Sinha, A. N., Verma, N., Lal, C. S., Gupta, A. K., Siddiqui, N. A., & Kar, S. K., (2001). A randomized clinical trial of low dosage combination of pentamidine and allopurinol in the treatment of antimony unresponsive cases of visceral leishmaniasis. *J. Assoc. Physicians India, 49*, 609–613.

Duarte, M. C., Tavares, G. S., Valadares, D. G., Lage, D. P., Ribeiro, T. G., Lage, L. M., Rodrigues, M. R., et al., (2016). Antileishmanial activity and mechanism of action from a purified fraction of *Zingiber officinalis Roscoe* against *Leishmania amazonensis*. *Exp. Parasitol., 166*, 21–28.

Esquenazi, D., Wigg, M. D., Miranda, M. M. F. S., Rodrigues, H. M., Tostes, J. B. F., Rozental, S., Da Silva, A. J. R., & Alvianod, C. S., (2002). Antimicrobial and antiviral activities of polyphenolics from *Cocos nucifera* Linn. (*Palmae*) husk fiber extract. *Research in Microb.*, *153*, 647–652.

Falcao, R. A., Do Nascimento, P. L., De Souza, S. A., Da Silva, T. M., De Queiroz, A. C., Da Matta, C. B., Moreira, M. S., et al., (2013). Antileishmanial phenylpropanoids from the leaves of *Hyptis pectinata* (L.) poit. *Evid. Based Complement Alternat. Med.*, 460613.

Farokhzad, O. C., & Langer, R., (2009). Impact of nanotechnology on drug delivery. *ACS Nano.*, *3*(1), 16–20.

Feise, K., Müllerschön, C., Steigleder, C., & Keller, J., (2010). Old world cutaneous leishmaniasis After a stay in Spain, topical therapy with intralesional glucantine and paromomycin ointment. *Akt. Dermatol.*, *36*, 316–319.

Firenzuoli, F., & Gori, L., (2007). Herbal medicine today: Clinical and research issues. *Evid. Based Complement Alternat. Med.*, *4*(1), 37–40.

Fokialakis, N., Kalpoutzakis, E., Tekwani, B. L., Skaltsounis, E. L., & Duke, S. O., (2006). Antileishmanial activity of natural diterpenes from *Cistus* sp. and semisynthetic derivatives thereof. *Biol. Pharm. Bull.*, *29*(8), 1775–1778.

Fonseca-Silva, F., Inacio, J. D., Canto-Cavalheiro, M. M., & Almeida-Amaral, E. E., (2011). Reactive oxygen species production and mitochondrial dysfunction contribute to quercetin induced death in *L. amazonensis*. *PloS One*, *6*(2), e14666.

Fournet, A. B., Barrios, A. A., Munoz, V., Hocquemiller, R., Cave, A., & Bruneton, J., (1993). 2-substituted quinoline alkaloids as potential antileishmanial drugs. *Antimicrob. Agents. Chemother.*, *37*(4), 859–863.

Garcia, A. R., Amaral, A. C. F., Azevedo, M. M. B., Corte-Real, S., Lopes, R. C., Alviano, C. S., Pinheiro, A. S., et al., (2017). Cytotoxicity and anti-*Leishmania amazonensis* activity of Citrus sinensis leaf extracts. *Pharm. Biol.*, *55*(1), 1780–1786.

Garcia, M., Monzote, L., Montalvo, A. M., & Scull, R., (2010). Screening of medicinal plants against *Leishmania amazonensis*. *Pharm. Biol.*, *48*(9), 1053–1058.

Gontijo, V. S., Judice, W. A., Codonho, B., Pereira, I. O., Assis, D. M., Januario, J. P., Caroselli, E. E., et al., (2012). Leishmanicidal, antiproteolytic and antioxidant evaluation of natural biflavonoids isolated from *Garcinia brasiliensis* and their semisynthetic derivatives. *Eur. J. Med. Chem.*, *58*, 613–623.

Goto, H., & Lindoso, J. A., (2010). Current diagnosis and treatment of cutaneous and mucocutaneous leishmaniasis. *Expert Rev. Anti. Infect. Ther.*, *8*(4), 419–433.

Gutierrez, V., Seabra, A. B., Reguera, R. M., Khandare, J., & Calderon, M., (2016). New approaches from nanomedicine for treating leishmaniasis. *Chem. Soc. Rev.*, *45*(1), 152–168.

Handman, E., (2001). Leishmaniasis: Current status of vaccine development. *Clin. Micro. Rev.*, 229–243.

Hassane, I., Vincent, L. V., Mayeule, L., Deborah, L., Eric, C., & Gilbert, D., (2001). ABT 378/r: A novel inhibitor of HIV-1 protease in haemodialysis. *AIDS*, *15*(5), 662–664.

Houel, E., Gonzalez, G., Bessiere, J. M., Odonne, G., Eparvier, V., Deharo, E., & Stien, D., (2015). Therapeutic switching: From antidermatophytic essential oils to new leishmanicidal products. *Mem. Inst. Oswaldo Cruz.*, *110*(1), 106–113.

Ibrahim, S. R., Abdallah, H. M., Mohamed, G. A., & Ross, S. A., (2016). Integracides H-J: New tetracyclic triterpenoids from the endophytic fungus *Fusarium* sp. *Fitoterapia*, *112*, 161–167.

Italia, J. L., Sharp, A., Carter, K. C., Warn, P., & Kumar, M. N., (2011). Peroral amphotericin B polymer nanoparticles lead to comparable or superior *in vivo* antifungal activity to that of intravenous AMBISOME (R) or fungizone. *PloS One*, *6*(10), e25744.

Jha, T. K., Sundar, S., Thakur, C. P., Bachmann, P., Karwang, J., Fisher, C., Voss, A., & Berman, J., (1999). Miltefosine, an oral agent, for the treatment of Indian visceral leishmaniasis. *The New England J. Med.*, *341*(24), 1795–1800.

Jha, T. K., Sundar, S., Thakur, C. P., Felton, J. M., Sabina, A. J., & Horton, J., (2005). A Phase II dose-ranging study of sitamaquine for the treatment of visceral leishmaniasis in India. *Amer. J. Trop. Med. Hyg.*, *73*(6), 1005–1011.

Karioti, A., Skaltsa, H., Kaiser, M., & Tasdemir, D., (2009). Trypanocidal, leishmanicidal and cytotoxic effects of anthecotulide-type linear sesquiterpene lactones from *Anthemis auriculata*. *Phytomedicine*, *16*(8), 783–787.

Kaye, P., & Scott, P., (2011). Leishmaniasis: Complexity at the host-pathogen interface. *Nat. Rev. Microbiol.*, *9*(8), 604–615.

Khedr, A. I., Ibrahim, S. R., Mohamed, G. A., Ahmed, H. E., Ahmad, A. S., Ramadan, M. A., El-Baky, A. E., et al., (2016). New ursane triterpenoids from *Ficuspandurata* and their binding affinity for human cannabinoid and opioid receptors. *Arch. Pharm. Res.*, *39*(7), 897–911.

Kim, H. S., (2005). Do not put too much value on conventional medicines. *J. Ethnopharmacol.*, *100*(1/2), 37–39.

Kolodziej, H., Kayser, O., Kiderlen, A. F., Hatano, H. I., Yoshida, T., & Foo, L. Y., (2001). Antileishmanial activity of hydraolyzable tannins and their modulatory effects on nitric oxide and tumor necrosis factor-α release in macrophages *in vitro*. *Planta. Med.*, *67*, 825–832.

Kumar, V. D., P. R. P., & Singh, S. K., (2015). Development and evaluation of biodegradable polymeric nanoparticles for the effective delivery of quercetin using a quality by design approach. *LWT-Food Science and Technology*, *61*(2), 330–338.

Kumar, V. D., Verma, P. R., Singh, S. K., & Viswanathan, S., (2015). LC-ESI-MS/MS analysis of quercetin in rat plasma after oral administration of biodegradable nanoparticles. *Biomedical Chromatography: BMC*, *29*(11), 1731–1736.

Laborin, L. R., & Vargas, C. M. N., (2009). Amphotericin B: Side effects and toxicity. *Rev. Iberoam. Micol.*, *26*(4), 223–227.

Ladurner, P., Rieger, R., & Baguna, J., (2000). Spatial distribution and differentiation potential of stem cells in hatchlings and adults in the marine *Platyhelminth macrostomum* sp.: A bromodeoxyuridine analysis. *Dev. Bio.*, *226*(2), 231–241.

Lala, S., Pramanick, S., Mukhopadhyay, S., Bandyopadhyay, S., & Basu, M. K., (2004). Harmine: Evaluation of its antileishmanial properties in various vesicular delivery systems. *J. Drug Target*, *12*(3), 165–175.

Larghi, E., Bracca, A., Arroyo, A. A., Heredia, D., Pergomet, J., Simonetti, S., & Kaufman, T., (2015). Neocryptolepine: A promising indoloisoquinoline alkaloid with interesting biological activity. Evaluation of the drug and its most relevant analogs. *Cur. Topics Med. Chem.*, *15*(17), 1683–1707.

Leishmaniasis (2020). https://www.who.int/news-room/fact-sheets/detail/leishmaniasis (accessed on 25 June 2020).

Lopes, R. M., Gaspar, M. M., Pereira, J., Eleutério, C. V., Carvalheiro, M., Almeida, A. J., & Cruz, M. E. M., (2014). Liposomes versus lipid nanoparticles: Comparative study of lipid-based systems as oryzalin carriers for the treatment of leishmaniasis. *J. Biomed. Nanotechnol.*, *10*, 1–11.

Machumia, F., Samoylenkob, V., Yenesewa, A., Dresea, S., Midiwoa, J. O., Wiggersb, F. T., Jacobb, M. R., et al., (2010). Antimicrobial and antiparasitic abietane diterpenoids from the roots of *Clerodendrumeriophyllum*. *Nat. Prod. Commun.*, *5*(6), 853–858.

Maltezou, H. C., (2010). Drug resistance in visceral leishmaniasis. *J. Biomed. Biotech.*, 617521.

Manjolin, L. C., Dos Reis, M. B., Maquiaveli, C. C., Santos-Filho, O. A., & Da Silva, E. R., (2013). Dietary flavonoids fisetin, luteolin and their derived compounds inhibit arginase, a central enzyme in *Leishmania amazonensis* infection. *Food Chem.*, *141*(3), 2253–2262.

Maregesi, S. M., Hermans, N., Dhooghe, L., Cimanga, K., Ferreira, D., Pannecouque, C., Vanden, B. D. A., et al., (2010). Phytochemical and biological investigations of *Elaeodendron schlechteranum*. *J. Ethnopharmacol.*, *129*(3), 319–326.

Mazoir, N., Benharref, A., Bailén, M., Reina, M., González-Coloma, A., & Martínez-Díaz, R. A., (2011). Antileishmanial and antitrypanosomal activity of triterpene derivatives from latex of two euphorbia species. *ZeitschriftfürNaturforschung C,66*, 0360.

Medda, S. M. S., & Basu, M. K., (1999). Evaluation of the *in-vivo* activity and toxicity of amaogentin, an antileishmanial agent, in both liposomal and niosomal forms. *J. Antimicro. Chem.*, *44*, 791–794.

Misra, P., Sashidhara, K. V., Singh, S. P., Kumar, A., Gupta, R., Chaudhaery, S. S., Gupta, S. S., et al., (2010). 16alpha-hydroxycleroda-3,13(14) Z-dien-15,16-olide from *Polyalthialongifolia*: A safe and orally active antileishmanial agent. *Br. J. Pharmacol.*, *159*(5), 1143–1150.

Moraes, A. R. D. P., Tavares, G. D., Soares, R. F. J., De Paula, E., & Giorgio, S., (2018). Effects of nanoemulsions prepared with essential oils of copaiba-and andiroba against *Leishmania infantum* and *Leishmania amazonensis* infections. *Exp. Parasitol.*, *187*, 12–21.

Moura, D. C. D. F., Amaral, A. C., Machado, G. M., Leon, L. L., & Silva, J. R., (2012). Chemical and biological analyses of the essential oils and main constituents of Piper species. *Molecules*, *17*(2), 1819–1829.

Muhammad, I., Dunbar, D. C., Khan, S. I., Tekwani, B. L., Bedir, E., Takamatsu, S., Ferreira, D., & Walker, L. A., (2003). Antiparasitic alkaloids from *Psychotriaklugii*. *J. Nat. Prod.*, *66*(7), 962–967.

Narender, T., Shweta, & Gupta, S., (2004). A convenient and biogenetic type synthesis of few naturally occurring chromeno dihydrochalcones and their *in vitro* antileishmanial activity. *Bioorg. Med. Chem. Lett.*, *14*(15), 3913–3916.

Neva, F. A., (1990). Immunotherapy for parasitic disease. *The New England J. Med.*, *322*(1), 55–57.

Nour, A. M., Khalid, S. A., Kaiser, M., Brun, R., Abdalla, W. E., & Schmidt, T. J., (2010). The antiprotozoal activity of methylated flavonoids from *Ageratum conyzoides* L. *J. Ethnopharmacol.*, *129*(1), 127–130.

Oghumu, S., Varikuti, S., Saljoughian, N., Terrazas, C., Huntsman, A. C., Parinandi, N. L., Fuchs, J. R., et al., (2017). Pentalinonsterol, a constituent of *Pentalinonandrieuxii*, possesses potent immunomodulatory activity and primes T-cell immune responses. *J. Nat. Prod.*, *80*(9), 2515–2523.

Pearson, R. D., & Sousa, A. D. Q., (1996). Clinical spectrum of leishmaniasis. *Clin. Inf. Dis.,22*, 1–13.

Perez, A. P., Casasco, A., Schilrreff, P., Tesoriero, M. V., Duempelmann, L., Pappalardo, J. S., Altube, M. J., et al., (2014). Enhanced photodynamic leishmanicidal activity of hydrophobic zinc phthalocyanine within archaeolipids containing liposomes. *Int. J. Nanomed.*, *9*, 3335–3345.

Pierrot, H. A. D., Nathalie, N., Michel, T., Louise, P., Denis, B., & Michel, B. G., (1995). Lymphoid tissues targeting of liposome-encapsulated 2,'3'-dideoxyinosine (ddl) by encapsulation in liposomes. *AIDS, 95*, 21–28.

Polonio, T., & Efferth, T., (2010). Leishmaniasis: Drug resistance and natural products (Review). *Int. J. Mol. Med., 22*, 277–286.

Pulivarthi, D., Steinberg, K. M., Monzote, L., Piñón, A., & Setzer, W. N., (2015). Antileishmanial activity of compounds isolated from *Sassafras albidum. Nat. Prod. Commun., 10*(7), 1229–1230.

Radwan, M. M., Elsohly, M. A., Slade, D., Ahmed, S. A., Khan, I. A., & Ross, S. A., (2009). Biologically active cannabinoids from high-potency *Cannabis sativa. J. Nat. Prod., 72*(5), 906–911.

Rafferty, J., (2005). Curing the stigma of leprosy. *Lepr. Rev., 76*, 119–126.

Rafiee, A., Riazi-Rad, F., Darabi, H., Khaze, V., Javadian, S., Ajdary, S., Bahrami, F., & Alimohammadian, M. H., (2014). Ferroportin-encapsulated nanoparticles reduce infection and improve immunity in mice infected with *Leishmania* major. *Int. J. Pharm., 466*(1/2), 375–381.

Rahman, L., Shinwari, Z. K., Iqrar, I., Rahman, L., & Tanveer, F., (2017). An assessment on the role of endophytic microbes in the therapeutic potential of *Fagonia indica. Ann. Clin. Microbiol. Antimicrob., 16*(1), 53.

Rebolledo, G. A. G., Drier-Jonas, S., & Jimenez-Arellanes, M. A., (2017). Natural compounds and extracts from Mexican medicinal plants with anti-leishmaniasis activity: An update. *Asian Pac. J. Trop. Med., 10*(12), 1105–1110.

Regueira-Neto, M. D. S., Tintino, S. R., Rolon, M., Coronal, C., Vega, M. C., De Queiroz, B. V., & De Melo, C. H. D., (2018). Antitrypanosomal, antileishmanial and cytotoxic activities of Brazilian red propolis and plant resin of *Dalbergiaecasta phyllum* (L) Taub. *Food Chem. Toxicol., 119*, 215–221.

Reina, M. R. M., L., Ruiz-Mesia, W., Sosa-Amay, F. E., Arevalo-Encinas, L., González-Coloma, A., & Martínez-Díaz, R., (2014). *Antiparasitic indole* alkaloids from *Aspidospermades manthum* and *A. spruceanum* from the *Peruvian Amazonia. Nat. Prod. Commun., 9*(8), 1075–1090.

Reithinger, R. D. J. C., Louzir, H., Pirmez, C., Alexander, B., & Brooker, S., (2007). Cutaneous leishmaniasis. *Lancet Infect. Dis., 7*, 581–596.

Rodrigues, I. A., Ramos, A. S., Falcao, D. Q., Ferreira, J. L. P., Basso, S. L., Silva, J. R. A., & Amaral, A. C. F., (2018). Development of nanoemulsions to enhance the antileishmanial activity of *Copaifera paupera* Oleoresins. *Biomed. Res. Int.*, 9781724.

Rottini, M. M., Amaral, A. C., Ferreira, J. L., Silva, J. R., Taniwaki, N. N., Souza, C. S., D'escoffier, L. N., et al., (2015). *In vitro* evaluation of (–) alpha-bisabolol as a promising agent against *Leishmania amazonensis. Exp. Parasitol., 148*, 66–72.

Roy, P., Das, S., Bera, T., Mondol, S., & Mukherjee, A., (2010). Andrographolide nanoparticles in leishmaniasis: Characterization and *in vitro* evaluations. *Int. J. Nanomed., 5*, 1113–1121.

Sacks, D., & Noben-Trauth, N., (2002). The immunology of susceptibility and resistance to *Leishmania major* in mice. *Nat. Rev. Immunol., 2*(11), 845–858.

Sairafianpour, M., Christensen, J., Stærk, D., Budnik, B. A., Kharazmi, A., Bagherzadeh, K., & Jaroszewski, J. W., (2001). Leishmanicidal, antiplasmodial, and cytotoxic activity of novel diterpenoid 1,2-Quinones from *Perovskia abrotanoides*: New source of tanshinones. *J. Nat. Prod., 64*, 1398–1403.

Salem, M. M., & Werbovetz, K. A., (2006). Natural products from plants as drug candidates and lead compounds against leishmaniasis and trypanosomiasis. *Cur. Med. Chem.*, *13*, 2571–2598.

Sarkar, S., Mandal, S., Sinha, J., Mukhopadhyay, S., Das, N., & Basu, M. K., (2002). Quercetin: Critical evaluation as an antileishmanial agent *in vivo* in hamsters using different vesicular delivery modes. *J. Drug Target*, *10*(8), 573–578.

Sartorelli, P., Andrade, S. P., Melhem, M. S., Prado, F. O., & Tempone, A. G., (2007). Isolation of antileishmanial sterol from the fruits of cassia fistula using bioguided fractionation. *Phytother. Res.*, *21*(7), 644–647.

Sidana, J., Singh, S., Arora, S. K., Foley, W. J., & Singh, I. P., (2012). Terpenoidal constituents of *Eucalyptus loxophleba* ssp. *lissophloia*. *Pharm. Biol.*, *50*(7), 823–827.

Silva, A. M., Tavares, J., Silvestre, R., Ouaissi, A., Coombs, G. H., & Cordeiro-da-Silva, A., (2012). Characterization of *Leishmania infantum* thiol-dependent reductase 1 and evaluation of its potential to induce immune protection. *Parasite Immunol.*, *34*(6), 345–350.

Singh, N., Kumar, M., & Singh, R. K., (2012). Leishmaniasis: Current status of available drugs and new potential drug targets. *Asian Pac. J. Trop. Med.*, 485–497.

Singh, R. K., Pandey, H. P., & Sundar, S., (2006). Visceral leishmaniasis (kala-azar): Challenges ahead. *Indian J. Med. Res.*, *123*(3), 331–344.

Sundar, S., & Chatterjee, M., (2006). Visceral leishmaniasis-current therapeutic modalities. *Indian J. Med. Res.*, *123*(3), 345–352.

Sundar, S., Jha, T. K., Thakur, C. P., Bhattacharya, S. K., & Rai, M., (2006). Oral miltefosine for the treatment of Indian visceral leishmaniasis. *Trans. R. Soc. Trop. Med. Hyg.*, *100*(1), 26–33.

Sundar, S., Sinha, P. K., Rai, M., Verma, D. K., Nawin, K., Alam, S., Chakravarty, J., et al., (2011). Comparison of short-course multidrug treatment with standard therapy for visceral leishmaniasis in India: An open-label, non-inferiority, randomized controlled trial. *Lancet*, *377*, 477–486.

Takahashi, M., Fuchino, H., Sekita, S., & Satake, M., (2004). *In vitro* leishmanicidal activity of some scarce natural products. *Phytother. Res.*, *18*(7), 573–578.

Teles, C. B., Moreira-Dill, L. S., Silva, A. A., Facundo, V. A., De Azevedo, W. F. Jr., Da Silva, L. H., Motta, M. C., et al., (2015). A lupane-triterpene isolated from *Combretum leprosum* Mart. fruit extracts that interferes with the intracellular development of *Leishmania* (L.) amazonensis *in vitro*. *BMC Complement Altern. Med.*, *15*, 165.

Thakur, B. B., (2003). Breakthrough in the management of visceral leishmaniasis. *JAPI*, *51*, 649–651.

Thakur, C. P., Kanyok, T. P., Pandey, A. K., Sinha, G. P., Messick, C., & Oliiaro, P., (2000). Treatment of visceral leishmaniasis with injectable paramomycin (aminosidine). An open-label randomized phase-II clinical study. *Trans. R. Soc. Trop. Med. Hyg.*, *94*, 432–433.

Tiuman, T. S., Ueda-Nakamura, T., Alonso, A., & Nakamura, C. V., (2014). Cell death in amastigote forms of *Leishmania amazonensis* induced by parthenolide. *BMC Microbiology*, *14*(152), 1–12.

Tiuman, T. S., Ueda-Nakamura, T., Garcia, C. D. A., Dias, F. B. P., Morgado-Diaz, J. A., De Souza, W., & Nakamura, C. V., (2005). Antileishmanial activity of parthenolide, a sesquiterpene lactone isolated from *Tanacetum parthenium*. *Antimicrob. Agents. Chemother.*, *49*(1), 176–182.

Ulloa, J. L., Spina, R., Casasco, A., Petray, P. B., Martino, V., Sosa, M. A., Frank, F. M., & Muschietti, L. V., (2017). Germacranolide-type sesquiterpene lactones from *Smallanthus*

Biomarkers as Targeted Herbal Drug Discovery

sonchifolius with promising activity against *Leishmania mexicana* and *Trypanosoma cruzi*. *Parasit. Vectors*, *10*(1), 567.

Von, S. E., & Udey, M. C., (2004). Requirements for Th1-dependent immunity against infection with *Leishmania major*. *Microbes Inf.*, *6*(12), 1102–1109.

Vyas, S. P., & Gupta, S., (2006). Optimizing efficacy of amphotericin B through nanomodification. *Int. J. Nanomed.*, *1*(4), 417–432.

Want, M. Y., Islammudin, M., Chouhan, G., Ozbak, H. A., Hemeg, H. A., Chattopadhyay, A. P., & Afrin, F., (2017). Nanoliposomal artemisinin for the treatment of murine visceral leishmaniasis. *Int. J. Nanomedicine*, *12*, 2189–2204.

Want, M. Y., Islamuddin, M., Chouhan, G., Ozbak, H. A., Hemeg, H. A., Dasgupta, A. K., Chattopadhyay, A. P., & Afrin, F., (2015). Therapeutic efficacy of artemisinin-loaded nanoparticles in experimental visceral leishmaniasis. *Colloids Surf. B. Biointerfaces.*, *130*, 215–221.

Wasunna, M. K., Rashid, J. R., Mbui, J., Kirigi, G., Kinoti, D., Lodenyo, H., Felton, J. M., Sabin, M. A., & Horton, J., (2005). A Phase II dose-increasing study of sitamaquine for the treatment of visceral leishmaniasis in Kenya. *Amer. J. Trop. Med. Hyg.*, *73*(5), 871–876.

Wink, M., (2012). Medicinal plants: A source of anti-parasitic secondary metabolites. *Molecules*, *17*(11), 12771–12791.

World Health Organization (2020). First WHO Report on Neglected Tropical Diseases. http://whqlibdoc.who.int/publications/2010/9789241564090_eng.pdf (accessed on 25 June 2020).

CHAPTER 6

Delivery of Herbal Cardiovascular Drugs in the Scenario of Nanotechnology: An Insight

KUMAR ANAND,[1] SUBHABRATA RAY,[2] MD. ADIL SHAHARYAR,[1]
MAHFOOZUR RAHMAN,[3] RUDRANIL BHOWMIK,[1]
SANMOY KARMAKAR,[1] and MONALISHA SEN GUPTA [1]

[1]*Department of Pharmaceutical Technology, Jadavpur University,
Kolkata – 700032, West Bengal, India,
E-mail: sanmoykarmakar@gmail.com (S. Karmakar)*

[2]*Dr. B. C. Roy College of Pharmacy and Allied Health Sciences, Durgapur,
West Bengal – 713206, India*

[3]*Department of Pharmaceutical Sciences, Faculty of Health Science,
SHUATS-Allahabad, Uttar Pradesh, India*

ABSTRACT

Abundant adverse effects following the administration of synthetic drugs mainly in the case of chronic diseases have led the human life to a faceless threat for a healthy lifestyle. Medicaments from herbal sources have emerges as a safe choice and a better alternative. History of herbal drugs in the health care system is almost as old as human civilization and herbs more than thousand in numbers have been listed under the traditional system for treatment of various cardiovascular problems. Many of these plants have been found to provide desired pharmacological actions but their clinical use is very less due to their low bioavailability and other related profiles. According to WHO about 80% of the population still believe that drugs from natural sources has potential for advancement on clinical platform. Nanotechnology bears much hope for the development of many of these poor bioavailable herbal drugs. Converting herbal drugs to the nanoscale delivery system using various fabrication approaches can result in the improvement of many pharmacokinetic profiles as well as *in vivo* stability and controlled absorption of the drug at the desired site. Aim of the present review is to focus on many facts related to cardiovascular diseases (CVDs) and the role of herbal drugs in treatment with nanotechnology driven delivery system.

6.1 INTRODUCTION

In the history of the health care system, cardiovascular diseases (CVDs) are one of the most serious concerns and are emerging as a worldwide threat. It includes many diseases such as myocardial infarction, angina, chronic heart failure (CHF), stroke, hypertension (HTN), arrhythmia, hyperlipidemia, hardening of the arteries, and many more circulatory system disorders. In recent studies, it has been found that in the United States (US) every 33 seconds claims one death due to CVDs (Heart Disease and Stroke Statistics, 2018). Even 40% of total annual deaths are caused by only CVDs. As far the global effects of CVDs are concerned it is found to be the leading cause of death and accounted for around 18 million deaths per year in 2015 which is expected to increase to 23.6 million by 2030 (Heart Disease and Stroke Statistics, 2018). Despite of having highly developed health care systems, till date cardiovascular system-related diseases poses a major challenge and need proper investigation of related factors.

6.2 CARDIOVASCULAR RISK AND POSSIBLE REASONS

It can be well understood that a health care problem related to heart and circulatory systems will have innumerable reasons such as diet, obesity, lifestyle, genetics, etc. Amongst all these, nowadays in developed as well as in developing countries diet and obesity are two of the major factors for various non-communicable diseases, primarily including many of the CVDs.

In many proofs of concept studies related to diet and obesity both in developed countries like US and UK (United Kingdom) and developing countries such as India, it has been found that these two factors play a major role in inducing various cardiovascular disorders either directly or indirectly (Yusuf et al., 2001; Eilat-Adar, 2013; Kochar et al., 2011; Lavie et al., 2009; Shabana and Vijay, 2010).

Food consumption is an unique and classified habit of various categories of population depending on the availability and geographical conditions. As far as the basic ingested food is concerned, it is same in terms of chemistry such as fat, carbohydrate, and many other energy supplements. However, there are innumerable controversies related to the diet system which further leads to various aspects of health. Undoubtedly, there has been a great change worldwide in food systems since lifestyle change has occurred rapidly throughout the modern world. Processed and packaged foods are having a major contribution in this change (Ng et al., 2012). This tradition of the packaged food system has vastly increased the caloric supply and in parallel provides low-cost feed to livestock which further induces cheap inputs in processed foods mainly for profiteering (Connor and Schiek, 1997). It is also a fact that these packaged and processed foods contain various unsaturated fats and other materials, long term intake of which can trigger CVDs, mainly atherosclerosis (Eman et al., 2012; Reddy and Katan, 2004). Now with all recent innovative technologies of food processing and easy availability from farm to fork, there is a significant enhancement of food consumption of various qualities (Welch and Mitchell, 2000; Fellows, 2009; Burch and Lawrence, 2007). It has also been found in some recent studies that the production of foods from animal sources has been increased multiple times as compared to coarse grains and other natural veggies such as roots, legumes, etc. (Schaffer, Hunt, and Ray, 2007; Weis, 2013).

Now if we consider all the above factors it might be easier to under-stand the relation between food habits and cardiovascular and other clinical precipitates both in developed and developing nations. As the major basic food, constituents are the same across the globe, the consumption and effect of the same can be generalized depending on many proof of concept studies and various field works. As an outcome of various studies, it can be observed that fruit-rich diets, unrefined grains, vegetables, dairy products of low-fat content, and a diet containing low saturated fats and sodium can result in lowering CVDs (Aldana et al., 2007). Diets containing mono and polyun-saturated fats, sterols from plant sources, brans, various nuts, soy proteins, isoflavones, etc., are found to be beneficial for the health of the heart and reduces various risk to CVDs (Frank et al., 2006; Jensen et al., 2004). On other side diets containing trans-fat, added sugar, refined grains, red meat, and processed meat, etc., can accelerate cardiovascular risk enhancing factors (Mensink et al., 2003; Pan et al., 2013; Micha, Michas, and Mozaffarian, 2012).

Obesity also has an indistinguishable role towards many of the CVDs. An unhealthy lifestyle and nutritional disorders can lead to obesity and it further precipitates diverse clinical situations such as atherosclerosis, renal disorders, HTN, etc. (John et al., 2002). Many circulatory system disorders can be possibly caused by obesity such as diabetes and dislipidemia which further leads to stiffness of blood vessels and stroke like conditions. So diet and obesity or both of these in combination (which happens frequently in a sedentary lifestyle) can lead to many serious cardiovascular disorders.

Now as these CVDs are getting generalized and emerging to be a common health care problem, in long term, management of these diseases is a challenge and demands best screening processes related to medicines and various other factors. Science and technology has introduced innumerable active pharmaceutical ingredients for prevention and cure of more or less all CVDs. These active moieties can be categorized as antihypertensive, anti-anginal, antiarrythmic, diuretics, blood thinning, antioxidants, etc. In spite of many complex clinical conditions, these agents are found to be successful in manifestation of CVDs. But it has also been observed that in the long term these synthetic drugs can precipitate some undesired effect which further compels us to think of other options.

Inspite of lacking significant data related to clinical effects many herbal cardiovascular agents are proven to be comparatively safer than synthetic agents and can be used as an alternative to many synthetic drugs (Nick et al., 1998). Unlike the synthetic medicinal drugs, the herbal drugs exert very little, if any adverse effects. Adverse effects of synthetic drugs is a potential threat and according to a study about 8% of hospital admission in America is due to adverse effect of the drugs (Karimi et al., 2015). However, toxicity of any herbal drug can be possible due to misidentification (Karimi et al., 2015). As Herbal drugs have been used in medical treatments since the times of ancient civilizations, various drugs have become the mainstay of human pharmacotherapy. In cardiovascular system, herbal drugs are used in many disorders such as congestive heart failure (CHF), angina pectoris, atherosclerosis, cerebral insufficiency, systolic HTN, venous insufficiency (Nick et al., 1998) (Figure 6.1).

6.3   HERBAL REMEDIES OF CVDS

In the list of available herbs for such disorders, there are many sources such as *Commiphora mukul, Crataegus oxycantha, Inula racemosa, Terminalia arjuna*, digitalis, garlic, etc. In many research works related to CVDs many

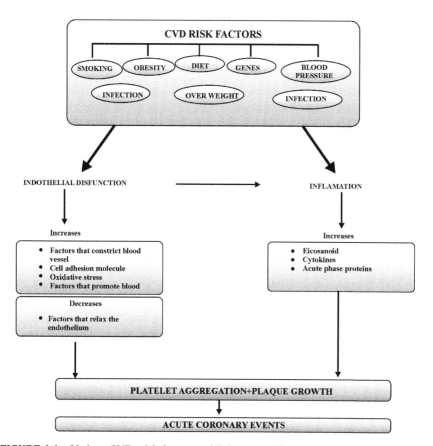

FIGURE 6.1   Various CVDs risk factors and links among them.

other herbs are being noticed to be useful for various CVDs (Jahan et al., 2016; Rachel and Michael, 2009). Many of the traditional herbs are also used in diet for betterment of heart as well as to reduce obesity (Hannah and Parameswari, 2010). The mechanism of action of these herbs and natural ingredients for keeping a heart-healthy may differ from product to product and sometimes exert multiple effects in a way to modulate cardiovascular system (Frishman, Sinatra, and Moizuddin, 2004). Ginger, garlic, curcumin, black pepper, coriander, and cinnamon are natural herbs which are used for a good cardiac health. Apart from the other global claims of these herbs, in traditional Indian system, i.e., Ayurveda, and Siddha all these species of herbs are described as medicinal plants for cardiac health and having properties such as antithrombic, hypolipidemic, antiatherosclerotic, etc. (Srivastava, Bordia, and Verma, 1995). A brief description of these medicinal herbs can be given as follows:

1. **Garlic:** It is well known as *Allium sativam* and believed to be originated from Central Asia. Garlic is used worldwide as a food ingredient mainly as flavoring agent to enhance physical and mental health. As a cardiovascular agent, garlic is claimed to prevent heart diseases and can also be used as a heart tonic by maintaining the fluidity of heart (Fenwick and Hanley, 1985; Mykolas, 2009). Garlic as a part of diet or alone is advocated to exert a positive role in preventing or delaying the CVDs by reducing blood lipid content by inhibiting enzymes involved in lipid synthesis, decreasing plate-lets aggregation, reducing HTN, preventing lipid per-oxidation of oxidized erythrocytes and inhibiting angiotensin converting enzymes (Rahman, 2001; Khalid et al., 2006).

2. **Ginger:** It is well known as *Zingiber officinale* and belongs to family Zingiberacae. Ginger is a very famous herbal medicine and is commonly used in Chinese, Tibb-Unani, and Ayurvedic herbal medicinal system. Since ancient age ginger is a part of diet and supposed to be useful for a wide range of health effects such as rheumatism, arthritis, sprains, muscular aches, pains, sore throats, cramps, HTN, constipation, indigestion, vomiting, dementia, fever, infectious diseases and helminthiasis (Ali et al., 2008). As far as the cardiovascular effects of the ginger are concerned, in an experi-mental study ginger is noticed to decrease coronary artery diseases by significant reduction in platelet aggregation (Bordia, Verma, and Srivastava, 1997). In a different proof of concept studies on various kinds of animals like rabbits and rats it has been concluded that ginger and its extracts can be useful for maintaining the lipid profiles (Sharma, Gusain, and Dixit, 1998; Bhandari, Kanojia, and Pillai, 2005).

3. **Cinnamon:** It is extensively used spices of India, Sri Lanka, Australia, Egypt, and China. The leaves and bark of cinnamon is used to produce essential oil (EO). The EO is believed to have some cardiovascular effects (Kawatra and Rathai, 2015). Cinnamon extracts are found to decrease cholesterol synthesis by inhibiting HMG-CoA reductase, an enzyme which catalyzes cholesterol biosynthesis. Cinnamon by activating $PPAR_\gamma$ results in improved

insulin resistance which further reduced fasted LDL-c, and managed obesity-related hyperlipidemia and also increased NO levels, which acts as a potent Vasodilator (Kamal, Thanaa, and El-Twab, 2009).

4. **Coriander:** It is one of the most common spices used in India. *Coriandrum sativam* or coriander as a traditional drug has a long history. In cardiovascular health, coriander is used to decreased cholesterol and lipid. Even it has been reported that the coriander is responsible for a significant decrease of LDL and VLDL and enhancement of HD L. Thus, in overall effect, *Coriandrum sativam* is responsible for good cardiac health.

Other than these all herbal medicine turmeric, black pepper, etc., are also found to improve cardiac health and useful in CVDs.

There are innumerable allopathic drugs available for the management of many serious cardiovascular disorders and many of the CVDs are chronic in nature. In the same context if we consider the safety of entire human physiology it will be better to consider that use of allopathic system can be a need of emergency but if we have time then there are other better ways such as treatment with herbal medicines. As far as the herbal medicines are concerned other than the above-mentioned herbal products there are many other herbs, extract, or parts of the same which can be used as medicine for the treatment of many acute or chronic CVDs like HTN, CHF, atherosclerosis, cerebral, and peripheral vascular disease, angina pectoris, venous insufficiency, arrhythmia, etc. Various medicinal plants such as *Crataegus oxycantha*, *Rauwolfia serpentina*, *Inula racemosa*, *Terminalia arjuna*, *Commiphora mukul*, *Digitalis*, *Astragalus*, *Aesculus hippocastan*, *Ginkgo biloba*, etc., are found to be useful for many cardiovascular disorders. Each of these herbs has their own property for treating CVDs.

Many herbs are found to contain potent cardioactive glycosides having serious cardiovascular effects showing positive inotropic actions. Digitalis purpurea is one of the famous herbs containing cardioactive glycosides used successfully for cardiac arrhythmia leading to CHF since many decades. Digoxin and Digitalis are the responsible cardioactive glycosides found in *Digitalis pupurea*. Digitalis lanata contains only digoxin. As a drawback of the drug, the therapeutic index of digitalis and digoxin is very low which makes the dose of the drug a subject of concern (Amine et al., 2016).

Another famous herb used for cardiovascular disease mainly for HTN is *Rauwolfia serpentina*. The root of Rauwolfia is used for this purpose. The main responsible drug used as antihypertensive is Reserpine. It was one of the most famous drugs used on a large scale in that period of time as a systemic antihypertensive. Mechanism of action of reserpine as antihypertensive includes decrease in vascular peripheral resistance and cardiac output, lowering heart rate as well as decreasing renin secretion (Charles et al., 1963).

Panax ginseng is also an important source of drug from herbal arena used for CVDs mainly HTN, myocardial ischemia and dyslipidemia. Ginseng is one of the older and traditional drugs used from natural sources. Part of the ginseng responsible for the drug action is known as ginsenoside. As far as the pharmacological actions are concerned as there are innumerable types of ginsenoside identified, it may have various pharmacological actions involve in the therapy. About 40 ginsenosides has been identified till 2012 depending on the method of separation and analysis (Fuzzati, 2004). In a proof of concept study, it has been found that the Korean red ginseng increases blood pressure (BP) in case of low BP while it works as an antihypertensive in the condition of higher BP (Jeon et al., 2000).

Breviscapine is one of the most significant drugs used for the treatment of cardiovascular and cerebrovascular disorders. It is a crude extract of many flavonoids of *Erigeron breviscapus* (Vant.). Hand.-Mazz., containing at least 85% of scutellarin, which is a famous traditional herbal drug used in China as a cerebrovascular medicine to improve cerebral blood supply. According to various *in vivo* and *in vitro* proofs of concept studies, it has been observed that breviscapine exerts a wide range of cardiovascular pharmacological effects, such as vasodilation, anticoagulat, antithrombotic, endothelial protector. Apart from that, it helps to reduce smooth muscle cell migration and proliferation and helps in anticardiac remodeling, antiarrhythmia, and blood lipid reduction. Further many clinical studies have reported that breviscapine could be used in conjunction with Western medicine for CVDs including coronary heart disease, myocardial infarction, atrial fibrillation, HTN, viral myocarditis, hyperlipidemia, pulmonary heart disease, and chronic heart failure.

Many other herbal drugs which are used as drugs for various CVDs can be seen as given in Table 6.1.

Regardless of having so many herbal drugs for variety of cardiovascular disorder both for acute and chronic in nature there are, many issues related to dose and efficacy of the drugs along with some toxicological concerns. These all herbal drugs are limited to their respective clinical manifestation because of their high dose and related toxic effects. Therefore, to overcome these problems and to make the herbal drugs more clinical significant, nanotechnology is a real need. This nanosized dependent technology where it is defined as techniques aimed to conceive, characterize, and produce material at the nanometer scale, represent a fully expanding domain, where one can predict without risk that production and utilization of nanosize materials will increase exponentially in near future.

TABLE 6.1   Herbal Drugs Used in Cardiovascular Disease

Sl. No.	Herbal Source	Cardiovascular Use	References
1.	Asian ginseng	Hypertension, hypercholesterolemia	Catherine et al., 2006
2.	Astragalus	Hyperhomocysteinemia, vascular protection	QIU et al., 2017
3.	Flaxseed oil	Hypercholestrolemia	Rodriguez-Leyva et al., 2010; Ankit et al., 2014
4.	Grape (*Vitis vinifera*) seeds	Atherosclerosis, hypertension, hypercholesterolemia, chronic venous insufficiency	Mustali and Joseph, 2009
5.	Hawthorn	Mild to moderate heart failure (NYHA I-II).	Mary et al., 2010
6.	Black pepper	Hypolipidemic effect, myocardial infarction, pressure overload-induced hypertrophy.	Shenuarin and Fukunaga, 2009
7.	*Inula racemosa*	Cardiac ischemia, pressure overload-induced hypertrophy	Chabukswar et al., 2010
8.	*Terminalia arjuna*	Cardioprotective, hypercholesterolemia	Shridhar, 2007

On conversion to nanoscale the surface area of parent molecule increases to a great extent which enables the formulation to achieve significantly enhanced pharmacokinetic parameters such as solubility, permeability, and hence bioavailability.

In recent decades with the help of many proofs of concept studies, it has been proven that herbal drug delivery using nanotechnology is better than the conventional herbal deliveries.

6.4   CONVENTIONAL DELIVERY PROBLEM OF HERBAL DRUGS

In the process of establishment of therapeutic efficacy and safety of herbal drugs, clinical studies are either not performed or scant from the studies.

In recent studies, it has been observed that in-spite of being therapeutically active many herbal drug shows clinical limitation and precipitates various toxicity problems depending on the dose and dosage of the drug. Many of the herbal drugs which are useful in various cardiovascular therapies are drawing attention towards their clinical use due to low therapeutic index which further signifies the dose of the drug and indicates the need of novel delivery system.

6.5 USE OF NANOTECHNOLOGY FOR OVERCOMING VARIOUS DELIVERY PROBLEMS

Novel drug delivery systems are emerging to be a necessity for herbal medicinal system for the purpose of increasing the efficacy of drug and reducing the side effects of many herbal compounds. The integration of the novel drug delivery system and innumerable herbal medicines is supposed to combat more serious diseases. Since decades regardless of established therapeutic and pharmacological effects, herbal medicines were not considered for the development of novel formulations due to lack of scientific justification and processing difficulties, like, extraction, standardization, and identification of individual drug components in mixed polyherbal systems. However, with the help of newer outcomes in research and technology in phytopharmaceutical field it seems to solve the problems related to delivery of herbal medicines and other pharmacokinetic problems such as determination of pharmacokinetics (PKs), mechanism of action, site of action, accurate dose required, etc., by incorporating the drugs in novel drug delivery system, such as microemulsions, nanoparticles, solid dispersions, matrix systems, liposomes, solid lipid nanoparticles (SLNs), etc. Recently used novel drug delivery systems for the incorporation of herbal drugs and compounds can be briefly described as:

1. **Liposome:** These are nanosized spherical lipoidal delivery systems capable of entrapment and delivery of both hydrophilic and hydrophobic drug candidates because of its specialized structural characteristics. Liposomal vesicles may composed of natural and/ or synthetic surface active agents like phospho or sphingo-lipids. These are natural surfactant and can arrange themselves in tail to tail manner forming a bilayer flexible membrane containing some water. Liposomes can vary from 0.5 μ to 5 μ in size and are unique delivery

system for drugs with highly variable lipophilicities. Liposomes with herbal drug are known as herbosomes. In CVDs, herbosomes can be used as a potential delivery system (La Grange et al., 1999). Other than herbosomes these systems are also known as planterosomes. In this word, planterosomes 'plantero' stands for herb and 'some' stand for cell-like structure. These are the novel formulation which offers comparatively significant and better bioavailability of hydrophilic herbal drugs and flavonoids and are absorbed through skin or gastrointestinal tract. Here the phosphatidylcholine molecules in the herbosomal or planterosomal complex act by pushing the phytochemical constituents through the outer membrane of gastrointestinal epithelial cells which further enters into the bloodstream (Athira et al., 2014).

2. **Microemulsion:** According to the definition of Danielsson and Lindman, "a microemulsion is a system of water, oil, and an amphiphile which is a single optically isotropic and thermodynamically stable liquid solution." These are transparent or translucent formulation and categorized as water in oil (w/o) or oil in water (o/w) systems in the size range of 5 to 50 nm (Danielsson and Lindman, 1981). Microemulsion system is usually much different than emulsion (with a size range of >0.1 µm) and nanoemulsion (thermodynamically unstable). According to IUPAC, in an emulsion liquid droplets and/or liquid crystals, are dispersed in a liquid. So As for the characteristics of the microemulsion is concerned, microemulsion is excluded from this definition if the word "dispersed" is explained as non-equilibrium and opposite to "solubilized," a term which can be applied to microemulsion and micellar systems. Unlike microemulsion, the latter ones are not thermodynamically stable.

3. **Nanoemulsion:** In recent decades, the branch of science dealing with fast screening of material and unique ability of combinatorial chemistry has gifted the idea of nanoemulsion formulation. Approaches for nanoemulsion remain more or less similar in comparison to microemulsion. It also requires a synthetic and/or natural oil, with surfactants and co-surfactants for fabrication into an oil in water (o/w) or water in oil (w/o) emulsion system having a droplet size of 5 to 500 nm (Kale et al., 2017). The membrane stability and flexibility of the system come as the result of the used surfactant and co-surfactant mixture. Nanoemulsion is thermodynamically unstable but has long term kinetic stability. The drug loading (DL) capacity

of nanoemulsion is quite high because of its increased surface area. Micro and nanoemulsion bear much hope for the successful delivery of hydrophobic drug candidates.

4. **Solid Lipid Nanoparticles (SLNs):** These deal mainly with particle science and can be seen as an alternative approach for nano/micro-emulsions and liposomes. In the SLN drug delivery system, the lipid droplets convert themselves in a crystallized state and orient themselves in highly ordered structures with the drug molecules present with them. The particles presented in nanoemulsion are mainly lipid in nature and hence the delivery system will be as advantageous as nano/microemulsions. SLNs can be viewed as submicron carriers ranging 50–1000 nm in size and are made up of biocompatible and biodegradable lipids capable of incorporating both lipophilic and hydrophilic drugs (Ekambaram, Sathali, and Priyanka, 2012). SLNs have been extensively studied as carriers for the delivery of antidepressants, cardiovascular, anticancer agents, (Dasam et al., 2016; Palanivel et al., 2018), and antioxidants. SLNs are particularly useful in enhancing the bioavailability of drugs that are used in treating CNS disorders. These SLNs can be coated with hydrophilic molecules which can improve the bio-distribution, stability, and other important pharmacokinetic parameters like bioavailability of incorporated drug moieties.

5. **Nanostructure Lipid Carriers (NLCs):** These are the modified form of SLNs. In SLNs, the lipid droplets are made to fully crystal-lize containing the therapeutic material in the core of it. It is seen that after a level of crystallization or re-crystallization the solubility of drug molecule present in the core of formulation starts to decline. NLCs thus contain a mixed form of lipid, i.e., solid, and liquid both. As recently approved lipophilic drug molecules are concerned, similar to the nanoemulsion and microemulsion formulations, the loading capacity of NLCs is also more because of oils in the formulation. In a recent carried research work, NLCs are used for Breviscapine isolated from the Chinese herb Erigeron breviscapus. In this experimental work it has been prove that isolated breviscapine loaded NLCs significantly enhance the various pharmacokinetic profiles in comparison to the conventional one (Mei et al., 2013).

Now as far as the drug delivery benefits of the nanotechnology-based dosage forms are a concern which is briefly described above, it can be clearly understood that nanosize particles or any form of structure which encloses the drug actually increases the surface area and volume ratio, and it results in the enhancement of basic pharmacokinetic functions such as absorption, solubility, dissolution, and finally results in the significant improvement of the bioavailability. Many advantages of the nanotechnology and nano carrier in herbal drug delivery are:

- Ability to deliver maximum concentrations of drugs to the sites of action due to their nanosize range and high loading efficiency.
- These nanocarriers enable the drug to be delivered in a very small size which results in significant enhancement of the entire surface area of the loaded herbal drugs and causes a fast release in the blood.
- Sustained release of the drug is possible which further reduces the frequent dosage regimen.
- Enhanced permeation and retention effect is possible, i.e., enhanced permeation through the barriers due to small size and retention because of poor lymphatic drainage such as in tumor.
- Shows passive targeting to the site of action without any addition of particular ligand moiety.
- Reduction in the dose of the drug.
- Reduction in side effects as well as toxicity due to significant dose reduction.
- Beneficial for the herbal drugs whose therapeutic index is low.

In the case of CVDs, many forms of herbal drugs are used depending on the nature of disease and the site of action. Regardless of favorable pharmacological actions these drugs are clinically unfit or facing some trouble due to conventional dosage forms. Digoxin ad digitoxin both are one of the oldest (about 200 years old) and probably the least expensive drugs for CHF. Digitoxin and digoxin are most famous cardiac glycosides and are used in case of CHF. Generally, both of these drugs are used in the form of tablets and liquid dosage form. This conventional dosage forms sometimes caused problems due to drug's narrow therapeutic index and requires better therapeutic monitoring. Digoxin is suggested not to be given with a loading dose in case of stable patients with sinus rhythm. A single daily dose of 0.25 mg for maintenance is commonly employed in adults with normal renal function. In the case of the elderly and the patients with renal impairment, a reduced dose of 0.125 or 0.0625 mg/day should be used (Amine et al., 2016). There are innumerable problems faced in the process to choose an effective dose for a drug such as digoxin and it is difficult because of many components showing narrow therapeutic index which further causes difficulty to define therapeutic endpoints, patients' variability, and varying effects of pathological states and drugs on digoxin disposition. Thus to reduce the dose with care to maintain the minimum therapeutic effect nanotechnology can be a better approach in comparison to the conventional one. In a recent experimental study, Ping Luo et al. has developed a SLN of digoxin (Ping and Yangwu, 2017). Here the aim of the study is to develop a polyethylene glycol-based nanoparticle of digoxin solid lipid and to enhance the absorption and bioavailability of the drug moiety. With this effect, it is also aimed to decrease the dose of the drug and hence the related toxicity and side effects. In this study, the diameter of digoxin SLN is about 275 nm where particle size again decreases with modification in PEG. *In-vitro* release of the digoxin SLN shows a sustained release with effect to 72-hour and cumulative release of 48.67%, further when its release rate slows with the increase of modification proportion of polyethylene glycol. With the same drug digoxin, Norah A Albekairi et al. has developed polymeric nanoparticle for transport across BoWocells (Norah et al., 2015). Biodegradable digoxin-loaded PEGylated poly (lactic-co-glycolic acid) nanoparticles are supposed to increase digoxin transport through BeWo b30 cell monolayers (an *in vitro* model of trophoblast in human placenta) by reducing the drug's interaction with P-gp (P-glycoprotein). Taking fetal cardiac arrhythmia as an important concern, this is a fine approach in health science to formulate such dosage form.

Depending on various reports and studies fetal cardiac arrhythmias is found to occur in 1% of pregnancies and can result in fatal heart failure (Thakur et al., 2013; Huhta, 2005). This kind of arrhythmias can also represent a leading cause of fetal hydrops, i.e., effusions in more than one fetal compartment, which has an incidence of 1 in 2500 pregnancies (Thakur et al., 2013; Parker, 2006). Digoxin is the drug of choice for the treatment of fetal tachyarrhythmias as well as fetal CHF (Mongiovì et al., 2010). As digoxin is a substrate for the efflux transporter P-gp, transplacental transfer of digoxin to the fetus is limited because P-gp is highly expressed in human placenta (Petropoulos, Gibb, and Matthews, 2010), and is also well expressed in BeWo cells (Utoguchi et al., 2000). So as a result, higher, and more frequent doses of digoxin are required during pregnancy to maintain therapeutic concentrations (Kleinman and Nehgme, 2004). Use of digoxin for prenatal therapy can lead to undesirable side effects for the mother, because the majority of the dose remains in the maternal circulation (Ward, 1996). These side effects can be seen as palpitations, second-degree atrioventricular block, and hypotension like serious effect (Ward, 1996). Now observing these situations, it's a great need to improve the delivery of digoxin to the fetus and simultaneously minimize maternal drug exposure. It is only possible by novel drug delivery systems which has the potential for better efficiency of DL with reduced dose and hence reduction in overall toxicity. As a result of these studies, it has been demonstrated that polymeric (PEGylated PLGA) nanoparticles is possible to be loaded successfully with digoxin with significant high encapsulation efficiency with the help of modified solvent displacement method. These developed nanoparticles will show sustained drug release kinetics, and further these nanoencapsulation is made to protect the loaded digoxin from P-gp-mediated efflux in the placental trophoblast layer, resulting in increased maternal-to fetal transfer of the drug, which is desired to optimize fetal drug therapy. Here delivery of digoxin is increased to the fetus which results in lower levels of the drug in the maternal circulation, which should result in reduced risks for the aforementioned maternal side effects (Norah et al., 2015). Here as a conclusion, use of polymeric nanoparticles encapsulated digoxin is to treat fetal cardiac arrhythmia and it has significantly improved outcomes for both the mother and her fetus.

In a different study of novel drug delivery, breviscapine is developed into PLGA microparticle (Hong et al., 2017). In this proof of concept study, nanocrystal technology along with a water-soluble polymer template method were used to develop nanocrystal-loaded microparticles with enhanced DL capacity and encapsulation efficiency for sustained delivery of breviscapine. Here using precipitation ultrasonication method nanocrystals were prepared and further the same is loaded into PLGA microparticles by casting in a mold from a water-soluble polymer. Applying both the methods, i.e., nanocrystal, and template methods the DL was significantly enhanced and jumped from 2.4% to 15.3%. Similarly, the encapsulation efficiency also increased from 48.5% to 91.9%. But with an increase in the DL here loading efficiency was found to be reduced. As far as the release pattern is concerned, all microparticles showed an initial burst release, and then a slow release period of 28 days followed by an erosion-accelerated release phase. This release pattern of the dosage form provides a sustained delivery of drugs over a month. A Stable serum drug level for more than 30 days was observed by using intramuscular injection of microparticles using rats. As a conclusion, it can be said that PLGA microparticles loaded with nanocrystals of poorly soluble drugs can be useful as a promising approach for long-term therapeutic products characterized with preferable *in vitro* and *in vivo* performance (Hong et al., 2017).

Genistein, a soybean derivative and 5,7,4, triatomic isoflavone, are supposed to improve cardiovascular risk profile in postmenopausal women carrying metabolic syndrome (MetS), but unfortunately only few literature records are available revealing genistein effects on cardiac system in humans (Cesare et al., 2017). This herbal drug is poorly aqueous soluble due to which it shows low serum level after administration (Aleksandra et al., 2010). Due to its low solubility the resulting bioavailability is low and this condition requires the emergence of a novel delivery system for improved PKs parameters. In these process nanoparticles of genistein has been prepared using Eudragit E. These nanoparticles have been prepared by nanoprecipitation method. Eudragit E are cationic polymers and widely used for improving the solubility of poor aqueous soluble drugs. Actually, Eudragit contains a tertiary amine group which ionizes in the G.I fluid. This tertiary amine group helps the dosage form to dissolve easily in gastric environment. In this present proof of concept study use of eudragit and nanoparticle form significantly enhances the bioavailability by improving genistein solubility. As a result of nanoparticle fabrication the relative bioavailability is found to be 241.8% as compared to the Genistein alone (Tang et al., 2011).

Since ancient age, Green tea has been considered as healthy beverage and included in daily food list. According to East Asian medicine, Consumption of green tea has been suggested for headaches, body aches and pains, depression, digestion, and detoxification as well as an energizer. Generally, green tea is believed to prolong life (Cabrera, Artacho, and Gimenez, 2006). Epigallocatechin-3-gallate (EGCG) is the major component of green tea. EGCG of tea catechins is found to exert many cellular and molecular effects related to the health-promoting actions. In various research studies, it has been found that oral consumption of green tea may give protection against obesity-related disorders such as atherosclerosis, HTN, and diabetes. As a very important fact, it has been observed that only purified EGCG (50–100 mg/kg), and not any other green tea catechins, significantly reduced or prevented an increase in body weight (BW) in lean and obese Zucker rats (Kao et al., 2000). These above effects are appeared to be reversible and associated with a reduction in food intake.

In recent decades many proofs of concept studies as well as various scientific and medical experiments has been subjected to green tea for the determination of its potential health benefits. As a result of these studies, it has been found that consumption of green tea includes the possibility of extending the human life span. As a conclusion, it can be understood that green tea drinkers are very less prone to die from stroke (Keli et al., 1996) and coronary heart diseases (Hertog et al., 1997). Many clinical parameters are unable to study due to the low bioavailability of green tea. This low bioavailability of green tea can be due to its limited intestinal absorption. Now as to enhance the bioavailability, it is an emerging need to deliver the green tea as a novel delivery.

One possible way to enhance the intestinal uptake of green tea catechins is to introduce a nanoemulsified capsule. Here nano-emulsification could improve bioavailability by enhancing intestinal uptake. The use of nano-emulsified capsule as a result significantly enhances the Protein expression of LDL receptor in the livers of both the GTE (green tea extract)- and NGTE (nanoemulsified green tea extract)-treated groups (+234.1%, P<.01 and +274.7%, P<.001), with a greater effect in the NGTE than in the GTE group. Cholesterol 7α-hydroxylase gene expression was also increased in both the GTE and NGTE groups. As a result, it can be concluded that delivery of green tea catechins through a nanoemulsified capsule can be a better way to increase bioavailability (Young et al., 2012).

6.6   LIMITATION OF HERBAL DRUGS

Despite using herbal drugs for more than 200 years and achieving innumerable pharmacological activities it is also true that maximum of these herbs are not clinically established for their concerned pharmacological properties. Clinical data related to innumerable and countless herbs are either scant or non-existent to date. As the clinical processes consist of determination of dose for different age groups such as pediatric and geriatric, the dose-less consumption of herbs and plant-related medicines can be an erroneous approach. Lacking of these clinical establishments many of the above-mentioned and various other herbal drugs that are prominently showing their pharmacological actions are showing many adverse actions (Nick et al., 1998). Because of such undesired and unwanted effects, it is going to be vital to inquire about such herbal medications and also to verify all related clinical information about the concerned herbal drug therapy.

6.7   CONCLUSION

In recent decades, general acceptability towards herbal drugs and plant-related medicines has been increased for the sake of a good lifestyle. Understanding the possible risks related to synthetic drugs, herbal drugs should be an important concern towards the health care system, especially for those diseases which are chronic in nature. In a similar context, as many of the CVDs are chronic in nature, it should be necessary to treat them with herbal drugs. As far as the clinical data are concerned, it is an important subject to be considered in order to enhance the various dimensions of safety-related facts. Further, in order to include plants and natural resources as an important part of modern medicine and to contribute largely to the commercial drug manufacturing industry today, it is an immediate necessity of the scientific world to clinically establish all the herbal drugs. Conclusively treatment of CVDs with the help of herbal drugs is an extremely important field and requires more interest in a better lifestyle.

ACKNOWLEDGMENT

We express our sincere thanks to the DST-Inspire fellowship program, Govt. of India, DST-SERB, UGC-UPE II, and AICTE-RPS, for providing financial support which was utilized for the present study.

KEYWORDS

- bioavailability
- cardiovascular problems
- congestive heart failure
- herbal drugs
- metabolic syndrome
- nanotechnology

REFERENCES

Aldana, S. G., Greenlaw, R., Salberg, A., Merrill, R. M., Hager, R., & Jorgensen, R. B., (2007). The effects of an intensive lifestyle modification program on carotid artery intima media thickness: A randomized trial. *American Journal of Health Promotion, 21*(6), 510–516.

Aleksandra, R., et al., (2010). Synthetic derivatives of genistein, their properties, and possible applications. *Acta Biochemical Polonica, 57*(1), 23–34.

Ali, H. B., Blunden, G., Tanira, O. M., & Nemmar, A., (2008). Some phytochemical, pharmacological and toxicological properties of ginger (*Zingiber officinale* Roscoe): A review of recent research. *Food Chem. Toxicol., 46*, 409–442.

Amine, B., et al., (2016). Evidence based digoxin therapeutic monitoring: A lower and narrower therapeutic range. *Mediterranean BioMedical Journals International Journal of Medicine and Surgery*, 3(1), 23–26.

Ankit, G., et al., (2014). Flax and flaxseed oil: An ancient medicine and modern functional food. *J. Food Sci. Technol., 51*(9), 1633–1653.

Athira, P. P., et al., (2014). Exploring potential of planterosomes as a novel drug delivery system: Reviewing decades of research. *Int. Res. J. Pharm., 5*(4), 254–258.

Bhandari, U., Kanojia, R., & Pillai, K. K., (2005). Effect of ethanolic extract of *Zingiber officinale* on dyslipidaemia in diabetic rats. *J. Ethnopharmacol., 97*, 227–223.

Bordia, A., Verma, S. K., & Srivastava, K. C., (1997). Effect of ginger (*Zingiber officinale* Roscoe) and fenugreek (*Trigonella foenum-graecum* L.) on blood lipids, blood sugar and platelet aggregation in patients with coronary artery disease. *Prostaglandins Leukot. Essent. Fatty Acids, 56*, 379–384.

Burch, D., & Lawrence, G., (2007). *Supermarkets and Agri-Food Supply Chains: Transformations in the Production and Consumption of Foods*. Cheltenham UK: Edward Elgar Publishing Ltd.

Cabrera, C., Artacho, R., & Gimenez, R., (2006). Beneficial effects of green tea: A review. *J. Am. Coll. Nutr., 25*, 79–99.

Catherine, B., et al., (2006). Systematic review of the effects of ginseng on cardiovascular risk factors. *The Annals of Pharmacotherapy, 40*, 83–95.

Cesare, D. G., et al., (2017). Genistein supplementation and cardiac function in postmenopausal women with metabolic syndrome: Results from a pilot strain-echo study. *Nutrients, 9*, 584. doi: 10.3390/nu9060584.

Chabukswar, A. R., et al., (2010). Cardio protective activity of *Inula racemosa. Int. J. Chem. Sci., 8*(3), 1545–1552.

Charles, A., et al., (1963). Myocardial norepinephrine concentration in man. *New England Journal of Medicine, 269*(13), 653–658.

Connor, J., & Schiek, W., (1997). *Food Processing: An Industrial Powerhouse in Transition*. NYC: John Wiley and Sons.

Danielsson, I., & Lindman, B., (1981). *Colloids Surf. A, 3*, 391.

Dasam, J. M., Natarajan, J., Karri, V. V. S. R., Wadhwani, A. D., & Antony, J., (2016). Targeting efficacy of simvastatin for hormone dependent carcinomas through solid lipid nanoparticles. *Journal of Nanomedicine and Nanotechnology, 7*(6), 1–7.

Eilat-Adar, S., (2013). Nutritional recommendations for cardiovascular disease prevention. *Nutrients, 5*, 3646–3683. doi: 10.3390/nu5093646.

Ekambaram, P., Sathali, A. A. H., & Priyanka, K., (2012). Solid lipid nanoparticles: A review. *International Journal of Applied Pharmaceutics*, 2(1), 80–102.

Eman, M. A., et al., (2012). Functional foods and nutraceuticals in the primary prevention of cardiovascular diseases. *Journal of Nutrition and Metabolism*, 16. Article ID: 569486, doi: 10.1155/2012/569486.

Fellows, P., (2009). *Food Processing Technology: Principles and Practice*, 3. Cambridge, UK: Woodhead Publishing.

Fenwick, G. R., & Hanley, A. B., (1985). The genus allium. *Crit. Rev. Food Sci. Nutr., 22*, 199–271.

Frank, M. S., et al., (2006). Soy protein, isoflavones, and cardiovascular health. *Circulation,* *113*(7).

Frishman, H. W., Sinatra, T. S., & Moizuddin, M., (2004). The use of herbs for treating cardiovascular disease. *Semin. Integr. Med., 2,* 23–35.

Fuzzati, N., (2004). Analysis methods of ginsenosides. *J. Chromatogr B. Analyt. Tecnol.* *Biomed. Life Sci., 812,* 119–133.

Hannah, R. V., & Parameswari, R. P., (2010). Indian spices for healthy heart: An overview. *Current Cardiology Reviews, 6,* 274–279.

Heart Disease and Stroke Statistics, (2018). *At-a-Glance.* Available at: http://www. americanheart.org (accessed on 25 June 2020).

Hertog, M. G., Sweetnam, P. M., Fehily, A. M., Elwood, P. C., & Kromhout, D., (1997). Antioxidant flavonols and ischemic heart disease in a Welsh population of men: The Caerphilly study. *Am. J. Clin. Nutr., 65,* 1489–1494.

Hong, W., et al., (2017). Enhanced encapsulation and bioavailability of breviscapine in PLGA microparticles by nanocrystal and water-soluble polymer template techniques. *European* *Journal of Pharmaceutics and Biopharmaceutics, 115,* 177–185.

Huhta, J. C., (2005). Fetal congestive heart failure. *Semin. Fetal Neonatal Med., 10,* 542–552.

Jahan, N., et al., (2016). Formulation and characterization of nanosuspension of herbal extracts for enhanced antiradical potential. *Journal of Experimental Nanoscience, 11*(1), 72–80.

Jensen, M. K., Koh-Banerjee, P., Hu, F. B., et al., (2004). Intakes of whole grains, bran, and germ and the risk of coronary heart disease in men. *American Journal of Clinical Nutrition,* *80*(6), 1492–1499.

Jeon, B. H., Kim, C. S., Park, K. S., Lee, J. W., Park, J. B., Kim, K. J., Kim, S. H., et al., (2000). Effect of Korea red ginseng on the blood pressure in conscious hypertensive rats. *Gen. Pharmacol., 35,* 135–141.

John, E. H., et al., (2002). Mechanisms of obesity-associated cardiovascular and renal disease. *The American Journal of the Medical Sciences, 324*(3), 127–137.

Kale, et al., (2017). Emulsion, micro-emulsion, and nano emulsion. *Sys. Rev. Pharm., 8*(1), 39–47.

Kamal, A., Thanaa, A., & El-Twab, M. A., (2009). Oxidative markers, nitric oxide, and homocysteine alteration in hypercholesterolemic rats, role of atorvastatin and cinnamon. *Int. J. Clin. Exp. Med., 2,* 254–265.

Kao, Y., et al., (2000). Modulation of obesity by a green tea catechin. *Am. J. Clin. Nutr., 72,* 1232–1241.

Karimi, A., et al., (2015). Herbal versus synthetic drugs; beliefs and facts. *J. Nephropharmacol.,* *4(*1), 27–30.

Kawatra, P., & Rathai, R., (2015). Cinnamon: Mystic powers of a minute ingredient. *Pharmacognosy Research, 7*(1), S1–6.

Keli, S. O., Hertog, M. G. L., Feskens, E. J. M., & Kromhout, D., (1996). Dietary flavonoids, antioxidant vitamins, and incidence of stroke—the Zutphen Study. *Arch Intern. Med., 156,* 637–642.

Khalid, R., et al., (2006). Garlic and cardiovascular disease: A critical review. *The Journal of* *Nutrition, 136*(3), 736S–740S.

Kleinman, C. S., & Nehgme, R. A., (2004). Cardiac arrhythmias in the human fetus. *Pediatr.* *Cardiol., 25,* 234–251.

Kochar, J., et al., (2011). Dietary factors and the risk of coronary heart disease. *Aging and* *Disease* (Vol. 2, No 2, pp. 149–157).

La Grange, L., Wang, M., Watkins, R., Ortiz, D., Sanchez, M. E., Konst, J., Lee, C., & Reyes, E., (1999). Protective effects of the flavonoids mixture, silymarin, on fetal rat brain and liver. *J. Ethnopharmacol., 65*, 53–61.

Lavie, et al., (2009). Obesity and heart disease. *Journal of the American College of Cardiology, 53*(21).

Mary, C. T., et al., (2010). Hawthorn (*Crataegus* spp.) in the treatment of cardiovascular disease. *Pharmacogn. Rev., 4*(7), 32–41.

Mei, L., et al., (2013). Development of ionic-complex-based nanostructured lipid carriers to improve the pharmacokinetic profiles of breviscapine. *Acta Pharmacol. Sin., 34*(8), 1108–1115.

Mensink, R. P., Zock, P. L., Kester, A. D., & Katan, M. B., (2003). Effects of dietary fatty acids and carbohydrates on the ratio of serum total to HDL cholesterol and on serum lipids and apolipoproteins: A meta-analysis of 60 controlled trials. *Am. J Clin. Nutr., 77*, 1146–1155. [PubMed: 12716665]

Micha, R., Michas, G., & Mozaffarian, D., (2012). Unprocessed red and processed meats and risk of coronary artery disease and type 2 diabetes-an updated review of the evidence. *Curr. Atheroscler. Rep., 14*, 515–524. [PubMed: 23001745]

Mongiovi, M., Fesslova, V., Fazio, G., Barbaro, G., & Pipitone, S., (2010). Diagnosis and prognosis of fetal cardiomyopathies: A review. *Curr. Pharm. Des., 16*, 2929–2934.

Mustali, M. D., & Joseph, A., (2009). Vita. Grapes and cardiovascular disease. *The Journal of Nutrition, 139*, 1788S–1793S.

Mykolas, A., (2009). In: Danik, M. M., (ed.), *Functional Foods for Chronic Diseases* (Vol. 4, pp. 234–241). D & A Inc/FF Publishing.

Ng, S. W., Slining, M. M., & Popkin, B. M., (2012). Use of caloric and noncaloric sweeteners in US consumer packaged foods, 2005–2009. *J. Acad. Nutr. Diet., 112*, 1828–1834. [PubMed: 23102182]

Nick, H. M., et al., (1998). Herbal medicine for the treatment of cardiovascular disease. *Arch Intern. Med., 158*, 2225–2234.

Norah, A. A., et al., (2015). Transport of digoxin-loaded polymeric nanoparticles across BeWo cells, an *in vitro* model of human placental trophoblast. *Ther. Deliv., 6*(12), 1325–1334.

Palanivel, G., et al., (2018). SLN delivery systems for oral delivery of phyto-bioactive compounds. *International Journal of Nanomedicine, 13*, 1569–1583.

Pan, A., Sun, Q., Bernstein, A. M., Manson, J. E., Willett, W. C., & Hu, F. B., (2013). Changes in red meat consumption and subsequent risk of type 2 diabetes mellitus: Three cohorts of US men and women. *JAMA Intern. Med., 173*, 1328–1335. [PubMed: 23779232]

Parker, L. A., (2006). *Hydrops fetalis. Newborn Infant Nurs. Rev., 6*, e1–e8.

Petropoulos, S., Gibb, W., & Matthews, S. G., (2010). Developmental expression of multidrug resistance phosphoglycoprotein (P-gp) in the mouse fetal brain and glucocorticoid regulation. *Brain Res., 1357*, 9–18.

Ping, L., & Yangwu, L., (2017). Preparation of nanoparticles of digoxin solid lipid. *Chemical Engineering Transactions, 62*, 1285–1290 doi: 10.3303/CET1762215.

QIU, et al., (2017). Vasoprotection by *Astragalus membranaceus*. In rats with hyperhomocysteinemia. *Experimental and Therapeutic Medicine, 14*, 2401–2407.

Rachel, N., & Michael, Y. H., (2009). Ginger (*Zingiber officinale* Roscoe): A hot remedy for cardiovascular disease? *International Journal of Cardiology, 131*(3), 408–409.

Rahman, K., (2001). Historical perspective on garlic and cardiovascular disease. *J. Nutr., 131*, 977S–979S.

Reddy, K. S., & Katan, M. B., (2004). Diet, nutrition and the prevention of hypertension and cardiovascular diseases. *Public Health Nutrition, 7*(1), 167–186.

Rodriguez-Leyva, et al., (2010). The cardiovascular effects of flaxseed and its omega-3 fatty acid, alpha-linolenic acid. *Can J. Cardiol., 26*(9), 489–495.

Schaffer, H. D., Hunt, D. B., & Ray, D. E., (2007). *US Agricultural Commodity Policy and its Relationship to Obesity* (p. 31). Agricultural Policy Analysis Center University of Tennessee; Knoxville.

Shabana, T., & Vijay, V., (2010). Effect of obesity on cardiovascular risk factors in urban population in South India. *Heart Asia*, 145e149. doi: 10.1136/ha.2009.000950.

Sharma, I., Gusain, D., & Dixit, V. P., (1998). Hypolipidaemic and antiatherosclerotic effects of *Zingiber officinale* in cholesterol-fed rabbits. *Phytother. Res., 10*, 517–518.

Shenuarin, B., & Fukunaga, K., (2009). Cardioprotection by vanadium compounds targeting Akt-mediated signaling. *J. Pharmacol. Sci., 110*, 1–13.

Shridhar, D., (2007). *Terminalia arjuna* Wight & Arn.: A useful drug for cardiovascular disorders. *Journal of Ethnopharmacology, 114*, 114–129.

Srivastava, K. C., Bordia, A., & Verma, S. K., (1995). Curcumin, a major component of food spice turmeric (*Curcuma Longa*) inhibits aggregation and alters eicosanoid metabolism in human blood platelets. *Prostaglandins Leukot. Essent. Fatty Acids, 52*, 223–227.

Tang, J., et al., (2011). Edragit nanoparticle containing Genistein formulation, development, and bioavailability assessment. *Int. J. Nanomed., 6*, 2429–2435.

Thakur, V., Fouron, J. C., Mertens, L., & Jaeggi, E. T., (2013). Diagnosis and management of fetal heart failure. *Can. J. Cardiol., 29*, 759–767.

Utoguchi, N., Chandorkar, G. A., Avery, M., & Audus, K. L., (2000). Functional expression of P-glycoprotein in primary cultures of human cytotrophoblasts and BeWo cells. *Reprod. Toxicol., 14*, 217–224.

Ward, R. M., (1996). Pharmacology of the maternal-placental-fetal-unit and fetal therapy. *Prog. Pediatr. Cardiol., 5*, 79–89.

Weis, T., (2013). *The Ecological Hoof Print: The Global Burden of Industrial Livestock.* London: Zed Books.

Welch, R., & Mitchell, P., (2000). Food processing: A century of change. *Br. Med. Bull., 56*, 1–17. [PubMed: 10885101]

Young, J. K., et al., (2012). Nanoemulsified green tea extract shows improved hypocholesterolemic effects in C57BL/6 mice. *Journal of Nutritional Biochemistry, 23*, 186–191.

Yusuf, et al., (2001). *Global Burden of Cardiovascular Diseases Part I: General Considerations, the Epidemiologic Transition, Risk Factors, and Impact of Urbanization* (pp. 2746–2753). Circulation.

CHAPTER 7

Nigella sativa Encapsulated Nano-Scaffolds and Their Bioactivity Significance

MOHAMMED ASADULLAH JAHANGIR,[1] ABDUL MUHEEM,[2]
SYED SARIM IMAM,[3] FARHAN JALEES AHMED,[3] and MOHD. AQIL [3]

[1] *Department of Pharmaceutics, Nibha Institute of Pharmaceutical Sciences, Rajgir, Nalanda – 803116, Bihar, India*

[2] *Dolcera ITES, Financial district, Hyderabad, Telangana – 500008, India*

[3] *Department of Pharmaceutics, College of Pharmacy, King Saud University, Riyadh, Saudi Arabia.*

[4] *Department of Pharmaceutics, School of Pharmaceutical Education and Research, Jamia Hamdard, New Delhi – 110062, India*

ABSTRACT

Recently the use of medicinal plants has attracted great attention and has gained its application instead of being a new synthetic chemical entity. Several literatures have reported that herbal medicines have been used traditionally and were clinically applied to cure and prevent several diseases. There lower toxicity and low price as compared to synthetic drugs make them an obvious selection in the treatment of many diseases. *Nigella sativa* L. (Ranunculaceae), commonly known as black cumin, has been utilized as a medicinal plant since ancient times. Volatile oils of *N. sativa* mainly contain thymoquinone (TQ) as one of the main active components. It is the most effected constituent and have several pharmacological properties like anti-tumor, anti-microbial, immunomodulatory, anti-inflammatory, and antioxidant effects. The encapsulation of herbal drug into the nanoscaffold makes them more effective than the traditional dosage form. The drug nanoscaffold able to enhance the therapeutic potential by enhancing the bioavailability and targeting. The present chapter highlights the application of *Nigella sativa*/thymoquinone loaded nanoscaffold by encapsulating to various delivery systems and also proven against several types of diseases.

7.1 INTRODUCTION

Humans had been using natural medicines for treatment of different ailments since the earliest civilizations. Many evidence and documents of ancient civilization support the use of herbs for its medicinal values. One natural medicine which have vastly used in the cultures of Africa, Asia, the Middle East, and Europe is *Nigella sativa*. It is known with different names like Black cumin, Black caraway, Black seed, Kalonji, etc. It is one of the few herbs which have been discussed in different Holy Scriptures too. The Easton Bible dictionary states that the Hebrew word ketsah refers to *N. sativa*. In Arabic approbation also, it has been described as "Habbatul Baraka" meaning the "seed of blessing" (Dajani et al., 2016). In Islamic literature, it is considered as one of the finest healing medicines and has been recommended to be used on regular basis in Tibb-e-Nabwi (Prophetic Medicine) (Ahmad et al., 2013). Many evidences suggest it to be a miracle herb. The family of *N. sativa* is Ranunculaceae. The plant is indigenous to Southern Europe, North Africa, the Middle Eastern Mediterranean region, Southwest Asia, India, Pakistan, Turkey, Syria, Saudi Arabia, and South Europe. The oil of the seeds has been used for centuries for different ailments. It also holds an important position in the Unani and Ayurvedic medicinal system (Sharma et al., 2005; Goreja, 2003).

7.1.1 PHARMACOGNOSTIC CHARACTERISTICS OF N. SATIVA

N. sativa can achieve a height of 20–90 cm and gives annual flowering with finely divided leaves. Different color of flowers is registered with *N. sativa* like yellow, pink, pale blue-white or pale purple. The flowers are very delicate and have 5–10 petals. The fruits are big and in the form of a capsule composing of 3–7 united follicles containing numerous seeds (Goreja, 2003; Warrier et al., 2004). The seeds are small with a black outer layer and white inside. The seeds are dicotyledonous and angular in shape. The seeds have a light aromatic odor and the taste is usually bitter (Ahmad et al., 2013).

7.1.2   CHEMICAL COMPOSITION OF N. SATIVA

The chief chemical constituents of *N. sativa* are thymoquinone (30–48%), thymohydroquinone, dithymoquinone, p-cymene, sesquiterpene longifolene, α-pinene and thymol, carvacrol, 4-tepineol, t-anethol, etc. Two different types of alkaloids are also found in the seeds, i.e., isoquinoline alkaloids, e.g., nigellicimine, and nigellicimine-N-oxide, and pyrazol alkaloids or alkaloid which bear an indazole ring, e.g., nigellidine, and nigellicine. Moreover, *N. sativa* seeds were also reported to contain alpha-hederin, which is a water-soluble pentacyclic triterpene and saponin, a potential anticancer agent (Atta-Ur-Rahman, 1995). Trace compounds like carvone, limonene, citronellol are also found. Quinine constituents possess pharmacological properties. Some vitamins and minerals like Cu, P, Zn, and Fe, etc., are also found.

7.1.3   PHARMACOLOGICAL POTENTIAL OF N. SATIVA

N. sativa is extensively researched in the past few decades and astonishingly positive results have been found for its application in the management and treatment of different ailments. It has found to be having antibacterial, antifungal, anti-inflammatory, analgesic activity, immunomodulatory activity, anti-schistosomiasis activity, antioxidant activity, antidiabetic activity, anticancer activity, cardiovascular activity, gastro-protective activity, hepatoprotective activity, nephroprotective activity, pulmonary-protective activity, and anti-asthmatic effects, testicular-protective activity, anticonvulsant activity, contraceptive, and anti-fertility activity, anti-oxytocic activity, dermatological, and cosmeceutical activity, etc. It has also been extensively studied to understand the toxicological effect of its use. The various pharmacological activities are listed in Table 7.1.

7.1.4   APPLICATIONS OF NIGELLA SATIVA LOADED NANOFORMULATIONS

N. sativa was an important component of the ancient system of medicine. Many active components have been extracted from *N. sativa* for instance, thymoquinone (TQ), thymohydroquinone, dithymoquinone, thymol, carvacrol, nigellimine-N-oxide, nigellicine, nigellidine, etc. The aqueous extract of *N. sativa* has various therapeutic actions although it has limited bioavailability and solubility in aqueous solution. The primary aim of developing nanoformulations is to achieve increased solubilization of TQ, a major component of *N. sativa* extract. The extract or TQ loaded nanoformulations should be prepared efficiently and possess required loading of the active components and should retain these for the required time period. Some nanoformulations aim for a prolonged release of drugs while others have additional mechanisms for cellular delivery or intracellular release. The seed extract of *N. sativa* is a remarkable herbal drug having a cure for various ailments and disorders such as inflammation, bacterial infection, genetic dysfunction, cancer, and treatment of nervous and hepatic disorders. Therefore, the review report focuses on the development of nanoformulations loaded with seed extracts of *N. sativa* using modern scientific techniques.

TABLE 7.1   Pharmacological Activities of *N. sativa*

Activity	Inference	References
Antibacterial	All tested strains of methicillin-resistant *Staphylococcus aureus* were found to be sensitive to ethanolic extract of *N. sativa; It was also found to* possess clinically useful anti-*H. pylori* activity which was comparable to triple therapy; clear inhibition of the growth of *Staphylococcus aureus* was reported at a concentration of 300 mg/mL with distilled water as a control. Researchers confirmed the inhibition by using the positive control Azithromycin, positive inhibition may be attributed to the two important active ingredients of *N. sativa*, TQ, and melanin.	Hannan et al., 2008; Salem et al., 2010; Bakathir et al., 2011
Antifungal	Ns-D1 and Ns-D2 are two novel antifungal defensins which were isolated from seeds of *N. sativa* and sequenced. The Ns-D1 and Ns-D2 defensins displayed strong divergent antifungal activity towards numerous phytopathogenic fungi; Another researcher reported that the antifungal effects of the quinones were comparable with those of preservatives commonly used in milk products at two pH levels (4.0 and 5.5), while thymohydroquinone and TQ possessed significant anti-yeast activity too.	Rogozhin et al., 2011; Halamova et al., 2010; Bita et al., 2012
Neuro-protective	The delivery system for NS with better drug release and GI permeation profiles and improved neuroprotective activity	Akhtar et al., 2014
Antioxidant	The oral administration of TQ resulted in significantly reduced the levels of pro-inflammatory mediators [IL-1β, IL-6, TNF-α, IFN-γ, and PGE (2)] and increased level of IL-10.	Umar et al., 2012
	The researcher suggested that *N. sativa* is a potent chemopreventive agent and suppresses Fe-NTA-induced oxidative stress, hyperproliferative response, and renal carcinogenesis in Wistar rats.	Bourgou et al., 2012

TABLE 7.1   *(Continued)*

Activity	Inference	References
Antidiabetic	The combination of α-LA, L-carnitine, and *N. sativa* may contribute significantly to improved carbohydrate metabolism and to less extent lipid metabolism in diabetic rats, thus increasing the success rate in the management of DM.	Salama et al., 2011
	The *in vivo* treatment with NSE exerts an insulin-sensitizing action by enhancing ACC phosphorylation, a major component of the insulin-independent AMPK signaling pathway, and by enhancing muscle Glut4 expression.	Bamosa et al., 2010
Anticancer	TQ has a beneficial effect in conditioning T-cells *in vitro* for adoptive T-cell therapy against cancer and infectious disease.	Salem et al., 2011
	Thymoquinone effectively inhibits tumor growth and angiogenesis both *in vitro* and *in vivo*.	Peng et al., 2013
	Thymoquinone can activate caspase-3 and caspase-9 and thus result in the chemosensitization of gastric cancer cells to 5-FU-induced cell death.	Lei et al., 2012
Anti-inflammatory and analgesic	TQ content of the callus of the leaf was 12 times higher than that measured in the seeds extract. A decrease in the TQ content of the callus was accompanied with an increase in its phenolic content and antioxidant ability.	Alemi et al., 2013
	N. sativa and TQ were shown to inhibit inflammatory cytokines such as interleukin-1 and 6 and the transcription factor, nuclear factor κB. Both NS and TQ have shown potential as an anti-osteoporotic agent	Shuid et al., 2012
Immuno-modulatory	In their research concluded that the aqueous extract of *N. sativa* significantly enhances NK cytotoxic activity against YAC-1 tumor cells.	Majdala-wieh et al., 2010
	The extract of *N. sativa* led to a significant decrease in pathological changes of the lung, but an increased IFN-γ. These results confirm a preventive effect of *N. sativa* extract on lung inflammation of sensitized guinea pigs.	Boskabady et al., 2011
Gastro-protective	TQ at a high dose level corrected the altered parameters in a comparable manner to that of the reference drug used, omeprazole. TQ has novel gastroprotective mechanisms via inhibiting proton pump, acid secretion, and neutrophil infiltration, while enhancing mucin secretion, and nitric oxide production.	Magdy et al., 2012
	Pups treated with NEC + NOS group had better clinical sickness scores and weight gain compared to the NEC group ($p < 0.05$). In the macroscopic assessment, histopathologic, and apoptosis evaluation (TUNEL), severity of bowel damage was significantly lower in the NEC + NOS group compared to the NEC group ($p < 0.05$).	Tayman et al., 2012

TABLE 7.1   *(Continued)*

Activity	Inference	References
Hepato-protective	TQ exerts modulatory influence on the antioxidant defense system on being subjected to toxic environment.	Zafeer, 2012
	TQ loaded formulation significantly inhibited the elevated levels of serum marker enzymes and showed improved histopathological deformities	Sayeed et al., 2017
Nephro-protective	TQ synergizes with its nephroprotective effect against cisplatin-induced acute kidney injury in rats.	Ulu et al., 2012;
	N. sativa seeds had nonsignificant effects on biochemical parameters, although the histopathologic properties of the kidneys relatively recovered after NS use.	Hadjzadeh et al., 2012
Testicular-protective	Thymoquinone use may decrease the destructive effects of methotrexate on testicular tissue of patients using this agent.	Gökçe et al., 2011
Neuro-pharma-cological	The *in-vivo* study result revealed that the higher amount of TQ reaches to the target region by showing higher levels of monoamines 5 hydroxytryptamines (5-HT), dopamine (DA) and norepinephrine (NE) as compared to thymoquinone suspension (TQS) in brain.	Alam et al., 2018
Anti-convulsant	Ezz et al. in their study showed promising anticonvulsant and potent antioxidant effects of curcumin and NSO in reducing oxidative stress, excitability, and the induction of seizures in epileptic animals and improving some of the adverse effects of antiepileptic drugs.	Ezz et al., 2011
Contra-ceptive and anti-fertility	The ethanolic extract of *N. sativa* seeds was found to possess an anti-fertility activity in male rats which might be due to inherent estrogenic activity of *N. sativa*.	Agarwal et al., 1990
Antioxytocic	*N. sativa* seeds inhibit the uterine smooth muscle contraction induced by oxytocin stimulation. The volatile oil of *N. sativa* seeds inhibited the spontaneous movements of rat and guinea piguterine smooth muscle and also the contractions induced by oxytocin stimulation which suggest the anti-oxytocic potential of *N. sativa* seeds oil	Aqel et al., 1996

7.1.4.1   EFFECT ON INFLAMMATION

The effect of *N. sativa* extracts and TQ have been studied on several inflammatory activities, *in vivo*. A number of pharmacological assays show that it has a potential anti-inflammatory action. Ravindran et al. enhance the effectiveness and bioavailability of TQ derived from *N. sativa* by exploiting polymer-based nanoparticles approach. The particle size range of prepared nanoparticles was 150–200 nm with 97.5% of entrapment efficiency of TQ. The finding from electrophoretic gel shift mobility assay confirmed that TQ encapsulated nanoparticles were more potent than TQ in inhibiting NF-kappaB activation and in suppressing the expression of cyclin D1, matrix metalloproteinase (MMP)-9, vascular endothelial growth factor (VEGF) consequently enhancing its anti-proliferative, and anti-inflammatory actions (Ravindran et al., 2010).

A biopolymer, poly (ε-caprolactone), based nanoparticles loaded with the *N. sativa* L. seeds essential oil (NSSEO), and indomethacin were first time synthesized, characterized, and evaluated for their anti-inflammatory and analgesic potential for the very first time. As reported, Particle size was ranged between 230 nm and 260 nm and zeta potential of nanoparticles range between -20 mV and -30 mV which leads to enhanced entrapment efficiency of 70% and 84% and drug loading (DL) of 14% and 5.63% for indomethacin and NSSEO, respectively. Both the drugs were successfully encapsulated into the nanoparticles and provided enhanced anti-inflammatory and analgesic effects (Badri et al., 2018). A unique amalgamation of marigold extract (ME), azelaic acids (AzA), and two plant-derived oils rich in ω-3 and ω-6 fatty acids (black caraway oil-Bco and rosehip seed oil-Ro) were encapsulated into lipid nanocarriers aimed to evaluate its anti-inflammatory action. The lipid nanocarriers comprising of a surfactant shell and lipid core, guarantees a high encapsulation efficiency of lipid as well as water-soluble and herbal extracts. *In-vitro* cell viability studies suggested no cytotoxic effects at 5–400 µg/mL concentrations of NLC on L929 cells. The ELISA results clearly revealed that the best results were obtained with the treatment of 400 µg/mL NLCBco/Ro that co-encapsulate both natural actives-ME and AzA (Lacatusu et al., 2017). Overall studies concluded that encapsulation of TQ or *N. sativa* extract into nanoformulations is a promising delivery system.

7.1.4.2   EFFECT ON BACTERIAL INFECTION

It has been reported that *N. sativa* possesses potential antibacterial activities against gram-positive (*Staphylococcus aureus*) as well as gram-negative (*Pseudomonas aeruginosa* and *Escherichia coli*) species. Jufri et al. fabricated black cumin oil encapsulated nanoemulsion gels for the determination of the antibacterial effect. The nanoemulsion gel was found to be highly stable at room temperature and low temperature as well and a significant difference was observed between the inhibiting zone of blank and black cumin oil entrapped nanoemulsion gel (P < 0.01) suggesting potent antibacterial action of the black cumin oil (Jufri et al., 2014). Gold nanoparticles (NsEO-AuNPs) were formulated with the essential oils (EOs) of *N. sativa* in an attempt to increase the antibacterial activity. In TEM analysis, gold nanoparticles were depicted spherical shape and size range of 15.6–28.4 nm, which may be enhanced the bioavailability of EO. The antibacterial assay of NsEO-AuNPs confirmed the enhanced inhibitory action against *Staphylococcus aureus* MTCC 9542 (16 mm) (gram-positive) than *Vibrio harveyi* MTCC 7771 (5 mm) (gram-negative) at the concentration level of 10 µg/mL. Gold nanoparticles decreases the hydrophobicity index and thus inhibits the biofilm formation of *S. aureus* and *V. harveyi* (Manju et al., 2016).

7.1.4.3 EFFECT ON IMMUNE SYSTEM AND CANCERS

Cancer stands as a major cause of death worldwide, characterized by the abnormal cell growth which has potential to invade or spread to other parts of the body. The invention of novel cytotoxic drugs with minimal adverse effects on the immune system is crucial for cancer treatment. From centuries, *N. sativa* and its oil are used as a tonic to boost the immunity and prevent diseases. It has been reported to possess immune potentiating, immune-modulating, and interferon (IFN)-like activities (Hailat et al., 1995). The preventive action of *N. sativa* seeds on the oxidative stress and carcinogenesis induced using methynitrosourea was also evaluated in the study by Mabrouk et al. in a murine model. It was shown to produce around 80% action against oxidative stress, inflammation, and carcinogenesis (Mabrouk et al., 2002). Human breast adenocarcinoma cell lines were exploited for a comparative anticancer activity study of thymoquinone and nanothymoquinone (NTQ). TQ loaded self-assembled, Myristic acid-chitosan (MA-chitosan) based nanogel was formulated by self-assemble technique followed by TQ was loaded into nanogel. *In vitro* cytotoxic activity of TQ and nano-based TQ were examined on human breast adenocarcinoma cell line (MCF7). It concluded that TQ loaded self-assembled, MA-chitosan nanogel exhibited a significant reduction in IC_{50} value demonstrating enhanced cytotoxicity compared to free TQ. It was found that TQ loaded nanogel based nanoparticles proved more effective compared to TQ (Dehghani et al., 2015). Haron et al. overcome the low hydrophobicity of TQ by formulating a nanocarrier system. TQ loaded nanostructured lipid carrier (TQ-NLC) was studied with the aim to evaluate the antiproliferative effects on liver cancer cells which are integrated with hepatitis B genome, Hep3B. While performing MTT assay, the Hep3B was treated with TQ or TQ-NLC for 24, 48, and 72 hours. Hence, the results suggested that TQ or TQ-NLC potentially inhibits the growth of Hep3B at IC_{50} <16.7 μM for 72 hours. TQ-NLC also induced apoptosis via activation of caspases-3/7 (Haron et al., 2018).

In another study by Bhattacharya et al. TQ loaded polymeric nanoparticles were formulated using biodegradable, hydrophilic polymers like polyvinylpyr-rolidone (PVP) and polyethyleneglycol (PEG) to overcome the low aqueous solubility, thermal, and light sensitivity issue of TQ, to enhance its efficacy in cancer treatment. The surface morphological features of TQ-Nps were found to be 50 nm particle sizes, spherical in shape, smooth surface texture, and negative zeta potential which facilitate their cellular uptake of TQ-Nps. PEG4000-TQ-Nps demonstrated potent anti-migratory properties by increasing the expression of miR-34a via p53. Moreover, TQ-Nps mediated miR-34a regulation directly disrupts the actin cytoskeleton which facilitates the reduction of cell migration (Bhattacharya et al., 2015). A literature search report on *N. sativa* or TQ loaded nanoformulations is showed in Table 7.2 for cancer treatment.

7.1.4.4   EFFECT ON OXIDANT ACTIVITIES

An antioxidant activity of *N. sativa* oil (NSO) on the antioxidant enzyme status and myocardium of cyclosporine-A-treated rats was investigated (Muheem et al., 2017). Prophylactic administration of NSO reduced the cyclosporine A induced heart injury in the rat, evident by cardiac histopa-thology, decreased lipid peroxidation (LPO) level, and enhanced antioxidant enzyme status (Ebru et al., 2008). Ismail et al. studied the therapeutic effects of thymoquinone rich fraction (TQRF) and TQ in both nano and conven-tional emulsions forms on LPO, total antioxidant status, antioxidants genes expression, memory deficit and soluble β-amyloid (Aβ) levels in high-fat cholesterol diet (HFCD) fed rats for 6 months. Supplementation of TQRF nanoemulsion could improve memory deficit, LPO, and soluble Aβ level and ameliorated the total antioxidant status and antioxidants genes expression levels (Ismail et al., 2017). HFCD or streptozotocin (STZ) induced diabetic rats were exploited to study the effects of alone and concurrent supplementa-tion of natural nano-sized clinoptilolite (NCLN) and *Nigella sativa* (NS) on anti-oxidative parameters and body weight (BW). The HFD or STZ induced diabetic rats were divided into four different groups viz., diabetic control (Group 1), NS 1%/food (Group 2), NCLN 2%/food (Group 3), NS 1%/food

TABLE 7.2 A Recent Research Summary of *N. sativa* Extract or TQ Loaded Nanoformulations for the Treatment of Various Types of Cancers

Nanoformulation	Drug	Excipients	Cell Line Types	Conclusive Remarks	References
Nanogel-based nanoparticle	Thymoquinone (TQ)	Myristic acid-chitosan (MA-chitosan)	Human breast adenocarcinoma cell line (MCF7)	High drug-targeting potential and efficiency demonstrates anticancer activity.	Dehghani et al., 2015
Nanoparticles	Thymoquinone (TQ)	Poly (lactide-co-glycolide) (PLGA), stabilizer-polyethylene glycol (PEG)-5000	Colon (HCT-116), breast (MCF-7), and prostrate cancer cells (PC-3) and multiple myeloma (U-266) cells	TQ into nanoparticles enhances its anti-proliferative, and chemosensitizing effects	Ravindran et al., 2010
Nanoemulsion	*N. sativa* extracts + doxorubicin	Phosphate-buffered saline (pH 7.4) + lipid aliquots	Human MCF-7 breast cancer cells	Promising and potential therapeutic modality	Mahmoud et al., 2013
Nanostructured Lipid Carrier (NLC)	Thymoquinone (TQ)	Mixture of solid lipid and liquid lipid	Liver Cancer Cell-Hep3B	Anticancer effects on the Hep3B	Haron et al., 2018
Nanoemulsion	*N. sativa* essential oil	Non-ionic surfactant + emulsifier polysorbate 80	MCF-7 breast cancer cells	Potential application in breast cancer therapy	Periasamy et al., 2016
Nanocarrier	Thymoquinone (TQ)	Pluronic F127 (5.0 wt.%) and Pluronic F68	MCF7 cells	Sustained delivery of TQ for cancer	Shaarani et al., 2017
PEGylated nanoparticles	Thymoquinone (TQ)	Polyvinylpyrrolidone (PVP) + polyethylene glycol (PEG) 4000	Mammary carcinoma cell lines (MCF-7, HBL-100)	Non-toxicity and effectivity of PEG4000-TQ-Nps against cancer cell migration.	Bhattacharya et al., 2015

+ NCLN 2%/food (Group 4), normal control (Group 5). Administration of NCLN and NCLN+NS for 7 weeks, decreased malondialdehyde (MDA) level compared to the diabetic control. Moreover, in the untreated diabetic control and NS groups, the level of total antioxidant capacity (TAC) was increased when compared to the normal control group. Additionally, the level of superoxide dismutase (SOD) decreased in the NS+NCLN group in comparison to the NS and NCLN groups ($p < 0.01$). It was concluded that discrete supplementation of NS and NCLN produced more efficient anti-oxidative effects when compared to the combined supplementation of NS and NCLN (Omidi et al., 2017). Table 7.3 describes about various antioxidant studies, which has been conducted on *N. sativa* extract or TQ loaded nanoformulation such as nanoemulsion, nanoparticles, etc.

7.1.4.5 EFFECTS ON NERVOUS DISORDERS

Alcoholic extract of *N. sativa* is a strong antidepressant. Moreover, the anxiolytic activity was demonstrated with the increase in serotonin (5-HT) and decrease in hydroxyindole acetic acid (5-HIAA) levels in the rat brain. The increased level of 5-HT in rats improved learning and memory capacity and augmented the tryptophan levels. The neuroprotective effects were due to the antioxidant, free radical scavenging and anti-inflammatory capacities of *N. sativa*. It may also act as anticonvulsant (Ahmad et al., 2013). The results of thymoquinone rich fraction nanoemulsion (TQRFNE), thymoquinone nanoemulsion (TQNE), and the conventional emulsion were studied on the high fat or cholesterol diet (HFCD) fed rats. Various proteins and enzymes levels such as amyloid-β (Aβ) generation; amyloid-β precursor protein (APP) processing, γ-secretases of presenilin 1 (PSEN1), β-secretase 1 (BACE1), and presenilin 2 (PSEN2), Aβ degradation; Aβ transportation; insulin-degrading enzyme (IDE), receptor for advanced glycation end products (RAGE) and low-density lipoprotein receptor-related protein 1 (LRP1) was estimated in brain tissues. TQRFNE were found to reduce the brain Aβ fragment length 1–40 and 1–42 (Aβ40 and Aβ42) levels, which could further improve the AD pathogenesis (Ismail et al., 2017).

7.1.4.6 EFFECTS ON HEPATIC DISORDERS

N. sativa extract effects on lactate dehydrogenase (LDH), TAC, catalase (CAT), myeloperoxidase (MPO), total oxidative status (TOS), aspartate

TABLE 7.3 A Recent Research Summary of Antioxidant Activities on *N. sativa* Extract or TQ Loaded Nanoformulations

Nanoformulations	Drug	Excipients	Study Conducted	Conclusive Remarks	References
Nanoemulsion	Thymoquinone (TQ)	Tween-80, triolein	high fat-cholesterol diet-induced rats	Improving total antioxidant status and antioxidants genes expression levels	Ismail et al., 2017
Nanoemulsions enriched with gold nanoparticle	*N. sativa* oil + Calendula officinalis extract	lipoic acid + gold (Chloroauric acid)	*In vitro* cellular investigations	Antioxidant and wound healing activity	Guler et al., 2014
Gold nanoparticles	Black seed extract	Hydrogen tetrachloroaurate tetrahydrate ($HAuCl_4 \cdot 4H_2O$)	NA	Antioxidant activities	Fragoon et al., 2012
Nanoparticles	Thymoquinone (TQ)	PAG (p-aminophenyl-1-thio-β-d-galactopyranoside) coated NIPAAM (N-isopropyl acrylamide)	CCl_4 mediated hepatotoxicity in rats	Benefit of the antioxidant property of TQ without any toxicity.	Verma et al., 2013
Solid lipid nanoparticles (SLN)	*N. sativa* essential oil	Hydrogenated palm oil Softisan 154 + sorbitol	NA	Acts as antioxidant, anti-inflammatory, anticancer, analgesic, antimicrobial activities.	Alhaj et al., 2010

aminotransferase (AST), alanine aminotransferase (ALT), and oxidative stress index (OSI) depicts that it has potent hepatoprotective activity (Adam et al., 2016). Hepatoprotective activity was observed by Verma et al. with NTQ, where optimized nanocarriers system exploits the beneficial antioxidant properties of TQ and minimizes its toxic effects. A targeted delivery system was designed by the encapsulation of TQ (NTQ) in their hydrophobic core of PAG (p-aminophenyl-1-thio-β-D-galactopyranoside) coated with NIPAAM (N-isopropyl acrylamide) nanoparticles. The serum and the biochemical analysis with the prepared nanoparticles (NTQ) showed superior hepatoprotective activity of NTQ as compared to TQ (Verma et al., 2013).

Another nanoformulation of TQ, (TQ-NLCs) was formulated using high-pressure homogenization with ultrasonication methodology. Entrapment efficiency was found to be between $84.6 \pm 5\%$ and $96.2 \pm 1.6\%$. An *in-vivo* study revealed that TQ AUC0-t values were higher in animals treated with NLCs, with a relative bioavailability of 2.03- and 3.97-fold higher than TQ suspension. Histopathological and enzyme levels studies revealed a significant decrease in both serum ALT and AST (305.0 ± 24.88 and 304.7 ± 23.55 U/mL, respectively) levels proving, the enhanced hepatoprotective effects of TQ in rats (Elmowafy et al., 2016).

7.1.4.7   EFFECT ON DIABETIC DISORDER

N. sativa was found to be a crucial herbal medicine in the attenuation of blood glucose levels with increased insulin and C-peptide level in animal models. TQ act as a potent antioxidant which plays a key role in the reduction of tissue MDA levels, DNA damage, preserves pancreatic β-cell integrity and mitochondrial vacuolization, and fragmentation. They exhibit an antihyperglycemic effect in rats although the effect of TQ loaded nanoformulation has not been reported in the literature.

Rani et al. studied the effect of TQ loaded nanoformulation against streptozotocin-nicotinamide induced type-2 diabetic rats and its comparative study was conducted with Thymoquinone (TQ) and standard marketed antidiabetic drugs, metformin. Nanoprecipitation technique and Box-Behnken statistical analysis tool was exploited for the formulation of TQ and metformin loaded polymeric nanocapsules (NCs) and optimization of a biocompatible polymer and other excipients as variables respectively. Different doses of metformin (150 mg/kg), TQ (20, 40, and 80 mg/kg) and their nanoformulations (80 mg/

kg for metformin and 20, 40, and 80 mg/kg for thymoquinone) were administered to type-2 diabetic-induced rats for 21 successive days. Blood glucose and BW were estimated every week for consecutively 3 weeks. Glycosylated hemoglobin and serum lipid were measured on 22 days. Oral administration of TQ loaded NCs reported better antihyperglycemic effect in type-2 diabetic rats at a half dose as when to thymoquinone alone demonstrating the profound utility of nanoformulations for dose reduction (Rani et al., 2018).

7.1.4.8   EFFECT ON FUNGAL INFECTION

N. sativa and its extract act against *Candida albicans* and *Madurella mycetomatis*. The activity of the extracts of *N. sativa* was claimed to be potentially more effective than antibiotics like amphotericin-B and griseofulvin against *Aspergillus niger*, *Fusarium solani*, and *Scopulariopsis brevicaulis*. Moreover, TQ confirmed potential activity against Trichophyton spp., Epidermophyton spp., and Microsporum spp. Aqueous extracts of *N. sativa* showed no antifungal activity. The plant extract of *N. sativa* caused a significant inhibition of the growth of the fungi, *Candida albicans* (Aljabre et al., 2015). Size reduction of Amphotericin-B, Ketoconazole, and Thymoquinone was attempted by the ball milling technique, and particle size was found to be 5 to 20 nm. The nanoparticulated drug and the conventionally available microstructured drug form were examined against Candida albicans yeast and candida biofilm. Prepared nanosized drug particles were found to be two or four times effective in both candida yeasts and candida biofilm (Randhawa et al., 2015).

7.2   CLINICAL TRIALS

The clinical trial search was performed in the official site of clinical trial.gov and found that there were no clinical trials conducted so far on the *N. sativa* extract or TQ loaded nanoformulations. The pharmacological activities of *N. sativa* are demonstrated in Table 7.4.

7.3   CONCLUSION AND FUTURE PROSPECTS

It has been more than half a century since TQ was extracted and identified from *N. sativa* although the limited study has been performed for the

TABLE 7.4 Various Clinical Studies and its Parameters of *N. sativa*

Clinical Trial No.	Title	Disease Conditions	Interventions	Collaborators	Age	Phases	References
NCT02816957	Benefits of *N. sativa* in children with Beta Thalassemia	Beta Thalassemia	*N. sativa*	Tanta Univ.	3–18 Years	Phase 1	https://clinicaltrials.gov assessed on 20th Dec 2018.
NCT01531062	Effect of *N. sativa* on lipid profiles in elderly	Dyslipidemia	*N. sativa* black sticky rice	Indonesia Univ.	60 Years and older	Phase 2	
NCT02307344	Effect of *N. sativa* on nonalcoholic Steatohepatitis and Steatosis	Nonalcoholic Steatohepatitis	*N. sativa* Placebo	Hillel Yaffe Medical Center	18 Years and older	Not Applicable	
NCT01393054	Effect of *N. sativa* seed extract on the blood pressure with Hypertension	Hypertension	*N. sativa* seed	Indonesia Univ	60 Years and older	Phase 3	
NCT01735097	Effect of *Nigella sativa* in the treatment of Palmer Arsenical Keratosis	Arsenical Keratosis	Vitamin E; *N. sativa* placebo	Bangabandhu Sheikh Mujib Medical Univ	18–60 Years	Not Applicable	
NCT00327054	Effectiveness of *Nigella sativa* in dyslipidemia	Hypercholesterolemia, diabetes mellitus Metabolic syndrome X	*N. sativa* seed	Aga Khan Univ	18–70 Years	Phase 2	

Biomarkers as Targeted Herbal Drug Discovery

TABLE 7.4 (Continued)

Clinical Trial No.	Title	Disease Conditions	Interventions	Collaborators	Age	Phases	References
NCT03270280	Comparison of salivary Interleukin-1î[2] and matrix Metalloproteinase-8 levels with chronic periodontitis	Chronic periodontitis	N. sativa oil	Univ of Lahore	19–40 Years	Phase 2	https://clinicaltrials.gov assessed on 20th Dec 2018.
NCT03175757	Effects of turmeric and black cumin seed formulation on cholesterol levels	Cholesterol Health	Turmeric and Black Cumin Seed placebo	Supplement Formulators, Inc	40–75 Years	Not Applicable	
NCT01360957	Effect of consumption of black cumin extract on weight loss in overweight women	Obesity	Black cumin water extract	Shahid Beheshti Univ.	16–60 Years	Not Applicable	
NCT02407262	Benefits of black seed oil on asthma inflammation and outcomes	Asthma	Black seed oil|Placebo	Univ College, London; King Abdulaziz Univ.	18–65 Years	Phase 2	
NCT03208790	Clinical evaluation of chemopreventive thymoquinone	Premalignant Lesion	Thymoquinone 200 mg|Placebo oral capsule	Cairo Univ	18–75 Years	Phase 2	

development and optimization of TQ loaded nanoformulations. *N. sativa* has demonstrated potent *in vitro* and *in vivo* activities for several human ailments. However, the low solubility and hence the bioavailability of the active components limit its therapeutic potential. Therefore, several nano-formulations of the active components of *N. sativa*, particularly, TQ have been developed to enhance their therapeutic usefulness. The nanoformulations demonstrated potent anti-inflammatory, antibacterial, anticancer, antioxidant, hepatoprotective, and neuroprotective effects. The various active components that have been isolated from *N. sativa* are thymoquinone, thymohydroquinone, dithymoquinone, thymol, carvacrol, nigellimine-N-oxide, nigellicine, nigellidine, etc., may cure various ailments and disorders. Thus, the primary aim of developing nanoformulations is to achieve increased solubilization of *N. sativa* or TQ. No clinical trials have been trailed on the *N. sativa* extract or TQ loaded nanoformulations. We assume this chapter will encourage to researchers for the development and optimization of *N. sativa* extract or TQ loaded nanoformulations to unfold its therapeutic potentials.

KEYWORDS

- **alanine aminotransferase**
- **antioxidant**
- **cancer**
- **nano-formulations**
- ***Nigella sativa***
- **thymoquinone**

REFERENCES

Adam, G. O., et al., (2016). Hepatoprotective effects of *Nigella sativa* seed extract against acetaminophen-induced oxidative stress. *Asian Pac. J. Trop. Med., 9*(3), 221–227.

Agarwal, C., et al., (1990). Effect of seeds of kalaunji on fertility and sialic acid content of the reproductive organs of male rat. *Geo Bios., 17*, 269–272.

Ahmad, A., et al., (2013). A review on therapeutic potential of *Nigella sativa*: A miracle herb. *Asian Pacific Journal of Tropical Biomedicine, 3*(5), 337–352.

Akhtar, M., et al., (2014). Neuroprotective study of *Nigella sativa*-loaded oral provesicular lipid formulation: *In vitro* and *ex vivo* study. *Drug Deliv., 21*(6), 487–494.

Alam, M., et al., (2018). Formulation and evaluation of nano lipid formulation containing CNS acting drug: Molecular docking, *in-vitro* assessment and bioactivity detail in rats, *Art. Cells, Nanomed. and Biotech.* doi: 10.1080/21691401.2018.1451873.

Alemi, M., et al., (2013). Anti-inflammatory effect of seeds and callus of *Nigella sativa* L. extracts on mix glial cells with regard to their thymoquinone content. *AAPS Pharm. Sci. Tech., 14*(1), 160–167.

Alhaj, N. A., et al., (2010). Characterization of *Nigella sativa* L. essential oil-loaded solid lipid nanoparticles. *Amer. J. Pharmacol. Toxicol., 5*(1), 52–57.

Aljabre, S. H. M., Alakloby, O. M., & Randhawa, M. A., (2015). Dermatological effects of *Nigella sativa. J. Dermatol Dermatologic Surgery, 19*(2), 92–98.

Aqel, M., & Shaheen, R., (1996). Effects of the volatile oil of *Nigella sativa* seeds on the uterine smooth muscle of rat and guinea pig. *J. Ethnopharm., 52*(1), 23–26.

Atta-Ur-Rahman, (1995). Nigellidine-a new indazole alkaloid from the seed of *Nigella sativa. Tetrahedron Lett., 36*(12), 1993–1994.

Badri, W., et al., (2018). Poly(ε-caprolactone) nanoparticles loaded with indomethacin and *Nigella sativa* L. essential oil for the topical treatment of inflammation. *J. Drug Del. Sci. Tech., 46*, 234–242.

Bakathir, H. A., & Abbas, N. A., (2011). Detection of the antibacterial effect of *Nigella sativa* ground seeds with water. *Afr. J. Tradit Complement Altern. Med., 8*(2), 159–164.

Bamosa, A. O., et al., (2010). Effect of *Nigella sativa* seeds on the glycemic control of patients with type 2 diabetes mellitus. *Indian J. Physiol. Pharmacol., 54*(4), 344–354.

Bhattacharya, S., et al., (2015). PEGylated-thymoquinone-nanoparticle mediated retardation of breast cancer cell migration by deregulation of cytoskeletal actin polymerization through miR-34a. *Biomat., 51*, 91–107.

Bita, A., et al., (2012). An alternative treatment for Candida infections with *Nigella sativa* extracts. *Eur. J. Hosp Pharm., 19*, 162.

Boskabady, M. H., et al., (2011). Potential immunomodulation effect of the extract of *Nigella sativa* on ovalbumin sensitized guinea pigs. *J. Zhejiang Univ. Sci. B., 12*(3), 201–209.

Bourgou, S., et al., (2008). Phenolic composition and biological activities of Tunisian *Nigella sativa* L. shoots and roots. *C R Biol., 331*(1), 48–55.

Dajani, E. Z., Shahwan, T. G., & Dajani, N. E., (2016). Overview of the preclinical pharmacological properties of *Nigella sativa* (black seeds): A complementary drug with historical and clinical significance. *J. Physiol. Pharmacol., 67*(6), 801–817.

Dehghani, H., et al., (2015). The comparison of anticancer activity of thymoquinone and nanothymoquinone on human breast adenocarcinoma. *Iran J. Pharm. Res., 14*(2), 539–546.

Ebru, U., et al., (2008). Cardio protective effects of *Nigella sativa* oil on cyclosporine A-induced cardiotoxicity in rats. *Basic Clin. Pharmacol. Toxicol., 103*(6), 574–580.

Elmowafy, M., et al., (2016). Enhancement of bioavailability and pharmacodynamic effects of thymoquinone via nanostructured lipid carrier (NLC) Formulation. *AAPS Pharm. Sci. Tech., 17*(3), 663–672.

Ezz, H. S., Khadrawy, Y. A., & Noor, N. A., (2011). The neuroprotective effect of curcumin and *Nigella sativa* oil against oxidative stress in the pilocarpine model of epilepsy: A comparison with valproate. *Neurochem. Res., 36*(11), 2195–2204.

Fragoon, A., et al., (2012). Biosynthesis of controllable size and shape gold nanoparticles by black seed (*Nigella sativa*) extract. *J. Nanosci. Nanotech., 12*(3), 2337–2345.

Gokce, A., et al., (2011). Protective effects of thymoquinone against methotrexate-induced testicular injury. *Hum. Exp. Toxicol., 30*(8), 897–903.

Goreja, W. G., (2003). *Black Seed: Nature's Miracle Remedy*. New York, NY: Amazing Herbs Press.

Guler, E., et al., (2014). Bio-active nanoemulsions enriched with gold nanoparticle, marigold extracts, and lipoic acid: *In vitro* investigations. *Colloids Surfaces B: Bioint., 121*, 299–306.

Hadjzadeh, M. A., et al., (2012). Effect of alcoholic extract of *Nigella sativa* on cisplatin-induced toxicity in rat. *Iran J. Kidney Dis., 6*(2), 99–104.

Hailat, N., et al., (1995). Effects of *Nigella sativa* volatile oil on jurkal T cell leukemia polypeptides. *Int. J. Pharmacog, 33*, 16–20.

Halamova, K., et al., (2010). *In vitro* antifungal effect of black cumin seed quinones against dairy spoilage yeasts at different acidity levels. *J. Food Prot., 73*(12), 2291–2295.

Hannan, A., et al., (2008). Antibacterial activity of *Nigella sativa* against clinical isolates of methicillin resistant *Staphylococcus aureus*. *J. Ayub. Med. Coll. Abbottabad., 20*(3), 72–74.

Haron, A. S., et al., (2018). Cytotoxic effect of thymoquinone-loaded nanostructured lipid carrier (TQ-NLC) on liver cancer cell integrated with hepatitis B genome, Hep3B. *Evid. Based Complemen. Alt. Med.,* 1–13.

https://clinicaltrials.gov (accessed on 25 June 2020).

Ismail, N., et al., (2017). Beneficial effects of TQRF and TQ nano-and conventional emulsions on memory deficit, lipid peroxidation, total antioxidant status, antioxidants genes expression, and soluble Aβ levels in high fat-cholesterol diet-induced rats. *Chem. Biol. Interact., 25*(275), 61–73.

Ismail, N., et al., (2017). Thymoquinone-rich fraction nanoemulsion (TQRFNE) decreases Aβ40 and Aβ42 levels by modulating APP processing, up-regulating IDE and LRP1, and down-regulating BACE1 and RAGE in response to high fat/cholesterol diet-induced rats. *Biomed. Pharmacother., 95*, 780–788.

Jufri, M., & Natalia, M., (2014). Physical stability and antibacterial activity of black cumin oil (*Nigella sativa* L.) nanoemulsion gel. *Int. J. of Pharm. Tech Res., 6*(4), 1162–1169.

Lacatusua, I., et al., (2017). Marigold extract, azelaic acid and black caraway oil into lipid nanocarriers provides a strong anti-inflammatory effect *in vivo*. *Ind. Crops and Prod., 109*, 141–150.

Lei, X., et al., (2012). Thymoquinone inhibits growth and augments 5-fluorouracil-induced apoptosis in gastric cancer cells both *in vitro* and *in vivo*. *Biochem. Biophys. Res. Commun., 417*(2), 864–868.

Mabrouk, G. M., et al., (2002). Inhibition of methynitrosourea (MNU)-induced oxidative stress and carcinogenesis by orally administered bee honey and Nigella grains in spraguedawley rats. *J. Exp. Clin. Cancer. Res., 21*, 341–346.

Magdy, M. A., El-A, H., & El-M, N., (2012). Thymoquinone: Novel gastro protective mechanisms. *Eur. J. Pharmacol., 697*(1–3), 126–131.

Mahmoud, S. S., & Torchilin, V. P., (2013). Hormetic/cytotoxic effects of *Nigella sativa* seed alcoholic and aqueous extracts on MCF-7 Breast cancer cells alone or in combination with doxorubicin. *Cell Biochem. and Biophys., 66*(3), 451–460.

Majdalawieh, A. F., Hmaidan, R., & Carr, R. I., (2010). *Nigella sativa* modulates splenocyte proliferation, Th1/Th2 cytokine profile, macrophage function, and NK anti-tumor activity. *J. Ethnopharmacol., 131*(2), 268–275.

Manju, S., et al., (2016). Antibacterial, antibiofilm and cytotoxic effects of *Nigella sativa* essential oil coated gold nanoparticles. *Microb. Pathog., 91*, 129–135.

Muheem, A., et al., (2017). A combinatorial statistical design approach to optimize the nanostructured cubosomal carrier system for oral delivery of ubidecarenone for management of doxorubicin-induced cardiotoxicity: *In vitro-in vivo* investigations. *J. Pharm. Sci., 106*(10), 3050–3065.

Omidi, H., et al., (2017). Effects of separate and concurrent supplementation of nano-sized clinoptilolite and *Nigella sativa* on oxidative stress, anti-oxidative parameters, and body weight in rats with type 2 diabetes. *Biomed. Pharmacother., 96*, 1335–1340.

Peng, L., et al., (2013). Antitumor and anti-angiogenesis effects of thymoquinone on osteosarcoma through the NF-κB pathway. *Oncol. Rep., 29*(2), 571–578.

Periasamy, V. S., Athinarayanan, J., & Alshatwi, A. A., (2016). Anticancer activity of an ultrasonic nanoemulsion formulation of *Nigella sativa* L. essential oil on human breast cancer cells. *Ultrasonics Sonochem., 31*, 449–455.

Randhawa, M. A., et al., (2015). Synthesis, morphology, and antifungal activity of nano-particulated amphotericin-B, ketoconazole and thymoquinone against Candida albicans yeasts and Candida biofilm. *J. Environ. Sci. Health A Tox Hazard. Subst. Environ. Eng., 50*(2), 119–124.

Rani, R., et al., (2018). Improvement of antihyperglycemic activity of nano-thymoquinone in rat model of type-2 diabetes. *Chem. Biol. Interact., 1*(295), 119–132.

Ravindran, J., et al., (2010). Thymoquinone poly(lactide-co-glycolide) nanoparticles exhibit enhanced anti-proliferative, anti-inflammatory, and chemosensitization potential. *Biochem. Pharmacol., 79*(11), 1640–1647.

Rogozhin, E. A., et al., (2011). Novel antifungal defensins from *Nigella sativa* L. seeds. *Plant Physiol. Biochem., 49*(2), 131–137.

Salama, R. H., (2011). Hypoglycemic effect of lipoic acid, carnitine and *Nigella sativa* in diabetic rat model. *Int. J. Health Sci. (Qassim), 5*(2), 126–134.

Salem, E. M., Yar, T., Bamosa, A. O., Al-Quorain, A., Yasawy, M. I., Alsulaiman, R. M., & Randhawa, M. A., (2010). Comparative study of *Nigella Sativa* and triple therapy in eradication of *Helicobacter pylori* in patients with non-ulcer dyspepsia. *Saudi J. Gastroenterol., 16*(3), 207–214.

Salem, M. L., Alenzi, F. Q., & Attia, W. Y., (2011). Thymoquinone, the active ingredient of *Nigella sativa* seeds, enhances survival and activity of antigen-specific CD8-positive T cells *in vitro*. *Br. J. Biomed Sci., 68*(3), 131–137.

Sayeed, S., et al., (2017). Nonionic surfactant based thymoquinone loaded nanoproniosomal formulation: *In vitro* physicochemical evaluation and *in vivo* hepatoprotective efficacy. *Drug Dev. and Ind. Pharm., 43*(9), 1413–1420.

Shaarani, S., Hamid, S. S., & Kaus, N. H. M., (2017). The Influence of pluronic F68 and F127 nanocarrier on physicochemical properties, *in vitro* release, and antiproliferative activity of thymoquinone drug. *Pharmacog. Res., 9*(1), 12–20.

Sharma, P. C., Yelne, M. B., & Dennis, T. J., (2005). *Database on Medicinal Plants used in Ayurveda* (pp. 420–440). New Delhi.

Shuid, A. N., et al., (2012). *Nigella sativa*: A potential antiosteoporotic agent. *Evid. Based Complement Alternat. Med.*, 696230.

Tayman, C., et al., (2012). Beneficial effects of *Nigella sativa* oil on intestinal damage in necrotizing enterocolitis. *J. Invest. Surg., 25*(5), 286–294.

Ulu, R., et al., (2012). Regulation of renal organic anion and cation transporters by thymoquinone in cisplatin induced kidney injury. *Food Chem. Toxicol., 50*(5), 1675–1679.

Umar, S., et al., (2012). Modulation of the oxidative stress and inflammatory cytokine response by thymoquinone in the collagen induced arthritis in Wistar rats. *Chem. Biol. Interact., 197*(1), 40–46.

Verma, S. K., et al., (2013). Nanothymoquinone, a novel hepatotargeted delivery system for treating CCl$_4$ mediated hepatotoxicity in rats. *J. Mat. Chem. B., 1*(23), 2956–2966.

Warrier, P. K., Nambiar, V. P. K., & Ramankutty, (2004). Chennai: Orient Longman Pvt. Ltd. *Indian Medicinal Plants-a Compendium of 500 Species* (pp. 139–142).

Zafeer, M. F., et al., (2012). Cadmium-induced hepatotoxicity and its abrogation by thymoquinone. *J. Biochem. Mol. Toxicol., 26*(5), 199–205.

CHAPTER 8

Phytoconstituent-Loaded Nanomedicines for Arthritis Management

SYED SALMAN ALI[1*], SNIGDHA BHARDWAJ[2], NAJAM ALI KHAN[1], SYED SARIM IMAM[3], and CHANDRA KALA[4]

[1]*Faculty of Pharmacy, IFTM University, Lodhipur Rajput, Delhi Road (NH-24), Moradabad – 244102, Uttar Pradesh, India*

[2]*Department of Pharmaceutical Science, SHALOM Institute of Health and Allied Sciences, Sam Higginbottom University of Agriculture, Technology and Sciences (SHUATS), Naini, Prayagraj, India*

[3]*College of Pharmacy, King Saud University, Riyadh, Saudi Arabia.*

[4]*Department of Pharmacology, Faculty of Pharmacy, Maulana Azad university, Jodhpur-342802, Rajasthan, India*

ABSTRACT

Arthritis is still a questionable for medical research in terms of effective treatment. A better knowledge of the pathophysiology of chronic inflammatory conditions, such as arthritis, nanomedicines are supposed to have improved penetration and prolonged retention mechanism and a ligand conjugation on a surface for active binding to the cell receptors, through which they can passively accumulate into inflammatory tissues resulting in increased efficacy and lesser systemic adverse effects. Currently available anti-arthritic synthetic treatment for the management of arthritis are found to have multiple disadvantages like serious side effects, high costs of treatment, requirement of parenteral administration and incomplete relief to patient in respect to pain intensity and joint movements. These problems encourage more research to provide a convenient, cost-effective therapy with minimum or no side effects.

Traditional herbal medicines are now extensively studied as a potential therapy of choice for arthritis patients because of their anti-inflammatory and immunomodulatory properties. Despite of the known fact, development of herbal drugs as novel drug delivery systems is not efficiently implemented by the scientists due to insufficient regulatory framework. The incorporation of herbal bioactives into nanocarriers like nanoparticles, metallic nanoparticles, liposomes, and phytosomes may overcome the existing problems of available treatment for arthritis in terms of improved bioavailability, stability, site-specificity, and fewer side effects. On the patient side, improved patient compliance may be achieved with the thought of lower side effects of natural's agents based medicines. Thus, the herbal nanomedicines can be an effective alternative medication for arthritis. This chapter highlights the research conducted, in recent years, using nanomedicines in combination with herbal drugs as an effective therapy in arthritis and concludes several important investigations with promising results for the treatment of chronic disease in an efficient way.

8.1 INTRODUCTION

8.1.1 CHRONIC INFLAMMATORY DISEASE: ARTHRITIS

Inflammation can be defined as a response generated towards infection or any injury. Under the extreme circumstances, the defensive mechanism of inflammation reverses and acts harmful with increasing response in respect to intensity and duration. Anaphylaxis and septic shock are conditions that lead to excessive and potentially chronic inflammatory responses. One of the main purposes of inflammation is to eradicate foreign pathogens such as bacteria. Through well-coordinated signaling, inflammation is involved in eliminating the initial cause of cell injury, clearing out damaged tissues while stimulating tissue repair. Although excessive inflammation can clearly be pathogenic. In chronic conditions of inflammation, like Crohn's disease and ulcerative colitis (collectively defined inflammatory bowel disease, IBD), rheumatoid arthritis (RA), ankylosing spondylitis, psoriatic arthritis and psoriasis, the coordination among cell is lost resulting in an unwanted inflammatory response, often distinguished by relapse-remission cycles with flares of increased activity (Philip et al., 2014).

Arthritis is not a single disease. It is joint inflammation. A joint may be referred as a point or junction where two bones join together. The edge of the bone is protected with a layer of tissue generally called cartilage (Harris et al., 1990; Semerano et al., 2016). This disease involves the breakdown of cartilage. Cartilage protects the joint and allows it move smoothly. Symptoms of this disease are joint pain, redness, swelling, stiffness. Arthritis occurs when the body's immune system attacks healthy tissue and cause inflammation. It leads to painful swelling in joints (Yarwood et al., 2016; Ruiz-Esquide et al., 2012; Okada et al., 2014). Osteoarthritis called degenerative joint disease as the shedding of the cartilage occurs at bone joints when rub together, resulting in pain, stiffness, and other symptoms (Majithia et al., 2007; Siddiqui et al., 2011). RA is a chronic disease it can affect many parts of body. RA is marked by symmetrical, peripheral polyarthritis, due to an inflammatory response that affects joints in the hands, feet, and wrists in particular (Erin et al., 2008; Pham et al., 2011). Similarly, ankylosing spondylitis refers to inflammation of the spinal joints. Psoriasis is an inflammatory skin disease, commonly indicative with plaque-type lesions on elbows, knees, and scalp. Generally, patients with psoriasis, (up to 30%) also develop psoriatic arthritis, in which, in addition to skin lesions, inflammation predominantly affects joints in the hands and in the spine (Firestein et al., 2003; Rathore et al., 2007). The pathogenesis of RA, ankylosing spondylitis, psoriasis, and psoriatic arthritis seem to be as multifactorial and involves causes such as genetic predisposition, reactivity to external pathogens and inappropriate activation of the immune system in the process (Afeltra et al., 2001; Alexandros et al., 2011) (Figure 8.1).

Inflammation is an immune system response that involves immune cells and small signaling proteins called cytokines. Of the inflammatory cytokines that mediate the inflammatory response, TNF is a central mediator to chronic inflammatory disease. The response mechanism of inflammatory may be subcategorized further into four general elements that indulge systemically in the inflammatory pathway (Daniel et al., 2012):

1. **Inflammatory Inducers:** These are generated signals that specifically work in stress, injury, and malfunction of tissues. The signals may be either exogenous (such as toxin, pathogens, etc.), or endogenous (such as urate crystals, ATP, etc.).
2. **Sensors:** Produce inflammatory mediators in response to inducer identification with their particular receptors, such as tissue-resident macrophages and mast cells. Production of mediators' combinations and amount may vary depending on the nature of the inducers, with

respect to the development of unique mediator impression for their specific inducer.

3.   **Inflammatory Mediators:** They work on targeted tissue resulting in the alteration their functional states. Apart from this, these mediators are also responsible for encouraging banishing of the inflammatory inducer, adjustment to the noxious condition, maintaining tissue homeostasis.

4.   **Target Tissues:** *Functio laesa* (disturbance of function) refers to potential of the inflammatory response in diseased conditions. With increasing alteration in target tissue due to inflammatory response, the endothelial adhesiveness and penetration of inflammatory cytokines like tumor necrosis factor (TNF) and interleukins are also increased which results in an increase in exudate and mucus production, promote host defense from infection.

In response to any inflammatory reaction, the change in the functional state of tissue represents the cost and pathological capacity of inflammation regardless of the intensity and duration of response generated. Thus, damage caused by extreme response to inflammatory site is considered to be the most common negative outcome observed during the process (Georg et al., 2018).

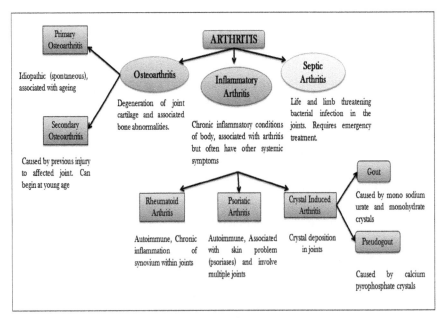

FIGURE 8.1   Common types of arthritis and their causes.

8.2 OVERVIEW OF NANOMEDICINE

Nanotechnology is a branch of technology that represents the field with fabrication of devices and tools of size less than 100 nanometers (nm) with modification at the atomic as well as molecular levels. After being in nanosize range, these particles possess distinctive structural, electronic, magnetic, and optical properties within the system which cannot be attained with large size molecules. The concept of nanotechnology using in clinical practice and medical investigation is referred as nanomedicines (Selvarajan et al., 2009).

Initially, a nanomedicine was described by European Science Foundation (ESF), as the technology designed to treat, diagnose, and prevent any disease, pain, or injury for achieving the improved human health provided with the proper understanding of these carrier performances within the human body. Further revision is done in the definition by the US NIH that explained nanomedicines as highly specific nano-carriers that intervene at the molecular level to cure the disease symptoms and repair tissue damage. The ESF mentioned five sub-areas of nanomedicines that are given below (Raj et al., 2009):

1. Investigative or analytical tools;
2. Imaging tools at nano level;
3. Properties and applications of nanomaterials (NMs) and nanodevices;
4. Clinical investigation and toxicity considerations clinical and toxicological issues;
5. Novel nano-drug carrier systems.

Nanomedicines present the medical use of nano-sized particles, nano-fiber, and nanodevices for delivering the active drug in the diagnosis and treatment of disease to the target cells in the human body thereby offers less damage to a healthy cell in the body. Nanomedicines are being assumed to have a great impact in medical research (public health) and offer several advantages such as nanoscale devices in medicine are of great use because of their prompt interaction at the molecular level on the cell surface of cells as well as penetration into and within cell. This approach offers noninvasive fabrication of devices that facilitate the entry of these devices to the interior of a target cell without damaging the normal one, which needs a better understanding of concepts like cell's biology and chemistry. Nano-carrier systems offer multiple advantages like improved bioavailability, dosing uniformity; speed up onset of action, and reduction in fasting and feeding variability as compared with traditional microparticulate systems. Nanomedicines represent advancement in drug delivery and types of delivery systems as well as the designing of miniaturized diagnostic and analytical methods (Moustafa et al., 2006).

8.2.1 FUNDAMENTALS OF NANOTECHNOLOGY-BASED TECHNIQUES

Nanomedicines include often hybrid multicomponent, nano-sized structures, and can be made using either both top-down or bottom-up manufacturing techniques. On the other hand, rising level of synthesizing those 'ultrafine' nanoparticles in the environment and/or workplace has been proved to be particularly hazardous during prolonged accidental human exposure. Thus using these NMs in a broad range of applications (from construction to aerospace materials, from environmental applications and electronic components to cosmetics and consumer products, etc.), has led to the birth of the field now termed 'nanotoxicology' (Ruth et al., 2012).

Drug designing using herbals at the nanoscale has been investigated and they offer several advantages to modify properties (solubility, release profile, penetration, bioavailability, etc.), that facilitates the development of suitable administration route with minimal toxicity, less side effects and improved biodistribution pattern of drug candidate to target site (receptor present on cell surface, lipid components of cell, proteins on cell, etc.). The nanostructures system consists of self-assembly, micellar structure which are formed from building blocks. Drug targeting is divided into active and passive targeting. In active targeting the moieties (such as protein, peptide, and antibody) serves as an anchor between delivery system and receptor at specific site, after being adhered to drug delivery system. Whereas in passive targeting, formed drug carrier complex, circulating via bloodstream is taken to target site by affinity (such as pH, temperature, site, etc.) (Jayanta et al., 2018).

8.3 HERBAL PHARMACOTHERAPY IN ARTHRITIS

Herbal remedies, after being an important research area and clinical practice in orthopedics and rheumatology, it is a key priority of physicians and their patients to understand the balance ratio of risk and benefits associated with herbal therapy for the proper management of arthritis, rheumatic conditions, and musculoskeletal pains. With increasing cases of various arthritic conditions (such as Osteoarthritis and other forms), recent studies suggest that available pharmacotherapy is not effective in terms of capability to retain the originality of bone structure and function in diseased conditions. Several problems like less relief of symptom, side-effects with prolonged treatment leads to chronic illness, makes less attractive approach towards conventional medical therapy for the proper treatment of arthritis, and other arthritic conditions indicate a straightforward approach for novel, innovative, safe, and effective alternative treatment for arthritic patients. Natural products may be an answer to the current problem in therapy as most of them have faith that herbals are a natural gift and moreover is a safer option as compared with synthetic drugs. Ethnopharmacology is a new and rapidly developing discipline and involves the study of the use of herbal and medicinal plants by particular cultural groups (Ali et al., 2012).

Herbal products belong to the ancient system of medicines such as traditional Chinese medicines, Indian Ayurveda medicines, Japanese traditional medicines Egyptian and other African traditional medicine; have a great collection of natural products for medical use. Medicinally active bioactives, extracted, and isolated from plants, have been developed as drug products as well as a delivery system and are consumed worldwide for treating diverse disorders (autoimmune disease, infectious disease, inflammatory conditions, and cancer) (Shivaprasad et al., 2016).

Some treatments and strategies for arthritis are fully satisfactory to patients because of the narrow safety window and less effective. So, it is required to design and develop new drug delivery systems that are specially targeted in flamed joints. The use of nanoparticles possible to increase bioavailability and enables selective targeting joints damaged (Ulbrich et al., 2010; Mitragotri et al., 2011).

8.4 CHALLENGES WITH HERBAL PHARMACOTHERAPY IN ARTHRITIS TREATMENT

Globally, many cases with age-related diseases associated with bone, joints, and muscles are gradually increasing day by day and affecting the physical and mental health of millions of people. According to United Nations (UN) and World Health Organization (WHO) reports that all types of arthritic condition is the leading cause of the disability and morbidity across the world and also affecting the people's work efficiency and healthcare expenses (Original Source: The Arthritis Foundation and WHO). Field of herbals and nutraceuticals are of great challenges at central as well as state government regulations (Mahfoozur et al., 2017).

8.4.1 THE CHALLENGES AND CONSTRAINTS IN HERBAL MEDICINES

Various challenges are to analyze the under dispute parameters like herbal toxicity and epidemiology. The key issues in using herbals in the formulations are as follows (Thillaivanan et al., 2014):

- Lack of planning in assessing risk management, improper communication on herbal developments as direct therapy.
- Non-availability of pharmacological, toxicity, and clinical data.
- In-effective pharmacovigilance;
- Poor availability of data on drug interaction;
- Improper measurement and constraints with clinical trials;
- Deficiency of standardization procedures;
- In-sufficient data on safety and efficacy parameters;
- Lack of information on developmental approach of high yielding plant species and their cultivation, etc.;
- Improper quality control measures;
- Poor GMP guidelines;
- Poor research and developmental standards establishment.

There are various medicines such as steroids, nonsteroidal anti-inflammatory drugs (NSAIDs), and immunosuppressant and widely used for controlling and suppressing inflammatory response but are associated with adverse effects. So, Herbal therapy is best suited as an alternate or complementary therapy to achieve increased pharmacological response with no or minimal side effects (Mona et al., 2016).

8.5 NANOTHERAPEUTIC APPROACHES TO ARTHRITIS TREATMENT

8.5.1 CARRIER SYSTEMS IN DRUG DELIVERY

Nanotechnology is the science and technology that have the ability to measure, design material at atomic, molecular, and supermolecular level. Development of NMs focuses on the treatment at cellular level in specific disease condition; reduce the toxicity and enhancing effectiveness. Targeted Release of bioactive from nanoparticles may follow active targeting and passive targeting process. These nanocarrier systems are biocompatible and degradable (Butoescu et al., 2009; Brennan et al., 2008).

Nanocarrier systems such as vesicles, liquid crystal nanoparticles, micelles as well as polymeric nanoparticles dispersions made up of very fine particles ranging in nano-scale (10–400 nm, depending upon type), offers wide scope for drug delivery and other applications like imaging, diagnosis, etc., (Figure 8.1). During the development of these nanoformulations, the ultimate aim remains is to formulate the drug delivery system with optimized drug entrapment, modified release profiles, low toxicity profiles, and prolonged shelf life (Sakuta et al., 2010) (Figure 8.2).

The active principle remains entangled within the core of the micellar structure and transported at concentrations with an increase in the intrinsic water-solubility profile. In the micellar structure, the hydrogen bonding generally takes place with the aqueous surroundings in the hydrophilic blocks which develops an intact covering layer around the micellar core. This provides nice protection to the hydrophobic contents of the core against chemical reactions such as hydrolysis and enzymatic degradation. Amphiphilic block copolymers can be easily changed their chemical composition of compounds, structural block length ration and molecular weight (total) which allows monitoring of surface morphology 9 (size, shape, and surface charge, etc.), of the micelles, represent extraordinary feature for drug delivery applications. Surface charge modification facilitates the functionalization of block copolymers with crosslinking groups (ligands), during micellar formation, resulting in high stability and site-selectivity of formed structure (Costas et al., 2006).

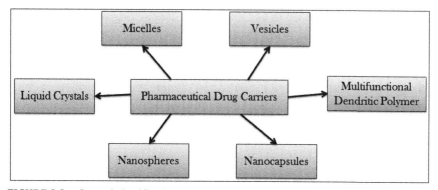

FIGURE 8.2   General classifications of pharmaceutical drug carriers.

8.5.2 NANOPARTICLES AS CARRIER SYSTEMS IN DRUG DELIVERY

By standard description, nanoparticles are nano-range sized polymeric colloids in which active medicament entrapped or dispersed (core) within the polymeric matrix or adsorbed or conjugate onto the surface (shell) and are considered to have at least one specific dimension of less than 100 nm. Depending on their respective micro and macro-scale counterparts, nanoparticles show different properties with the same chemical compositions. The more the surface energy of nanoparticles more will be the cohesion between nanoparticles. In addition, the progressive improvement in energy on nanoparticles surface may lead to alteration in crystal arrangement of nanoparticles, reactive nature at interface and intrinsic properties may be affected (Lee et al., 2012).

The polymers used to synthetically formulate the nanoparticles consist of biodegradable and nonbiodegradable. Currently, biodegradable polymers are often considered to be a more attracted approach towards the synthesis of nanoparticles. Nanoparticles may also be designed using different materials like silica, silver, gold, copper, zinc oxides, therapeutics, quantum dots, Nanotubes, and various contrast agents. Major improvements through these nanocarrier systems has been investigated in respect of their effectiveness in escaping multidrug resistance and targeted delivery via active targeting of drug (Biswajit et al., 2014).

There are different methods through which nanoparticles can be synthesized. The following aspects are involved in formulating nanoparticles are neutral pH, low cost, and environmental friendly approach (nontoxic). Nanoparticles production by plants is considered as more acceptable mode in terms of more stability and faster rate of synthesis as compared to other cases of organisms. Thus, suitable methods for synthesizing nanoparticles using herbs need to be developed in upcoming days, considering cost-effectiveness and maintenance issues. NMs are further classified into sub-groups which are depicted in Figure 8.3 (Heera et al., 2015).

Generally, multiple mechanisms that contribute to drug release from nanocarriers such as diffusion-controlled, degradation controlled, stimuli controlled and solvent controlled, though each and every mechanism has its own influence on drug release. For example, in polymeric nanogels, drug release is controlled by two mechanisms, i.e., swelling, and diffusion through the membrane. Nanoparticles are further designed and modified in several other ways to attain patterned monitoring on the drug release kinetics as given in Table 8.1 (Jinhyun et al., 2015).

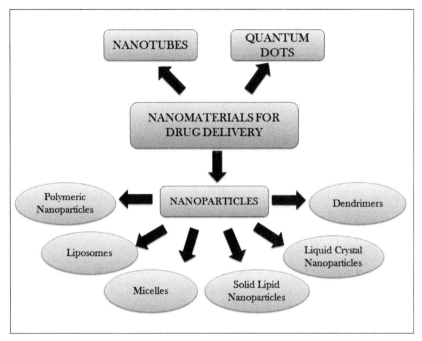

FIGURE 8.3   Types of nanomaterials for drug delivery.

8.5.3   THERAPEUTIC RELEASE FROM CARRIER SYSTEMS

Drug release from nanocarriers, with respect to its temporal control; focuses on maintaining drug levels in systemic circulation and target tissue effectively. Different mathematical models has been developed and can be used to analyze release kinetics (such as zero order, first order, Huguchi model, Hixson-Crowell, Korsmeyer-Peppas model, and regression model) from delivery systems. Several mechanisms involved in drug release from the carriers can control or modify system kinetics. For instance, release kinetics can be modified and is controlled by drug diffusion across the carrier matrix or a barrier. Different approaches like swelling of matrix and breakdown of drug-polymer linkage also are of concern in terms of controlling rate of drug release (Jinhyun et al., 2015).

8.6   CURRENT LANDSCAPE OF NANOMEDICINE FOR ARTHRITIS

Nanomedicine is an interdisciplinary technology which has become field of great importance worldwide, in respect to advancement in multiple branches

TABLE 8.1 Types of Nanomaterials Used in Drug Delivery of Pharmaceuticals

Types of Nanomaterials		Size Range	Description	Applications	References
Nanoparticles	Polymeric micelles	10–100 (nm)	Spherical colloidal particles with hydrophobic interior (core) and hydrophilic body (shell) amphiphilic copolymer micelles, high drug entrapment, and biostability	Useful in encapsulating water-soluble pharmaceuticals	Costas et al., 2006
	Polymeric nanoparticles	10–1000 (nm)	These are biocompatible and biodegradable systems and efficiently protect the drug from the surrounding environment.	Surface modified nano-carriers can be used for active and passive delivery of bioactive as well as carriers for controlled drug delivery.	Bhatia et al., 2016
	Metallic nanoparticles	<100 (nm)	Different metals used in the fabrication of these tiny particles (such as Gold, silver, and other heavy metals), Highly stable and functionalized in nature due to the availability of high surface area.	Metallic nanoparticles are biosensors and excellent carriers for therapeutics delivery in cancer treatment.	Biswajit et al., 2014
	Liposomes	50–200 (nm)	Bilayer vesicles consisting of phospholipids. Offers good drug entrapment and are biocompatible	Carrier for controlled delivery and also used for active and passive delivery of proteins, peptide, and genes.	Lee et al., 2012
	Dendrimers	<10 (nm)	Three dimensional, branched structures contain three moieties such as core part branched part and tight-packed surface.	Used as contrast agents, drug delivery for anti-cancerous drugs, and gene vectors.	Rye et al., 2013

Types of Nanomaterials	Size Range	Description	Applications	References
Solid lipid nanoparticles	50–1000 (nm)	Prepared by phospholipids (such as mono-di-tri-glycerides and fatty acids) dispersed in an aqueous medium containing surfactants.	Adjuvant for vaccines, targeted carrier for anticancer drug, lung infection, brain delivery, ultrasonic drug, and gene delivery, cosmetic, and dermatological preparations and agricultural purpose.	Ekambaram et al., 2012
Liquid crystals nanoparticles	2–9.5 (nm)	The ordered self-organization of rod-shaped structures, and are electrically charged. They exhibit both liquid and solid-state properties.	Applications in Photonic crystal paper or advanced composites.	Camila et al., 2018
Carbon nanotubes (CNT)	Diameter: 0.5–3 (nm) Length: 20–1000 (nm)	Two dimensional, made up of the third allotrope of carbon as crystalline carbon sheets and divided into single-walled or multi-walled types. Electrically charged, great mechanical strength but lightweight.	Biosensors for Proteins and DNA, Ion channel blocking agents, bioseparators, and biocatalysts. Coating for prosthetics and surgical implants (e.g., vascular stents)	Anna et al., 2015
Quantum dots	10–100 (Å)	Three dimensional, semiconductors, formulated with II, III-V, and VI column element. Offers intense fluorescence, fine emission, and high photostability.	Disease diagnosis and screening technologies like cellular imaging, real-time tracking of molecules and cells in sustained profiles and tumor targeting	Biswajit et al., 2014; Rye et al., 2013

of treatment towards high-level disorders due to advantages such as efficacy and efficiency. It is assumed that in the coming 10–15 years, the Indian market of nanomedicines is believed to expand the growth of USD 1.6 billion values and after that India would be able to be a ranker among the top three healthcare markets by 2020. The government of India is also supporting the research and development activities in the field of nanomedicines to fulfill the current societal needs.

Government departments involved in research activities also focus on the drug delivery advancement by setting new standards for these nanomedicines and their implementation in research organizations working on it. Few examples are the Department of Science and Technology (DST), in 2007, started a mission namely "nanomission" to boost fundamental research, designing of research infrastructure, to make better international collaborations, strengthen the platform for developing nano-based technologies. Other organizations such as the Council of Scientific and Industrial Research (CSIR), Defense Research and Development Organization (DRDO), Department of Biotechnology (DBT) and Indian Council of Medical Research (ICMR), also promoting and providing funds for the research-based related to nanomedicines associated with herbals.

Although with this progression in nanomedicines research in India, the involvement of Indian departments in the area of nanomedicines and innovations is currently not up to the level that may be difficult to provide a proper landscape on nanomedicines (Pooja et al., 2018). Another reason is that these nanomedicines affected by individual biological variation because of diseased conditions offer a restricted landscape as scale-up production as additional steps in the process may be required for surface conjugation of ligand moieties which makes the manufacturing process more complex (Bruno et al., 2017).

8.7   METHODS USED FOR PRODUCING NATURAL PRODUCT-BASED NANOMEDICINE

8.7.1   GREEN-SYNTHESIZED METAL NANOPARTICLES USING PLANTS FOR ARTHRITIS TREATMENT

The production of nanostructured system may be a serious issue with respect to toxicology as the high reactivity increases from the large surface-to-volume ratio of these nanosystems compared to bulk systems, which is a matter of concern. Any newly developed nanostructures system needs to be tested carefully with respect to its potential side effects within the human body and the environment.

Nanotechnology concepts for its clinical application also require for strict regulatory guidelines to ensure the safe and proper use of new nano-medical devices and drugs originating from nanoscience (Kristina et al., 2009).

Anti-inflammatory mechanism is an important wound healing mechanism responsible for the production of immune responsive agents like cytokines and interleukins, lymphocytes, and macrophages which are secreted from primary immune organs. These anti-inflammatory mediators induce the healing process and control the expansion of diseases after being involved in biochemical pathways. Some other inflammatory mediators (enzymes, antibodies, etc.), are secreted by endocrine system. Various studies on synthesis of gold nanoparticles attract the researcher to think over it as future therapy because these systems are compatible and have wide scope in drug delivery. It has also been studies that gold nanoparticles have been explored as effective therapy in wound repair and tissue generation in inflammatory conditions. Hence, this evidence strongly supports the fact that gold and other metal nanoparticles can be explored as an alternative therapy for the treatment of inflammatory conditions (Palaniselvam et al., 2016).

Green synthesis refers the process which uses natural source agents (plant, bacteria, fungi, etc.). As well, all know that plants are sustainable resources in nature and hence may be explored in the green synthesis of nanoparticles and other nanosystems along with these factors like wide distribution, easy availability and reproducibility make them a better candidate for nanomedicines. The green chemistry is an alternative approach to formulate biocompatible nanoparticles by a chemical process and represents the anchor between two emerging specializations such as material science and biotechnology (Nanobiotechnology). Green synthesis is the method of synthesizing nanoparticles from herbal resources. Several metallic nanoparticles using herbal bioactives have been synthesized by this process (Table 8.2). The metal nanoparticle-herb combination may show better efficacy against different inflammatory conditions.

8.7.2   INCLUSION OF HERBAL BIOACTIVE TO FORMULATE DIFFERENT TYPES OF NANOMEDICINES FOR CONTROLLED DELIVERY SYSTEMS

Several herbal bioactive has been explored for their therapeutic efficiency against the pathological conditions of arthritis. Incorporating these herbal compounds in the systems for synthesizing different nanostructured systems for biomedical applications has been produced in recent times. Several benefits attract herbals for the synthesis of nanosystems is availability, easy, and harmless handling as well as to the environment. Few plants are listed in Table 8.3 which has been used to formulate the different nanomedicines (Jayanta et al., 2014).

TABLE 8.2   Metal Nanoparticles Using Herbal Compounds for the Management of Arthritis

Sl. No.	Nanoparticles	Plant used	Part used	Treatment	References
1.	Ag-NP	Night Jasmine (*Nyctanthes arbor-tristis*)	Aqueous Extract	Rheumatoid Arthritis	Arumugam et al., 2013
2.	Ag-NP	*Tylophora ovata*	The leaves and roots	Arthritis	Joy et al., 2015
3.	CD Conjugated Au-NP	Curcumin	Rhizomes extract	Osteoarthritis	Murali et al., 2015
4.	Ag-NP	*Cardiospermum halicacabum*	The leaves extract	Rheumatism and arthritis	Mahipal et al., 2013
5.	Ag-NP	*Morinda tinctoria Roxb*	The leaves extract	Arthritis	Geetha et al., 2017
6.	Ag-NP	*Centratherum punctatum* Cass.	The leaves extract	Arthritis	Krithika et al., 2016
7.	Au-NP	*Achyranthes aspera* Linn	Seeds	Arthritis	Anand et al., 2014
8.	ZnO-NP	*Moringa oleifera*	Immature pods and flowers	Arthritis	Monakari et al., 2016
9.	Ag-NP	Caffeic acid	The plant source	Osteoarthritis	Qingyan et al., 2017
10.	Cu-NP	*Delonix elata*	Flower extract	Arthritis	Suganya et al., 2016

* Ag: Silver, Au: Gold, ZnO: Zinc Oxide, Cu: Copper, CD: Cyclodextrin.

8.8   NANOPARTICLE THERAPY IN ARTHRITIS

8.8.1   TARGETED APPROACH: MOLECULAR TARGETS FOR NANOMEDICINES IN ARTHRITIS

Site-specific delivery of drugs to target cells and tissues is considered to be an important application of engineered nanoparticles as medicines. Recent investigation for herbal drugs has been tested against various forms of arthritic conditions and indicates a significant decrease in the levels of IL-6 and TNF-α in the synovial fluid. Active medicaments derived from herbals exhibits a great impact in lowering amounts of cytokines in the Synovial fluid resulting in the relief from the diseased condition that may lead to better quality of life of patients. This aspect presents a promising approach of developing nanostructures systems using active drugs which enables drug release in surrounding environment at controlled rate, thereby, requires less drug dosages and avoids the non-specific side effects of the drugs (Li et al., 2010; Kowalski et al., 2013).

TABLE 8.3 Inclusion of Bioactive Compound in Different Forms of Nanomedicines

Sl. No.	Bioactive Group	Bioactive Component	Nano Carrier System	Type of Delivery System
1.	Polyphenols	Quercetin	Nanoparticles	Quercetin PLGA-NP
			Nanocapsule	Lipid coated NC
		Resveratrol	Nanoparticles	PLGA NP containing Resveratrol
			Solid lipid nanoparticles	Resveratrol loaded SLN
			Cyclodextrin nanosponge	CD-based nanosponge
		Ellagic acid	Nanoparticles	Ellagic acid-loaded PLGA NP
2.	Phytocanna-binoid	Δ-9-Tetrahydrocanna-binol	Lipid nanoparticles	NLC
			Nanoparticles	PLGA-NP
3.	Stanols	Phytosterols	Nanodispersion	Produced by emulsification-evaporation
				Suspension of submicron particles of phytosterols
4.	Carbohydrates	Mannose-6-phosphate	Nanocapsule	Polyamide NC
			Liposomes	Liposome containing Aloe vera gel
5.	Essential oil (EO)	Oregano and cassia EO	Nanoparticle	Corn zein NP
		Thymol and Carvacrol	Nanoparticle	Corn zein NP

TABLE 8.3   *(Continued)*

Sl. No.	Bioactive Group	Bioactive Component	Nano Carrier System	Type of Delivery System
		Cinnamon and Thyme EO	Cyclodextrins	Inclusion in CD
		Lippiasidoides EO	Nanoparticle	Alginate/Cashew gum NP
		Cumin and Basil EO	Nanocapsules	Polyamide NC
6.	Terpenoids	Squalene	Nanocapsules	Polyelectrolyte multilayer NC
		Lycopene	Nanoemulsion	Aquos propolis and lycopene
			Nanoparticles	SLN
			Cyclodextrins	Inclusion in CD
		p-Cymene	Cyclodextrins	Inclusion in CD
		Linalool	Cyclodextrins	Inclusion in CD
		Carvacrol	Cyclodextrins	Inclusion in CD

* NP: Nanoparticles; CD: Cyclodextrins; NC: Nanocarriers; SLN: Solid lipid nanoparticle; NLC: Nanostructured lipid carriers; PLGA: Poly (lactic-co-glycolic acid).

*Source:*Raffaele et al. (2017).

8.8.1.1   DESIGNING OF ACTIVE TARGETING NANOMEDICINES FOR ARTHRITIS TREATMENT

In active targeting, the modification or functionalization of the drug carries is done so that content can be delivered to the site corresponding to which the carrier is designed. Ideal active targeting nanomedicines for arthritis need suitable range between 10 to 100 nm and charge on their surface (Lee et al., 2014; Kim et al., 2013).

Active targeting nanomedicines need to overcome three barriers to achieve the optimal effects on arthritis:

1. Drug loaded nanocarriers were modified with PEG and active ligands to for the active targeting nanomedicine.
2. PEGlyation prolonged the duration of nanomedicines in blood circulation.
3. Modification at surface charge facilitated the active delivery of nanomedicines to inflamed tissues and cells (Lee et al., 2013; Kim et al., 2015).

8.8.1.2 APPLICATIONS OF ACTIVE TARGETING NANOMEDICINES

Nanomedicines are multidisciplinary domains and have been used for different purposes. Some of these applications are listed here (Rocco et al., 2003; Bindhani et al., 2013):

- As potential platform for therapeutic application;
- As diagnostic purpose with improved fluorescent for screening purpose;
- Delivery of antigens for vaccination;
- Drug delivery for targeted at specific sites in the body;
- Bioavailability issues improvisation with potential nanotechnology solution;
- Provides protection for agent susceptible to degradation.

Some of the literature studies indicate observation of multiple mechanisms in different types of arthritis. Some of the molecules has been identified and considered a potential targets by the upcoming therapies for arthritis or several inflammation conditions (Table 8.4).

TABLE 8.4 Molecular Targets for Nanomedicines in Arthritis and in Other Inflammatory Conditions

Target Group	Targets at Molecular Level	Occurrence	Description
Cytokines	Interleukin-1β (IL-1β)	Knee joint and synovial fluid	Prevent hyaline cartilage production
	Interleukin-6 (IL-6)	Synovial T-cells	Divergence of T helper cells as TH-1, TH-2, and TH-17 cells
	Interleukin-17 A (IL-17A)	Synovial fluids	Activation and expression of interleukins-1, 6 and 8
	Tumor necrosis Factor-α	Synovial fluids	Secretion of interleukins and matrix metalloproteinases (MMPs)
	Urokinase-type plasminogen (uPA)	Synovial cells	uPA/uPAR signaling provoke inflammation at joints.
	Cathepsin-B	During early degenerative phase of Osteoarthritis in synovial tissue	Promotes progression of Osteoarthritis by splitting aggrecan

TABLE 8.4   *(Continued)*

Target Group	Targets at Molecular Level	Occurrence	Description
	Matrix metalloproteinases -3 (MMP-3)	Synovial tissue	Develops osteoarthritis pathogenesis
	Oncostatin M	Synovial fibroblasts	Promote cartilage damage through synergistic effect with IL-1
Proteins	Type I collagen	Bone	Initiation of osteoblastic separation of cells in bone marrow
	Type II collagen	Cartilage	Support cartilage Strength
	Aggrecan	Synovium	Support cartilage Strength
Inflam–matory Cells	Prostaglandin E1	Osteocytes	Encourage bone resorption
	Forkhead box T-cells	Synovium	Maintain equilibrium among regulatory and helper (T-H-17) T-cells
Extracellular matrix glycoprotein	Osteopontin	Secreted by leukocytes, present in extracellular fluids and at the sites of inflammation.	Trigger cell adhesion, movement, invasion, and controls signaling function

Source: Kislay et al. (2015).

8.9   SCOPE OF HERBAL NANOMEDICINES IN ARTHRITIS PHARMACOTHERAPY

The concept of nanotechnology can be of great effectiveness for medicinal plants as well as for its biological active constituents. Herbal compounds (phytotherapeutics) delivery in form of nanoparticles likely to improve their pharmacokinetic and pharmacodynamics profiles. The purpose to combine the herbal medicine with nanotechnology is to design nanostructured systems that provoke the action potential of plant extractives, minimization of effective dose, dosing frequency, and lowering side effects (Newman et al., 2007). For instance, bioactive incorporate such as hesperidin, curcumin, celastrol, resveratrol results in high efficacy for the treatment of arthritis which opens up the door for new and effective drug delivery for arthritis as an alternate to low effective conventional therapy. Phytocontituents have immense potential in arthritis pharmacotherapy but hindrances associated with restricted use of herbals in medical research might be overcome using nanocarriers based drug delivery methods for their effective delivery (Allen et al., 2004).

In designing of a proper delivery system, the physicochemical parameters of natural therapeutics and the system are of great importance to understand drug absorption. These properties control the target site action and penetration across the skin due to the presence of metabolic enzymes and skin fencing. Currently, nanomedicines such as liposomes, microspheres, solid lipid nanoparticles (SLNs), nanoemulsions, and microemulsions have been developed to improve the absorption of such bioactive so as to avoid above-mentioned issues (Kostarelos et al., 2003). These systems offer several merits like controlled delivery of drugs (both hydrophobic and hydrophilic in nature), high drug loading (DL) capability, and better suitability in systemic and topical drug delivery. In addition, the nanostructured system provides higher surface area-to-volume ratio, which provides in significant improvement in the pharmacodynamic and pharmacokinetic properties of active drugs on the specific site. A system consisting of small size particles favors better skin interaction and permeation that contributes the extended circulation of drug molecule to specific site via active targeting (Allemann et al., 1999).

8.10   HERBS REPORTED FOR USE IN ARTHRITIS

Nowadays, researcher's interest is mainly concerned with the medicinal therapeutics extracted and isolated from plants as because the currently available therapy is considered to have some issues related to adverse effects as well as high expense. Currently in India, more than 2500 traditional plant species are using as herbal medicines for the treatment either as directly medication or indirectly as an ingredient of pharmaceutical preparation. Hence, from this perspective, thorough information of these potential herbals may help in finding innovative and economic drugs as an alternative therapy (Manjusha et al., 2015) (Table 8.5).

8.11   FUTURE OF NANOMEDICINE AND DRUG DELIVERY SYSTEM FOR ARTHRITIS

The science of nanomedicines is among the most interesting areas of research. In the last two decades, the filling of 1500 patents and completion of several dozens of clinical trials has already been conducted. In the nanomedicines approach, using an appropriate nano-delivery system facilitate the delivery of the accurate amount of drug to the affected cells without disturbing the physiology of the normal cells. The application of the nano-drug delivery system is currently the trend that will remain to be the future arena of research and development for the near future. Research on NMs has to be done on a higher level with more consistent uniformity and DL and release capacity. The incorporation of metals such as gold, silver, and copper within nanostructures systems provides advancement in diagnosis and therapy in various inflammatory conditions that could potentially lead to wider application of nanomedicines in the treatment of arthritis in coming decades (Raffaele et al., 2017).

Biochemical observations of the experimental studies clearly demonstrate the important role of herbals in the regulation of proinflammatory cytokines, although more clinical studies at large scales need to be performed to confirm the analysis as well as to dissolve some conflicts. The word "natural anti-inflammatory" refers to natural compounds, lifestyle, exercise, and sleep, and eating habits. Various studies on natural compounds and herbal medicines suggested variable outcomes and an inconsistent result which might be based on the method of extraction of chemical constituents because the pharmacological effect of each medicinal herb is the result of plenty of metabolites combination and their synergistic effects; perhaps, it is one of the reasons of contradictory results. There are several synthetic anti-arthritic drugs that have been used in arthritis therapy, but they suffer from several drawbacks which restrict their efficacy.

Herbal treatment approach is of great concern with respect to have great structural diversity, which has not usually seen with synthetic ones. Several synthetic anti-arthritic compounds, employed in arthritis therapy, have several limitations such as non-uniformity in dose and poor bioavailability and higher metabolism. Recent studies revealed that phytotherapeutics have been delivered by means of nanocarriers so as to achieve specific action in arthritis therapy by minimizing dose, and higher drug localization at the target site. For the effective delivery of bioactive, research data on nanocarriers needs to be established *in vitro* and *in vivo* along with safety data. In the near future, nanomedicine may become a first-line approach for an effective delivery system for targeted delivery of bioactive for better management of arthritis. To support the already available research data more investigations need to be done for further materialistic approach in respect to clinical trials and market approvals so as to reach to the desired population (Mona et al., 2016).

TABLE 8.5 Some Reported Herbs Used in the Management of Arthritis

Sl. No.	Plant Name	Biological Source	Family	Active Component	References
1.	Aloe vera	Aloe barbadensis	Liliaceae	Anthraquinones	Devis et al., 1986; Joshep et al., 2010
2.	Spicewood	Lindera aggregata	Lauraceae	Norisoboldine (NOR)	Wei et al., 2012
3.	Ginger	Zingiber officinale	Zingiberaceae	Sesquiterpenoids, sesquiterpene lactones	Rehman et al., 2011; Zaker et al., 2011
4.	Ashwagandha	Withania somnifera	Solanaceae	Withanolides	Grover et al., 2010
5.	Barringtonia	Barringtonia racemosa Linn.	Lecythidaceae	Bartogenic acid	Sun et al., 2008
6.	Panicled Erycibe	Erycibe obtusifolia	Convolvulaceae	Scopoletin	Pan et al., 2010
7.	Milk weed	Calotropis procera Linn	Asclepiadaceae	Benzoyllineolone, Benzolisolineolone	Vaidya et al., 2006
8.	Kalpanath	Andrographis paniculata	Acanthaceae	Andrographolide	Burgos et al., 2009
9.	Thunder god vine	Tripterygium wilfordii	Celastraceae	Triptolide	Kimura et al., 2011
10.	Day-blooming Jasmine	Cestrum diurnum	Solanaceae	Ursolic acid	Ahmad et al., 2006
11.	Chhotahalkusa	Leucasaspera Linn.	Lamiaceae	Ethanolic extract	Narendhirakannan et al., 2005
12.	Galangal	Alpinia officinarum	Zingiberaceae	Diarylheptanoids	Lee et al., 2009
13.	Ashoka	Saraca asoca Roxb.	Caesalpiniaceae	methanol extract	Prajapati et al., 2010

TABLE 8.5 (Continued)

Sl. No.	Plant Name	Biological Source	Family	Active Component	References
14.	Chinese peony	*Paeonia lactiflora*	Paeoniaceae	Gallic acid	Jiang et al., 2011
15.	Tinosporagulancha	*Tinospora cordifolia Linn.*	Menispermaceae	Tinosporine, tinosporide, cordifolide, heptacosanol.	Kumar et al., 2003
16.	Deodar cedar	*Cedrus deodara*	Pinaceae	Polyphenols	Rajan et al., 2011
17.	Indian sarsaparilla	*Hemidusmus indicus Linn.*	Asciepiadaceae	Coumarin	Bajpai et al., 2009
18.	Black adusa	*Gendarussa Linn.*	Acanthaceae	Ethanolic extract of leaves	Sheihk et al., 2011; Paval et al., 2009
19.	Indian white cedar,	*Dysoxylum binectariferum*	Meliaceae	Rohitukine	Jain et al., 2012
20.	Pink Arnebia	*Arnebia euchroma*	Boraginaceae	Hydroxy naphthaquinone	Fan et al., 2012

8.12 CONCLUSION

This chapter tried to highlight the potential of different herbs and herbal constituents which have been active and traditionally used in the treatment of arthritis as a main or supplementary medication. Though research on animal studies put interesting facts and observations but not much clinical and toxicological studies have been performed in this area to support the efficacy and potency of the treatment by herbals. Future opportunities for research in this area have a wide scope which may yield new drug candidates against arthritis, a major socio-economical medical problem among senior persons around the world. Nanotechnology has been already employed for drug delivery and tissue engineering of various natural compounds, as it offers the possibility to develop a therapy with improved therapeutic efficacy of natural bioactive molecules, increased drug bioavailability, site-specific targeted delivery and ultimately reducing toxic side effects. We are hopeful that natural compounds will be a complementary treatment against arthritis and bone-joint related disorder in the coming future.

KEYWORDS

- **arthritis treatment**
- **carbon nanotubes**
- **essential oil**
- **matrix metalloproteinases**
- **nanomedicines**
- **pharmacotherapy**

REFERENCES

Afeltra, A., (2001). Treatment of rheumatoid arthritis: New therapeutic approaches with biological agents. *Journal of Rheumatology, 1*(1), 45–65.

Ahmad, S. F., Khan, B., Sarangbani, Suri, K. A., Satti, N. K., & Qazi, G. N., (2006). Amelioration of adjuvant-induced arthritis by ursolic acid through altered Th1/Th2 cytokine production. *Pharmacol. Res., 53*, 233–240.

Alexandros, A., (2011). Abatacept: A biologic immune modulator for rheumatoid arthritis. *Informa Healthcare, 11*(8), 1113–1129.

Ali, M., (2012). Intersection of inflammation and herbal medicine in the treatment of osteoarthritis. *Curr. Rheumatol. Rep., 14*, 604–616.

Allemann, E., Gurny, R., & Doelker, E., (1999). Drug loaded nanoparticles: Preparation methods and drug targeting issues. *Eur. J. Pharm. Biopharm., 39*, 173–191.

Allen, T. M., & Cullis, P. R., (2004). Drug delivery systems: Entering the mainstream. *Science, 303*, 1818–1822.

Anand, M., Selvaraj, V., Alagar, M., & Ranjitha, J., (2014). Green phyto-synthesis of gold nanoparticles using *Achyranthes aspera* Linn seed epicotyls layer extracts and its anticancer activity. *Asian J. Pharm. Clin. Res., 7*(5), 136–139.

Anna, P. N., (2015). Nanotechnology and its applications in medicine. *Med. Chem., 5*(2), 81–89.

Arumugam, P., Imrankhan, K., & Sankarvyas, S., (2013). Green synthesis of nano-particles and its application in treatment of rheumatoid arthritis. *International Journal of Computing Algorithm, 2*, 450–457.

Bajpai, A., (2009). *Saraca asoca* (Ashoka): A review. *Journal of Chemical and Pharmaceutical Research, 1*(1), 62–71.

Bhatia, S., (2016). Nanoparticles types, classification, characterization, fabrication methods, and drug delivery applications. *Natural Polymer Drug Delivery Systems*.

Bindhani, B. K., Parida, U. K., Biswal, S. K., Panigrahi, A. K., & Nayak, P. L., (2013). Gold nanoparticles and their biomedical applications. *Rev. Nanosci. Nanotechnol., 2*, 247.

Biswajit, M., Niladri, S. D., Ruma, M., Priyanka, B., Pranab, J. D., & Paramita, P., (2014). *Current Status and Future Scope for Nanomaterials in Drug Delivery* (pp. 525–545). Intech.

Brennan, F. M., (2008). Evidence that cytokines play a role in rheumatoid arthritis. *J. Clin. Invest., 118*(11), 3537–3545.

Bruno, S., & Marco, S., (2017). Nanomedicines for increased specificity and therapeutic efficacy of rheumatoid arthritis. *EMJ. Rheumatol., 4*(1), 98–102.

Burgos, R. A., Hancke, J. L., Bertoglio, J. C., Aguirre, V., Calvo, M., & Caceres, D. D., (2009). Efficacy of an *Andrographis paniculata* composition for the relief of rheumatoid arthritis symptoms: A prospective randomized placebo-controlled trial. *Clin. Rheumatol., 28*, 931–946.

Butoescu, N., Jordan, O., & Doelker, E., (2009). Intra-articular drug delivery systems for the treatment of rheumatic diseases: A review of the factors influencing their performance. *Eur. J. Pharm. Biopharm., 73*(2), 205–218.

Camila, H. R., Claudius, L., Christina, S., Roland, S., Mikhail, A., Osipov, J. B., & Jan, P. F., (2018). *Fractionation of Cellulose Nanocrystals: Enhancing Liquid Crystal Ordering Without Promoting Gelation* (pp. 1–11). NPG Asia Materials.

Costas, K., Sofia, A., Katerina, K., & Sotira, C., (2006). Recent advances in novel drug delivery systems. *Azojomo Journal of Materials, 1*–17.

Daniel, O., & Ruslan, M., (2012). Evolution of inflammatory diseases. *Curr. Biol., 22*(17), R733–R740.

Devis, R. H., Agnew, P. S., & Shapiro, E., (1986). Anti arthritic activity of anthraquinones found in aloe for podiatric medicine. *Journal of the American Podiatric Medical Assoc., 76*(2), 61–66.

Ekambaram, P., Abdul, A. H. S., & Priyanka, K., (2012). Solid lipid nanoparticles: A review. *Sci. Revs. Chem. Commun., 2*(1), 80–102.

Fan, H., Yang, M., Che, X., Zhang, Z., Xu, H., Liu, K., & Meng, Q., (2012). Activity study of a hydroxylnapthoquinone fraction from *Arnebia euchroma* in experimental arthritis. *Fitoter, 83*, 1226–1237.

Firestein, G. S., (2003). Evolving concepts of rheumatoid arthritis. *Nature, 423*, 356–361.

Geetha, P., Revathy, K., Sugapriya, M. P., & Jeyaraj, P., (2017). Green synthesis of silver nanoparticles from *Morinda tinctoria* Roxb and scrutiny of its multi facet on biomedical applications. *Pharmaceutical and Biological Evaluations, 4*(5), 222–233.

Georg, S., & Markus, F. N., (2018). Resolution of chronic inflammatory disease: Universal and tissue-specific concepts. *Nature Communications, 9*(3261), 1–8.

Grover, A., Shandilya, A., Punetha, A., Bisaria, V. S., & Sundar, D., (2010). Inhibition of the NEMO/IKKβ association complex formation, a novel mechanism associated with the NF-kB activation suppression by *Withania somnifera's* key metabolite withaferin A. *BMC Genomics, 11*, 25.

Harris, E. D., (1990). Rheumatoid arthritis: Pathophysiology and implications for therapy. *N. Engl. J. Med., 322,* 1277–1289.

Heera, P., & Shanmugam, S., (2015). Nanoparticle characterization and application: An overview. *Int. J. Curr. Microbiol. App. Sci., 4*(8), 379–386.

Hunter, P., (2012). The inflammation theory of disease. *EMBO Reports, 13*(11), 968–970.

Jain, S. K., Bharate, S. B., & Vishwakarma, R. A., (2012). Cyclin-dependent kinase inhibition by flavoalkaloids. *Mini Rev. Med. Chem., 12,* 632–649.

Jayanta, K. P., & Kwang, H. B., (2014). Green nanobiotechnology: Factors affecting synthesis and characterization techniques. *Journal of Nanomaterials*, 1–13.

Jayanta, K. P., Gitishree, D., Leonardo, F. F., Estefania, V. R. C., Maria, D. P. R. T., et al., (2018). Nano based drug delivery systems: Recent developments and future prospects. *J. Nanobiotechnol., 16*(71), 1–33.

Jiang, D., Chen, Y., Hou, X., Xu, J., Mu, X., & Chen, W., (2011). Influence of *Paeonia lactiflora* roots extract on cAMP-phosphodiesterase activity and related anti-inflammatory action. *J. Ethanopharmacol., 137,* 914–920.

Jinhyun, H. L., & Yoon, Y., (2015). Controlled drug release from pharmaceutical nanocarriers. *Chem. Eng Sci., 125,* 75–84.

Joshp, B., & Raj, S., (2010). Pharmacognostic and pharmacology properties of Aloe Vera. *International Journal of Pharmaceutical Sciences Review and Research, 4*(2), 106–109.

Kim, H. J., Lee, S. M., Park, K. H., et al., (2015). Drug-loaded gold/iron/gold plasmonic nanoparticles for magnetic targeted chemo-photothermal treatment of rheumatoid arthritis. *Biomaterials, 61,* 95–102.

Kim, S. H., Kim, J. H., You, D. G., et al., (2013). Self-assembled dextran sulfate nanoparticles for targeting rheumatoid arthritis. *Chem. Commun., 49*(88), 10349–10351.

Kimura, K., Norni, N. Y. Z. H., Orita, T., & Nishida, T., (2011). Inhibition of poly(I:C)–induced matrix metalloproteinase expression in human corneal fibroblasts by triptolide. *Molecular Vision, 17,* 526–532.

Kislay, R., Rupinder, K. K., & Jagat, R. K., (2015). Molecular targets in arthritis and recent trends in nanotherapy. *International Journal of Nanomedicine, 10,* 5407–5420.

Kostarelos, K., (2003). Rational design and engineering of delivery systems for therapeutics: Biomedical exercises in colloid and surface science. *Adv. Colloid Interface Sci., 106,* 147–168.

Kowalski, P. S., Lintermans, L. L., Morselt, H. W., et al., (2013). Anti-VCAM-1 and anti-E-selectin SAINT-O-Somes for selective delivery of siRNA into inflammation-activated primary endothelial cells. *Mol. Pharm., 10*(8), 3033–3044.

Kristina, R., Stefan, W., Schneider, Thomas, A., Luger, Biana, G., Mauro, F., & Harald, F., (2009). Nanomedicine-challenge and perspectives. *Angew. Chem. Int. Ed., 48,* 872–897.

Krithika, S., Niraimathi, K. L., Narendran, R., Balaji, K., & Brinda, P., (2016). *Int. J. Rs. Ayurveda Pharma., 7*(2), 61–66.

Kumar, S. S. S., Pandey, S. C., Srivastava, S., Gupta, V. S., Patro, B., & Ghosh, A. C., (2003). Chemistry and medicinal properties of *Tinospora cordifolia. Indian Journal of Pharmacology, 35*, 83–91.

Lee, C., & Ventola, M. S., (2012). The nanomedicine revolution (Part 1: Emerging concept). *P & T, 37*(9), 512–525.

Lee, H., Lee, M. Y., Bhang, S. H., et al., (2014). Hyaluronate-gold nanoparticle/tocilizumab complex for the treatment of rheumatoid arthritis. *ACS Nano, 8*(5), 4790–4798.

Lee, J., Kim, K. A., Jeong, S., Lee, S., Park, H. J., Kim, N. J., & Lim, S., (2009). Antiinflammatory, anti-nociceptive, and anti-psychiatric effects by the rhizomes of *Alpinia officinarum* on complete Freund's adjuvant-induced arthritis in rats. *J. Ethnopharmacol., 126*, 258–264.

Lee, S. M., Kim, H. J., Ha, Y. J., et al., (2013). Targeted chemo-photothermal treatments of rheumatoid arthritis using gold half-shell multifunctional nanoparticles. *ACS Nano, 7*(1), 50–57.

Li, S. D., & Huang, L., (2010). Stealth nanoparticles: High density but sheddable PEG is a key for tumor targeting. *J. Control Release, 145*(3), 178–181.

Mahfoozur, R., Sarwar, B., Amita, V., Fahad, A., Al, A., Firoz, A., Sumant, S., Sohail, A., & Vikas, K., (2017). Phytoconstituents as pharmacotherapeutics in rheumatoid arthritis: Challenges and scope of nano/submicromedicine in its effective delivery. *Journal of Pharmacy and Pharmacology, 69*, 1–14.

Mahipal, S., Shekhawat, M., Manokari, N., Kannan, J., Revathi, R., & Latha, (2013). Synthesis of silver nanoparticles using *Cardiospermum halicacabum* L. leaf extract and their characterization. *The Journal of Phytopharmacology, 2*(5), 15–20.

Majithia, V., & Geraci, S. A., (2007). Rheumatoid arthritis: Diagnosis and management. *Am. J. Med., 120*(11), 936–939.

Manjusha, C., Vipin, K., Hitesh, M., & Surender, S., (2015). Medicinal plants with potential antiarthritic activity. *J. Intercult. Ethnopharmacol., 4*(2), 147–169.

Manokari, M., Mahipal, & Shekhawat, S., (2016). Zinc oxide nanoparticles synthesis from *Moringa oleifera* Lam. Extracts and their characterization. *World Scientific News*, 252–262.

Mitragotri, S., & Yoo, J. W., (2011). Designing micro-and nano-particles for treating rheumatoid arthritis. *Arch. Pharm. Res., 34*, 1887–1897.

Mona, G., Sina, O., & Mohammad, B. O., (2016). Review of anti-inflammatory herbal medicines. *Advances in Pharmacological Sciences*, 1–11.

Moustafa, M. A., (2006). An overview of nanomedicine. *JMRI, 27*(4), 248–254.

Murali, M., Yallapu, Prashanth, K., Bhusetty, N., Meena, J., & Subhash, C. C., (2015). Therapeutic applications of curcumin nanoformulations. *The AAPS Journal, 17*(6), 1341–1357.

Narendhirakannan, R. T., Subramanian, S., & Kandaswamy, M., (2005). Free radical scavenging activity of *Cleome gynandra* L. leaves on adjuvant induced arthritis in rats. *Molecular and Cellular Biochemistry, 276*(1, 2), 71–80.

Newman, D. J., & Cragg, G. M., (2007). Natural products as source of new drugs over the last 25 years. *J. Nat. Prod., 70*, 461–477.

Okada, Y., Wu, D., Trynka, G., Raj, T., Terao, C., Ikari, K., Kochi, Y., Ohmura, K., Suzuki, A., Yoshida, S., et al., (2014). Genetics of rheumatoid arthritis contributes to biology and drug discovery. *Nature, 506*, 376–381.

Palaniselvam, K., Mashitah, M., Yusoff, Gaanty, P. M., & atanamurugaraj, G., (2016). Biosynthesis of metallic nanoparticles using plant derivatives and their new avenues in pharmacological applications: An updated report. *Saudi Pharmaceutical Journal, 24*, 473–484.

Pan, R., Gao, X. H., LI, Y., Xia, Y. F., & Dai, Y., (2010). Anti-arthritic effect of scopoletin, a coumarin compound occurring in *Erycibe obtusifolia* Benth stems, is associated with decreased angiogenesis in synovium. *Fundam. Clin. Pharmacol., 24*, 477–490.

Paval, J., Kaitheri, S. K., Potu, B. K., Govindan, S., Kumar, R. S., Narayanan, S. N., & Moorkoth, S., (2009). Anti-arthritic potential of the plant *Justicia gendarussa Burm* F. *Clinics, 64*(4), 357–362.

Pooja, B., Suhas, V., & Anil, W., (2018). A landscape of nanomedicine innovations in India. *Nanotechnol. Rev.*

Prabu, H. J., & Johnson, I., (2015). Plant-mediated biosynthesis and characterization of silver nanoparticles by leaf extracts of *Tragia involucrata, Cymbopogon citronella, Solanum verbascifolium and Tylophora ovata. Karbala International Journal of Modern Science, 1*, 237–246.

Prajapati, M. S., Patel, J. B., Modi, K., & Shah, M. B., (2010). *Leucasaspera*: A review. *Pharmacognosy Review, 4*(7), 85–88.

Qingyan, L., Heqing, H., Liying, C., & Guixiu, S., (2017). Synthesis of caffeic acid coated silver nanoparticles for the treatment of osteoarthritis. *Biomedical Research, 28*(3), 1276–1279.

Raffaele, C., Valentina, M., Gianfranco, P., Anna, C., & Pierfrancesco, C., (2017). Recent advances in nanoparticle-mediated delivery of anti-inflammatory phytocompounds. *Int. J. Mol. Sci., 18*, 709–731.

Raj, B., (2009). *Nanopharmaceuticals for Drug Delivery: A Review.*

Rajan, S., Shalini, R., Bharathi, C., Aruna, V., & Elgin, A. S., (2011). An update on *Nyctanthes arbortristis* Linn. *International Pharmaceutica sciencia, 1*(1), 77–86.

Rathore, B., Mahdi, A. A., Paul, B. N., Saxena, P. N., & Das, S. K., (2007). Indian herbal medicines; possible potent therapeutic agents for rheumatoid arthritis. *J. Clin. Biochem. Nutri., 41*(1), 12–17.

Rehman, R., Akram, M., Akhtar, N., Jabeen, Q., Saeed, T., Shah, S. M. A., et al., (2011). *Zingiber officinale* roscoe (pharmacological activity). *Journal of Medicinal Plants Research, 5*(3), 344–348.

Rocco, M. C., (2003). Nanotechnology: Convergence with modern biology and medicine. *Curr. Opin. Biotechnol, 3*, 337–346.

Ruiz-Esquide, V., & Sanmarti, R., (2012). Tobacco and other environmental risk factors in rheumatoid arthritis. *Rheumatol. Clin., 8*, 342–350.

Ruth, D., (2012). Nanomedicine(s) and their regulation: An overview, Chapter 1. In: Bengt, F., (ed.),*Safety Assessment of Nanomaterials: Implications for Nanomedicine* (pp. 1–30). Pan Stanford Publishing.

Rye, S., (2013). *Nanomedicine New Solutions or New Problems*? Health Care Without Harm, Europe.

Sakuta, T., Morita, Y., Satoh, M., Fox, D. A., & Kashihara, N., (2010). Involvement of the renin-angiotensin system in the development of vascular damage in a rat model of arthritis: Effect of angiotensin receptor blockers. *Arthritis Rheum, 62*(5), 1319–1328.

Selvarajan, S., Steven, A. D., & Surendiran, A., (2009). Emerging trends of nanomedicine: An overview. *Fundamental and Clinical Pharmacology, 23*, 263–269.

Semerano, L., Minichiello, E., Bessis, N., & Boissier, M. C., (2016). Novel immunotherapeutic avenues for rheumatoid arthritis. *Trends Mol. Med., 22,* 214–229.

Shaikh, P. Z., (2011). Study of anti-inflammatory activity of ethanolic extract of *Hemidesmus indicus* roots in acute, subchronic and chronic inflammation in experimental animals. *International Journal of Pharmacy and Life Sciences, 2*(10), 1154–1173.

Shivaprasad, H., Venkatesh, Brian, A., Siddaraju, M., Nanjundaia, Hong, R. K., et al., (2016). Control of autoimmune arthritis by herbal extracts and their bioactive components. *Asian Journal of Pharmaceutical Sciences, 11,* 301–307.

Siddiqui, M. A., Amir, A., Vats, P., Rani, K., Malik, S. A., Arya, A., Kapoor, N., & Kumar, H., (2011). Arthritis database: A composite web interface for antiarthritic plants. *J. Med. Plant. Res., 5*(12), 2457–2461.

Suganya, M., & Valli, G., (2016). Green synthesis of copper nanoparticles using *delonix elata* flower extract. *Int. J. Nano Corr. Sci. and Engg., 3*(4), 156–165.

Sun, H. Y., Long, L. J., & Wu, J., (2008). Chemical constituents of mangrove plant *Barringtonia racemosa*. Anti-inflammatory and analgesic agents from Indian medicinal plants. *International Journal of Integrative Biology, 3*(1), 57–72.

Thillaivanan, S., & Samraj, K., (2014). Challenges, constraints, and opportunities in herbal medicines: A review. *International Journal of Herbal Medicine, 2*(1), 21–24.

Ulbrich, W., & Lamprecht, A., (2010). Targeted drug-delivery approaches by nanoparticulate carriers in the therapy of inflammatory diseases. *J. Roy. Soc. Interface., 7*(1), S55–S66.

Vaidya, A. D. B., (2006). Reverse pharmacological correlates of Ayurvedic drug action. *Indian Journal of Pharmacology, 38*(5), 311–315.

Wei, Z., Wang, F., Song, J., Lu, Q., Zhao, P., Xia, Y., Chou, G., et al., (2012). Norisoboldine inhibits the production of interleukin-6 in fibroblast-like synoviocytes from adjuvant arthritis rats through PKC/MAPK/NF-κB-p65/CREB pathways. *J. Cell Biochem., 113,* 2785–2795.

Yarwood, A., Huizinga, T. W., & Worthington, J., (2016). *The Genetics of Rheumatoid Arthritis: Risk and Protection in Different Stages of the Evolution of RA Rheumatology, 55,* 199–209.

Zaker, Z., Izadi, S., Bari, Z., & Soltani, F., (2011). The effects of ginger extract on knee pain, stiffness, and difficulty in patients with knee osteoarthritis. *Journal of Medicinal Plants Research, 5*(15), 3375–3379.

CHAPTER 9

Phytoconstituent-Based Nanotherapeutics as Ocular Delivery Systems

MOHAMMED JAFAR,[1*] SYED SARIM IMAM,[2] and
SYED AZIZULLAH GHORI[3]

[1]*Department of Pharmaceutics, College of Clinical Pharmacy,
Imam Abdulrahman Bin Faisal University, P.O. Box 1982,
Dammam-31441, Saudi Arabia. E-mail: e.mail: mjomar@iau.edu.sa*

[2]*Department of Pharmaceutics, Glocal School of Pharmacy,
Glocal University, Saharanpur-247121, Uttar Pradesh.*

[3]*Department Department of Pharmacy practice,
College of Clinical Pharmacy, Imam Abdulrahman Bin Faisal University,
P.O. Box 1982, Dammam-31441, Saudi Arabia.*

ABSTRACT

In the last few years, there has been a wide growth in the field of phyto-medicine and gaining popularity all over the globe because of their natural origin and lesser side effects. The applications of different phytoconstituents loaded nanoformulations have been widely accepted as delivery systems for various diseases. The application of nanoformulation opened the door in a disease like glaucoma, eye cancer, and other anterior ocular diseases by significantly modifying the properties of drugs and their carriers. It utilized various nanoformulations like nanoparticle, nanoemulsion, nano lipid structure, nano lipid vesicle to transport the different phytoconstituents like curcumin, quercetin, forskolin to the site of action. The greater stability of phytoconstituents loaded nanoformulation is due to the formation of chemical links between lipid molecules and active agents. There are several phytoconstituents loaded nanoformulation have depicted a novel delivery system to deliver active compounds to the target site of action, and at present, several nanoformulations are in clinical use. This chapter summarizes the latest research reports regarding the possible administration of phytoconstituents loaded nanoformulations for different ocular diseases.

9.1   INTRODUCTION

The eye is considered as an essential part of the body that comprises of two major anatomical parts: the anterior as well as the posterior region. The posterior region mainly composed of choroid, vitreous chamber, macula, and retina and importantly the posterior area of the sclera is located interior to the lens (Janagam et al., 2017). The majority of eye-related illnesses seem to be arisen from internal structures of the eye, hence raising the quantum and intensity in a consistent manner (Thrimawithana et al., 2011). If left untreated, these problems may cause permanent eye damage resulting in loss of complete vision. According to the recent data reports it was revealed that around 39 million people were affected because of age-associated macular degeneration (AMD), Retinopathy due to diabetes, and disease of glaucoma of the posterior region of the eye resulting in the complete visual loss (International Federation, 2013; McGrath et al., 2017).

Presently, the use of invasive procedures and topical administration of drugs in the form of ocular gel, ointment, etc., to the posterior and anterior regions of the eye is the only available option for managing these disorders. Yet, posterior side topical drug delivery abides a point of confrontation because of diverse effluence systems and organic impediments, like nasolacrimal drainage, tear clearance, the cornea, conjunctiva, and scleral barriers. The current advancement in the field of nanotechnology and nano-drug studies, laid down a great provision and access by overwhelming the restrictions of the conventional treatments, due to their protecting capability for encapsulated medications that ease their transport to a particular spot of tissue (Weng et al., 2017; Kaur and Kakkar, 2014). Additionally, nanoparticles aids as a favorable vehicle for topical drug delivery systems due to prolonged drug duration, higher drug absorbency beyond the barriers, and posterior area drug delivery via restrained rate (Delplace et al., 2015). Varied nano-vehicles such as lipid nanoparticles, liposomes, emulsions, spanlastics, micelles, polymeric nanoparticles, layered double hydroxides (LDH), dendrimers, cyclodextrins, and pro-active medication with built-in quality has been employed in order to achieve and devise a novel formulation optimization designs in case of topical administration of posterior eye (Madni et al., 2017).

As reported by World Health Organization (WHO), in southeast countries like India, China, and such other developing countries, the main health needs of approximately 80% of the population are met and/or complemented by traditional medicine (Robinson and Zhang, 2011). Since ancient times herbal extracts have been used in treating various eye diseases. Macerated fruit of Atropa belladonna was the plant-derived substance used by the Egyptians first time in the anterior region of the eye to treat ophthalmic disease (Duncan and Collison, 2003). Several new phytoconstituents have been studied exhaustively in order to find out constituents with the capacity to give greater advantages to eye tissue and the sight. Transpiring indications of wound-healing, anti-inflammatory, antioxidant, antimicrobial, antiangiogenic, and antineoplastic characteristics ascribed to herbal extracts has advocated larger speculations in investigation in this field. Regardless of technological progress in the manufacture of synthetic drugs, the pharmaceutical industry still look for novel active constituents from natural origin, moreover, often visiting previously accepted plant-derived compounds. Considering the above facts, this chapter aims to report different nano-based ocular drug delivery systems of phytoconstituents used in the effective treatment of vision-threatening posterior eye diseases.

9.2 PHYTOCONSTITUENTS BASED NOVEL OCULAR DRUG DELIVERY SYSTEMS

9.2.1 LIPID NANOMEDICINES

Solid lipid nanoparticles (SLN), as well as nanostructured lipid carriers (NLC), are considered to be regularly investigated lipid nanoparticles that are used for the ocular drug delivery. These nano-drugs usually contain a solid lipid core, which has potential in accumulating medications with hydrophilic and lipophilic nature into lipid fabric (Figure 9.1). SLN are accurately embraced with more than a single solid lipid, which shows a melting point of 40°C and even higher. Subsequently in the beginning of 1990s the benefits of control release property of SLNs has been emerged (Souto and Doktorovova, 2009), including cellular toxicity, augmented compatibility, and high *in vivo* tolerance (Doktorovova et al., 2014, 2016). Compared to SLN, NLCs which contain suitable blends of both liquid and solid lipids seem to possess the benefits of elevated medication carrying potential, improved storage steadiness, and efficient drug discharging characteristics (Das et al., 2012; Liu et al., 2017). Several phytoconstituents based lipid nanomedicines were developed for the effective treatment of vision-threatening diseases. Yu et al. (2018) designed a new nanostructured lipid carrier (NLC) embedded double-receptive hydrogel for ocular drug delivery of quercetin (QN). NLC loaded with quercetin (QN-NLC) was devised using melt emulsification combined with the ultra-sonication method. A three-factor five-level central composite design (CCD) was utilized to optimize the formulation of QN-NLC. The optimized QN-NLC presented a particle size of 75.54 nm with narrow size distribution and greater encapsulation efficiency (97.14%). QN-NLC was identified by differential scanning calorimetry (DSC) and scanning electron microscopy (SEM). Moreover, a pH and temperature double-receptive hydrogel consisting of carboxymethyl chitosan (CMCS) and poloxamer 407 (F127) was fabricated by a cross-linking reaction with a naturally occurring nontoxic crosslinking agent genipin (GP). FT-IR was used to exhibit that F127/CMCS hydrogel was successfully produced. The results of SEM analysis and swelling experiments demonstrated that F127/CMCS hydrogel was both pH, as well as temperature-receptive. Moreover, *In vitro* release studies exhibited dual temperature and pH responsiveness of the hydrogel, and 80.52% of total quercetin was released from the QN-NLC based hydrogel (QN-NLC-Gel) within 3 days, unfolding QN-NLC-Gel released drug sustainability. Collectively speaking, the produced NLC-based hydrogel was a promising drug delivery system for the application to the ophthalmic region.

Lakhani et al. (2018) were conducted a new study on preparation, optimization, and evaluation of curcumin-incorporated NLCs for their *in vitro* and *ex vivo* characteristics. A standard CCD was utilized in optimization of NLCs, which are formulated using hot-melt emulsification and ultrasonication methods, these NLCs were evaluated for their *in vitro* physicochemical characteristics. Their stability over an extended period of 3 months and transcorneal permeation across excised rabbit corneas (*ex vivo*) were examined for the optimized NLCs. The optimized NLC, with polydispersity index of 0.17 ± 0.05, particle size of 66.8 ± 2 nm, drug loading (DL) of $3.1 \pm 0.05\%$ w/w, and entrapment efficiency of $96 \pm 1.6\%$, was chosen using CCD. The optimized NLCs showed optimum *ex vivo* stability at 4°C for the study period and showed a significant improvement in curcumin permeation (2.5-fold) across the rabbit cornea in comparison to the control. Altogether, these studies demonstrated the successful designing and development of NLCs utilizing the design of experiment approach; the formulation improved curcumin permeation across excised corneas and did not show any harmful side effects.

Wang et al. (2017) prepared, optimized, and characterized a cationic lipid nanoparticle (CLN) system containing fractioned drugs utilizing a molecular dynamics model as a novel approach of optimizing and characterizing the formulations. Puerarin (PUE) and scutellarin (SCU) were used as model drugs. Melt-emulsion ultrasonication and low temperature-solidification methods were used in the preparation of CLNs. The characteristics of CLNs such as gross morphology, zeta potential, and particle size, DL, entrapment efficiency (EE), and *in-vitro* drug release performance were assessed. The CLNs were also evaluated by corneal permeation, preocular retention time, and pharmacokinetics (PKs) in the aqueous humor. Moreover, a molecular dynamics model was employed to assess the formulation. SEM results revealed that the nanoparticles were approximately spherical in shape. All other physical parameters results of these nanoparticles were satisfactory and most importantly the mathematical values calculated for these systems were statistically significant. The pharmacokinetic study performed collecting samples from the aqueous humor demonstrated that compared with the PUE and SCU solution, the area under the concentration-time curve (AUC) value of PUE was increased by two folds for PUE-SCU CLNs, and the SCU AUC was also enhanced by two folds. In the molecular dynamics model, PUE, and SCU passed through the POPC bilayer, with a clear cut difference in the free energy well depth. It was found that the maximum free energy required for PUE and SCU transmembrane movement was ~15 and 88 kJmol^{-1}, respectively. These findings indicated that compared with SCU, PUE easily passed through the membrane. The diffusion coefficient values obtained for PUE and SCU were also statistically significant. Data obtained from the molecular dynamics model were in accordance with the experimental data. All data showed that CLNs have a high capability for ocular administration and can be used as an ocular delivery system for multi-component drugs. Moreover, the molecular dynamics model can also be used as a novel method for assessing new formulations.

Li et al. (2014) prepared employing emulsion evaporation-solidification at low temperature method tetrandrine-loaded cationic solid lipid nanoparticles (TET-CNP) and solid lipid nanoparticles (TET-NP). The particle size, zeta potential, entrapment efficiency of TET-CNP, and TET-NP were determined. The results revealed that the TET-CNP and TET-NP had acceptable sizes with optimum zeta potentials and high entrapment efficiencies respectively. *In vitro* drug release studies showed that both the TET-CNP and TET-NP perpetuated the drug entity much better than tetrandrineoccular solutions (TET-SOL). In the PKs investigations, the AUC values of TET-CNP and TET-NP were almost two-fold greater than that of TET-SOL; the Cmax values of TET-CNP and TET-NP were also almost two and a half fold greater than that of the TET-SOL respectively. Cytotoxicity study revealed that TET-CNP and TET-NP had no significant cytotoxicity at minimum amounts. Flow cytometry studies and confocal microscopy analysis showed that calcein labeled NP (CA-NP) uptake by SRA 01/04 cells was much greater than those of calcein labeled CNP (CA-CNP) and calcein solution (CA-SOL).

Liu et al. (2011) prepared and evaluated the solid lipid nanoparticles of baicalin (BA-SLN) for ocular delivery. The method used to prepare BA-SLN was also an emulsification/ultrasonication technique. The advent of BA-SLN was assessed by the negative stain technique. The key physical parameters mean diameter and zeta potential of BA-SLN were evaluated using a Zetasizer. Another key feature entrapment efficiency of BA-SLN was also measured by using Sephadex-G50 column. Solid-state characterization of BA-SLN was performed by DSC and X-ray studies. The *in-vitro* drug release from BA-SLN was estimated using dialysis bag diffusion method. Isolated rabbit corneas were used to assess the effects of SLN on corneal permeability of baicalin. The *in-vivo* ocular irritation test for prepared BA-SLN was carried out on rabbits and the intensity of irritation to rabbit eye after application of the above nanoparticles was examined observing pathological sections of rabbit eye. The PKs studies were performed by microdialysis in the rabbit aqueous humors. The results revealed that the BA-SLN had a good particle size distribution with a positive zeta potential and the good entrapment efficiency. *In vitro* drug release studies clearly showed that the BA-SLN retained the drug entity better than the baicalin ophthalmic solutions (BA-SOL). In the PKs studies, the AUC value of BA-SLN was four-fold versus the BA-SOL, and the Cmax value of BA-SLN versus the BA-SOL was fivefold with very low p values. Thus, SLN can be used as a carrier to enhance the ocular bioavailability of baicalin.

9.2.2   LIPOSOMES

Liposomes are colloidal vesicular transporters, which are produced by the hydration of phospholipids. The nanosized liposomes are made up of phospholipids composed of the polar head as well as nonpolar fatty acid chains (Figure 9.1), which aids them accommodated in individual minor structural phospholipid units both the hydrophilic and hydrophobic drug molecules accessing their delivery to the targeted sites (Peptu et al., 2015). Phosphatidylcholine (PC), phosphatidylserine (PS), Soya phosphatidylcholine, and Phosphatidylethanolamine, containing indistinguishable nature with the lipid present on the surface of the cell membrane, generally opted for liposomal preparations that lead to enhance pre-corneal absorption (Agarwal et al., 2016). The newer generation surface-modified liposomes possessing both mucoadhesive and improved penetration properties, not only capable of entrapping the therapeutic agent but can also aims to specific sites through corneal binding (Fangueiro et al., 2016).

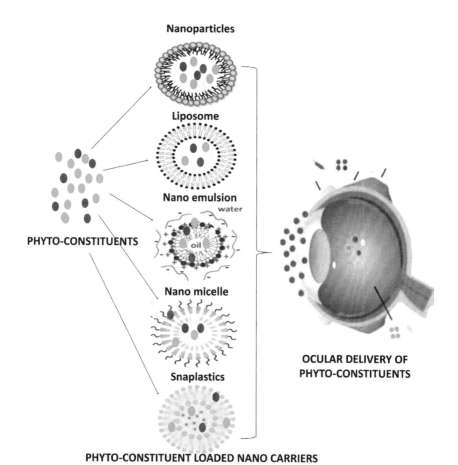

FIGURE 9.1 Ocular delivery of phytoconstituents through various nanocarriers.

Abdelkader et al. (2016) proved in their recent report that L-carnosine phytosomes could be the better substitute for N-acetyl-L-carnosine (a prodrug) as a novel drug carrier for the lens an anterior part of an eye. L-carnosine was incorporated into phytosomes prepared using phosphotidyl choline (in two molar ratios 1:1 and 1:2) and also in phytosomes prepared dispersing in them hyaluronic acid (HA) (in 1:2 molar ratio). The widely used solvent evaporation method was employed to prepare these phytosomes. In these phytosomes, preparation phospholipids were dispersed in either HA (0.1% w/v) in phosphate buffered saline or phosphate-buffered saline (pH 7.4) to obtain phytosomes. These phytosomal preparations were studied for physical characteristics such as gross morphology which includes size, zeta potential, spreading coefficient, contact angle, and viscosity of the drug carrier system. *Ex-vivo* transcorneal permeation studies and cytotoxicity studies were also carried out for both the phytosomes utilizing preliminary corneal cells of humans. L-carnosine-phospholipid (1:2) phytosomes were in the acceptable nanosize and also polydispersity index results were satisfactory. The viscosity of phytosome containing hayluronic acid increased up to 5-fold in comparison with plain HA solution and phytosome containing phospholipid respectively. Notably reduced surface tension, low contact angle, and consequently higher spreadability for both the types of phytosomes were noted. *Ex vivo* transcorneal, permeation study results demonstrated notably managed penetration of L-carnosine through the cornea by these novel drug carrier systems without any notable influence on preliminary corneal cell motility in humans. The results of another important parameter lens incubation study revealed that the lenses of porcine which were kept in incubator at standard conditions of incubation in high sugar media with and without L-carnosine demonstrated concentration-dependent marked inhibition of lens brunescence revealing the capacity for delaying changes that underlie cataractogenesis which may be directly linked to diabetic procedures.

In another interesting high-level study reported by Zhang et al. (2016) they designed and developed N-trimethyl chitosan (TMC)-coated liposomes of cyanidin-3-glycoside (C3G) (C3G-TCL) to attenuate oxidative stress produced by selenite sodium in rats. C3G-TCL were prepared by reverse-phase evaporation method and then coated with self-synthesized TMC. The physicochemical properties such as size, zeta potential, etc., were measured. The state of the art a gamma scintigraphy study was performed to evaluate the pre-corneal elimination of the radioactive preparations. The transcorneal visualization for fluorescence-labeled samples was determined by confocal laser scanning microscopy (CLSM). The *in vivo* anti-oxidative study using

C3G-TCL was carried out in rats with selenite-induced cataracts by topical administration. The round structural morphological characterization of the formulated vesicles was confirmed by TEM, with an acceptable size and a zeta potential of the above carrier systems. The encapsulation efficiency was $53.7 \pm 0.2\%$ as measured by ultrafiltration. C3G-TCL showed a 3.3-fold increment in precorneal residence time when compared with that of the 99 mTc-solution. A TMC coating enhanced the transepithelial transport of liposomes to a depth of 40-mm in the cornea. In addition, C3G-TCL could significantly enhance the activity of superoxide dismutase (SOD) and catalase (CAT) in lens and also demonstrate a considerable reversal of reduced glutathione activity. The lipid peroxidation (LPO) in lens was strongly prevented when compared with that of groups treated with uncoated C3G-loaded liposomes. The coating material TMC for liposomes helps enhance the antioxidative effect of C3G *in vivo* through prolonged residence time on the cornea and improved permeability in the corneal epithelium.

A vehicle with TMC has been developed by He et al. (2013), using various percentage of quaternization (DQ) as coating substance, vitamin A palmitate (VAP) incorporated cationic liposomes disseminated within heat-sensitive *in situ* gels (ISG) through a poloxamer. TMC-coated with DQ of 20, 40, and 60% respectively, was chosen and disseminated in P407 solution with the aid of film dispersion method, resulting in attainment of TMC-coated VAPL ISG VAP-loaded liposomes (VAPL). The physicochemical characteristics of the carrier systems such as gross morphology, zeta potential, particle size, DL efficiency, *in-vitro* drug release and drug retention in the eye were examined. *In vivo* parameters like, ocular retention, followed by irritation in eye and pharmacokinetic influence on aqueous humor of the system involving rabbits has been investigated and tested. With the aid of VAPL, smooth round surface with a nanosize and a negative zeta potential value has been identified. There was no significant changes seen in the morphology and entrapment efficiency after the TMC-coating process, however, the zeta potential was changed to positive, Increase in the mean size, and release of drug was further hold-up, the process in turns controlled by DQ of TMC. A small effect has been identified in relation to gel-forming temperature of Poloxamer solution, and at the P407 concentration of 25% (w/v), by TMC-coated VAPL that resembles the temperature of 34 C, which is just similar with that of the eye surface when it dissolves with artificial tears. The TMC-coated VAPL ISG showed highly detained drug liberation and gel corrosion with an adequate linear relation between them, and with an incremental DQ, the slow delivery of medication and gel corrosion has been exhibited when compared to that of the oculotect gel and an uncoated VAPL ISG. In both, *in vivo* as well as *in vitro* studies, the TMC-coated VAPL ISG ocular retention time, was found to be noticeably extended with a positive link with DQ of TMC. A prolonged tmax, enhanced Cmax and AUC (024) in aqueous humor of the rabbit eye, recommending the prolonged drug release with a desirable corneal penetration and absorption when compared with that of the marketed gels, has been executed by TMC60-coated VAPL ISG. The insignificant side effect like local irritation has been recognized with that of the TMC-coated VAPL ISG. The TMC-coated VAPL ISG shows significant features such as slow release of the medicament; prolonged retention in the eye, improved corneal permeation, and favorable bio-safety characteristics is proven to be effective and can be considered for future studies.

9.2.3   EMULSIONS

Micro- or nano-emulsions are some of the most rising liquid globules applied onto the ocular anterior surface with some exclusive nature (enhanced bioavailability, ocular tissue compatibility, high DL) (Kumar and Sinha, 2014). Emulsions can be defined as biphasic liquid drug delivery systems where two immiscible liquids are made to become miscible by adding an emulgent (surfactant or co-surfactant) (Figure 9.1). The emulsion droplets behave as a drug pool for liberating hydrophilic as well as hydrophobic agents in the corneal layer. Droplets of emulsions are formed by blending the oil phase with the aqueous phase and surface-active agents, which possess lower energy absorption (Vandammee, 2002). Microemulsions ranging between sizes of 5 nm to 200 nm show immense drug absorption and also improve the pre-corneal penetration. An effective medication for overcoming macular degeneration, using a nano-emulsion (NE) system comprising of isopropyl myristate, triacetin, Tween 80, and ethyl alcohol to enhance the solubility and permeability of lutein, has been discovered by Lim et al. (2016). To recognize the self-emulsifying area, a pseudo-ternary phase structure was established. Eight different formulations were identified and chosen to characterize each formulation. We notified physical characteristics including particle size, drug solubility, formulation stability, and turbidity. The transparent optimized formulations such as NE 5 (NE-5) and NE-8, has been chosen. The particle size of NE was ca. found to be in a range of 10–12 nm with a narrow size distribution. For about 7 days, there was no separation and change in the particle size was notified. The lutein loading NEs demonstrated a significant increase in lutein release and sustained release. In contradiction, lutein prepared using oil and starch shows restricted drug release profiles under 5%. The produced lutein NE formulation is proven to be a possible substituent for lutein delivery systems.

9.2.4 POLYMERIC NANOPARTICLES

Polymers show different characteristics in their composition. For attaining favorable ocular drug delivery to the targeted area, the best suitable option is the polymeric nanoparticles of colloidal nanosized systems (1 nm < d < 1000 nm) (Ghangoria et al., 2016). Based on the structural differences, the polymeric nanoparticles are classified as: nanospheres (NSs) and nanocapsules (NCs) (Figure 9.1). NSs generally consist of polymeric matrix with three drug-loading patterns: (i) to encapsulate drugs into the spheres; (ii) to absorb drugs onto the surface; (iii) to disperse drugs within the polymeric network. In contrast to nonospheres, nanocapsule score-shell possesses the ability to dissolve drugs in the core or to absorb drugs on the shell when present in drug-loading form (Meyer et al., 2012; Tekade et al., 2014).

A stimulus-amenable, *in situ*-forming, nanoparticle-laden hydrogel for controlled release of poorly bioavailable drugs into the aqueous humor of the eye has been established by Kabiri et al. (2018). A composite of HA and methylcellulose (MC) is used to formulate a hydrogel. Poly (ethylene oxide) (PEO) and poly (lactic acid) (PLA) are present in the amphiphilic nanoparticles. The hydrogel composition and nanoparticle content in the formulation, is recognized by an experimental design and the formulation accessibly switched between thixotropy and temperature-dependent rheopexy when it was examined in a rheometer under conditions that imitate the ocular surface, including blinking. These features need to assure that the formulation coats the cornea via blinking of the eyelid and eases for application of it as an eye drop instantly before the patient's bedtime. We eventually, examined the efficacy of our formulation in whole-eye experiments through loading the nanoparticulate with cannabigerolic acid (CBGA). Above 300% enhancement in transcorneal penetration over control formulation has been established with our formulation. This research laids the basic way for introduction of new products targeting treatment of ocular diseases to the market.

A newer nano-carrier formulation composed of Pluronic-F127 sustained D-Tocopherolpolyethene glycol 1000 succinate nanoparticlulate, which were employed for emulsifying greater curcumin concentrations (4.3 mg/mL) in a promising level has been reported by Davis et al. (2018) study. Characterization with x-ray diffraction and *in vitro* release studies resulted in restraining of curcumin to the nano-carrier interior, measuring <20 nm diameter for each particulate size. Curcumin-stacked nanocatalysts (CN) were found to be as mainstay of therapy for Cobalt chloride-induced hypoxia and glutamate-induced toxicity *in vitro*, with CN treatment prominently enhancing R28 cell feasibility. The topical application of CN twice-daily for three weeks that has the ability to reduce retinal ganglion cell loss compared to the controls has been prepared by employing glaucoma-related *in vivo* models of ocular hypertension (OHT) and partial optic nerve transaction (PONT). The above results revealed that the newer topical CN formulation research has been shown a promising effect for neuroprotective therapy in glaucoma and other related eye diseases with neuronal pathology. Epigallocatechin-3-gallate (EGCG), possessing antiangiogenesis activity acting as blocker for human vascular endothelial cells for corneal neovascularization (NV) therapy has been proposed by Chang et al. (2017).

In the current research, conjugated complex of arginine-glycine-aspartic acid (RGD) peptide HA-coating on the gelatin/EGCG self-assembly nanoparticles (GEH-RGD NPs) was formed to target V3 integrin on human umbilical vein endothelial cells (HUVECs) and a corneal NV mouse model was utilized in order to assess the clinical outcome of this nano-drug used as eye drops. H1NMR and FT-IR has been utilized to establish HA-RGD conjugation through COOH and amine grouping. The average size for GEH-RGD NPs was satisfactory to say it is in nanosize with a positive zeta potential, and EGCG-loading efficiency of almost 100%. Images of GEH-A spherical shape and shell structure in nanosize have been visible with RGD NPs obtained through a transmission electron microscopy method. At about 30% after 30 hours of duration, a slow-release design of nano-formulation was notified in the surface plasmon resonance assuring that the GEH-RGD NPs specifically binds to the integrin V3. The GEH-RGD effectively inhibits HUVEC proliferation, at a reduced EGCG concentration as compared to that of the EGCG or non-RGD-modified NPs, in the *in vitro* cell-viability studies. Besides, GEH-RGD NPs notably inhibits HUVEC migration lowers than 58%, lasting for 24 hours of duration. In the corneal NV mouse, model, minimal, and thinner vessels were found in the alkali-burned cornea after treatment with GEH-RGD NP eye drops. Ultimately, this research proved that the GEH-RGD NPs were favorably designed and produced as vascular endothelial cell inhibitors with a definite targeting capability. Furthermore, it can also be employed for eye drops to inhibit angiogenesis in corneal NV mice.

A novel penta block (PB) copolymer (PB-1: PCL-PLA-PEG-PLA-PCL) builded nano-forms suspended in a thermosensitive gelling copolymer (PB-2: mPEG-PCL-PLA-PCL-PEGm) termed as composite nano-formulation has been developed and synthesized by Agrahari et al. (2016). An insignificant shatter release effect has been notified by the composite nanoformulation that was synthesized to provide a sustained delivery of complex molecules over a longer duration. The posterior segment ocular diseases such as age-related (wet) macular degeneration, diabetic retinopathy, and diabetic macular edema are managed with the aid of such a delivery system. The novel PB copolymers were identified by FT-IR spectroscopy, 1H-NMR spectroscopy and gel permeation chromatography for identification of functional groups, molecular weight and purity respectively. To determine the crystallinity of copolymers, the X-Ray diffraction method was employed. The PB-1 nanoparticles (NPs) size distribution was found to be ~150 nm using nanoparticle tracking analysis, following an emulsification-solvent evaporation method. The encapsulation efficiency and DL percentage (%) were found to be as 66.64%} 1.75 and 18.17%} 0.39, respectively, (n = 3). For *in vitro* release studies of IgG-Fab from composite nanoforms, variant weight percentages (15 wt.% and 20 wt.%) of the PB-2 copolymer has been used. An insignificant shatter release with continuous near zero-order has been identified from the composite nanoforms analyzed up to 80 days of duration. The *in vitro* cell viability and biocompatibility studies carried out on ocular (human corneal epithelial and retinal pigment epithelium) and macrophage (RAW 264.7) cell lines, revealed that the produced PB copolymer-based composite nanoforms were safe and effective for clinical applications. Based on the above results, it can be concluded that the PB copolymer constructed composite nanoforms can provide a strong platform for therapeutic proteins ocular delivery. Moreover, the composite nanoformulations may also provide fewer side effects associated with frequent intravitreal injections.

9.2.5 SNAPLASTICS

Spanlastics are considered as newer elastic micro-vesicular carriers comprises of spans and non-ionic surfactants that possess considerable elasticity nature in structure and quantity. Hydrophilic, hydrophobic, and amphiphilic drugs can be loaded into its multi-lamellar micro-vesicles with the aid of snaplastics (Figure 9.1). Non-ionic surfactants like tweens play an eminent role in reducing interfacial tension, enhancing fluid nature, and deformability that results in improved diffusion of spanlastics (Deol et al., 2015). Broadly, the application of surfactants is encouraged for expanding the pores of the bio-membrane encouraging the temporary entry of huge spanlastics (Kakkar and Kaur, 2011). To facilitate the posterior eye segment drug delivery, spanlastics is highly recommended and considered favorable and efficient ophthalmic nanodevice.

9.2.6 MICELLES

Nano-micelles consisting of polymeric and surfactant nano-micelles are known to be as rising novel carrier systems for posterior eye drug delivery. Apart from their smaller size, improved drug solubility and stability (Alvarez et al., 2016), enhanced corneal permeation (Prosperi-Porta et al., 2016), lower adverse effects and high biocompatibility (Vadlapudi et al., 2014) aids them to become potential candidates for poorly aqueous soluble drug delivery system. Fewer amphiphilic molecules when added to special solvents adapt to self-assemble and results in core-shell monomers called nano-micelles (Cholkar et al., 2012) (Figure 9.1). A newer curcumin composed nanomicelle formulation utilizing a polyvinyl caprolactam-polyvinyl acetate-polyethylene glycol (PVCL-PVA-PEG) graft copolymer has been demonstrated by Li et al. (2017). Nanomicelle curcumin, formulated, and optimized, which was further assessed for *in-vitro* cytotoxicity, cellular uptake, and antioxidant activity followed by *in-vivo* ocular irritation, corneal permeation, and anti-inflammatory efficacy respectively. After the encapsulation process of the PVCL-PVA-PEG nanomicelles, the solubility, chemical stability, and antioxidant activity were drastically enhanced. The nanomicelle curcumin based ophthalmic solution was easy to produce and the nanomicelles possess adequate stability as well, it also contains better cellular tolerance. Excellent ocular tolerance in rabbits has been noticed by Nanomicelle curcumin. The usage of nanomicelles remarkably enhances the *in vitro* cellular uptake as well as the *in vivo* corneal permeation. Additionally, nanomicelles also intensify the anti-inflammatory efficacy when compared with that of a free curcumin solution. These findings reveal that the nanomicelles act as significant topical delivery systems for the ocular administration of curcumin.

The Flt1 peptidehyaluronate (HA) conjugates synthesization results in micelle-like nanoparticulates formation that were utilized to encapsulate genistein, an inhibitor of tyrosine-specific protein kinases, for the treatment of ocular NV has been described by Kim et al. (2012). The mean diameter of genistein-loaded Flt1 peptide HA conjugate micelles was found to be as 172.0 ± 18.7 nm, with a drug-loading efficiency of 4050%. The *in vitro* release tests of genistein through a genistein-loaded Flt1 peptide HA conjugate micelles shows the controlled release phenomena for more than 24 hrs. Furthermore, the *in-vitro* biological activity of genistein/Flt1 peptide HA micelles was authenticated via the synergistic anti-proliferation activity of HUVECs. Besides, we can also affirm the anti-angiogenic activity of genistein/Flt1 peptide HA micelles from the data revealing a statistically significant suppression of corneal NV in silver nitrate cauterized corneas of SD rats. In diabetic retinopathy rat models, the retinal vascular hyperpermeability was also found to be reduced upon treatment.

9.3 CONCLUSION AND FUTURE PROSPECTS

The use of phytocomponents in the treatment of ocular diseases has been widely accepted globally, since several decades. The advancement in the field of phytochemical and phytopharmacological sciences has permitted elucidation of the composition and biological activities of several medicinal plant products. The phytochemical potency majorly depends on the availability of active compounds. Several biologically active constituents are highly water-soluble, with a lower systemic absorption, because they are inaccessible to cross the corneal layer resulting in loss of bioavailability and efficacy. The phytochemical entrapment with nanoforms might result to ameliorate the action, thus reducing the desired dose and side effects, and in turn improving activity. Nanoforms, can deliver the active chemicals at an adequate concentration during the complete treatment duration, directing it to the desired targeted action site. Still, there have been many promising challenges for implementation of clinically viable ocular therapies in this area. The management of nanoform interactions with biological systems represents some of the current challenges mimicking our novel trial process. Fewer additional new challenges include probing of targeted efficiency of nanoforms and satisfying the international standards in relation with their toxicology and biocompatibility aspects (Table 9.1).

TABLE 9.1 Phytoconstituent-Based Nanoformulations and Their Biological Activity

Phyto constituent	Formulation	Inference	References
Rebaudioside A	Micelles	RA micelle formulations have shown potential to improve the bioavailability of hydrophobic drugs.	Song et al., 2018
Forskolin	NPs	Scintigraphy studies indicated longer retention of CS-PLGA NP's while increased effectiveness after single instillation in reducing the intraocular pressure was observed.	Khan et al., 2018
Quercetin	Nanostructured lipid carriers	80.52% of total quercetin was released from the QN-NLC based hydrogel (QN-NLC-Gel) within 3 days, revealing QN-NLC-Gel released drug sustainably.	Yu et al., 2018
Coumarin-6	Nanostructured lipid carriers	Increase in drug absorption was greater in the cornea than in the conjunctiva.	Liu et al., 2017
Curcumin	Nanostructured lipid carriers	Clearance of the formulations was significantly delayed in the presence of CS-NAC and the effect was positively related to the degree of thiolation.	Liu et al., 2017
Coumarin-6	Nanostructured lipid carriers	Promising oculardrug delivery systems to achieve prolonged precorneal retention, higher corneal permeability and enhanced ocular bioavailability.	Li et al., 2017
Tacrolimus	Proglycosomes	Studies in rabbits demonstrated prolonged precorneal retention (up to 8 h) and manifestly improved intraocular drug levels, well above therapeutic levels.	Garg et al., 2017
Curcumin	Nanostructured lipid carriers	CS-NAC-CUR-NLC possesses a greater potential as an oculardrug-delivery system	Li et al., 2016
L-carnosine	Phytosome	*Ex vivo* transcorneal permeation parameters showed significantly controlled corneal permeation of L-carnosine without any significant impact on primary human corneal cell viability.	Abdelkader et al., 2016

TABLE 9.1 *(Continued)*

Phyto constituent	Formulation	Inference	References
Curcumin	Nanogel	The maximal concentration (Cmax) was significantly improved (p<0.01). The prolonged mean residence time (p<0.01) indicated that CUR-CNLC-GEL is a controlled release formulation.	Liu et al., 2016
Tacrolimus	Niosomes	Pharmacokinetics test showed that area under curve of HA-coated niosomes was 2.3-fold and 1.2-fold as that of suspension and non-coated niosomes, respectively.	Zeng et al., 2016
Mangiferin	Nanostructured lipid carriers	Pharmacokinetic study suggested a 5.69-fold increase of ocular bioavailability compared with solution.	Liu et al., 2012
Curcumin	Nanoparticle	The *in vivo* study also revealed that the formulation could significantly increase curcumin bioavailability in the aqueous humor.	Lou et al., 2014

KEYWORDS

- **phytoconstituents**
- **nanoformulation**
- **ocular delivery**
- **liposomes**

REFERENCES

Abdelkader, H., Longman, M. R., Alany, R. G., & Pierscionek, B., (2016). Phytosome-hyaluronic acid systems for ocular delivery of L-carnosine. *Int. J. Nanomedicine, 11*, 2815–2827.

Afify, E. A. M., Elsayed, I., Gad, M. K., Mohamed, M. I., & Afify, M. A. R., (2018). Enhancement of pharmacokinetic and pharmacological behavior of ocular dorzolamide after factorial optimization of self-assembled nanostructures. *PLoS One, 13*(2), e0191415.

Agarwal, R., Iezhitsa, I., Agarwal, P., et al., (2016). Liposomes in topical ophthalmic drug delivery; An update. *Drug Deliv., 23*(4), 1075–1091.

Agrahari, V., Agrahari, V., Hung, W. T., Christenson, L. K., & Mitra, A. K., (2016). Composite nanoformulation therapeutics for long-term ocular delivery of macromolecules. *Mol Pharm., 13*(9), 2912–2922.

Alvarez-Rivera, F., Fernández-Villanueva, D., Concheiro, A., et al., (2016). α-Lipoic acid in soluplus® polymeric nanomicelles for ocular treatment of diabetes-associated corneal diseases. *J. Pharm. Sci., 105*(9), 2855–2863.

Chang, C. Y., Wang, M. C., Miyagawa, T., Chen, Z. Y., Lin, F. H., Chen, K. H., Liu, G. S., & Tseng, C. L., (2016). Preparation of arginine-glycine-aspartic acid-modified biopolymeric nanoparticles containing epigalloccatechin-3-gallate for targeting vascular endothelial cells to inhibit corneal neovascularization. *Int. J. Nanomedicine, 12*, 279–294.

Cholkar, K., Patel, A., Vadlapudi, A. D., et al., (2012). Novel nanomicellar formulation approaches for anterior and posterior segment ocular drug delivery. *Recent Pat. Nanomed., 2*(2), 82–95.

Das, S., Ng, W. K., & Tan, R. B., (2012). Are nano structured lipid carriers (NLCs) better than solid lipid nanoparticles (SLN): Development, characterizations and comparative evaluations of clotrimazole-loaded SLN and NLCs? *Eur. J. Pharm. Sci., 47*(1), 139–151.

Davis, B. M., Pahlitzsch, M., Guo, L., Balendra, S., Shah, P., Ravindran, N., & Malaguarnera, G., et al., (2018). Topical curcumin nanocarriers are neuroprotective in eye disease. *Scientific Reports, 8*, 11066.

Delplace, V., Payne, S., & Shoichet, M., (2015). Delivery strategies for treatment of age-related ocular diseases: From a biological understanding to biomaterial solutions. *J. Control Release, 219*, 652–668.

Deol, P., Kaur, I. P., Sharma, G., et al., (2015). Potential of nanomaterials as movers and packers for drug molecules. *Solid State Phenom., 222*, 159–178.

Doktorovová, S., Kovačević, A. B., Garcia, M. L., et al., (2016). Preclinical safety of solid lipid nanoparticles and nanostructured lipid carriers: Current evidence from *in vitro* and *in vivo* evaluation. *Eur. J. Pharm. Biopharm., 108*(Supplement C), 235–252.

Doktorovova, S., Souto, E. B., & Silva, A. M., (2014). Nanotoxicology applied to solid lipid nanoparticles and nanostructured lipid carriers: A systematic review of *in vitro* data. *Eur. J. Pharm. Biopharm., 87*(1), 1–18.

Duncan, G., & Collison, D. J., (2003). Role of the non-neuronal cholinergic system in the eye: A review. *Life Sci., 72*(18/19), 2013–2019.

Elsayed, I., & Sayed, S., (2017). Tailored nanostructured platforms for boosting transcorneal permeation: Box-Behnken statistical optimization, comprehensive *in vitro*, *ex vivo*, and *in vivo* characterization. *Int. J. Nanomedicine., 12*, 7947–7962.

ElShaer, A., Mustafa, S., Kasar, M., Thapa, S., Ghatora, B., & Alany, R. G., (2016). Nanoparticle-laden contact lens for controlled ocular delivery of prednisolone: Formulation optimization using statistical experimental design. *Pharmaceutics, 8*(2), 14.

Fangueiro, J. F., Veiga, F., Silva, A. M., et al., (2016). Ocular drug delivery-new strategies for targeting anterior and posterior segments of the eye. *Curr. Pharm. Des., 22*(9), 1135–1146.

Fouda, N. H., Abdelrehim, R. T., Hegazy, D. A., & Habib, B. A., (2018). Sustained ocular delivery of Dorzolamide-HCl via proniosomal gel formulation: *In-vitro* characterization, statistical optimization, and *in-vivo* pharmacodynamic evaluation in rabbits. *Drug Deliv., 25*(1), 1340–1349.

Garg, V., Suri, R., Jain, G. K., & Kohli, K., (2017). Proglycosomes: A novel nano-vesicle for ocular delivery of tacrolimus. *Colloids Surf B Biointerfaces, 157*, 40–47.

Ghanghoria, R., Tekade, R. K., Mishra, A. K., et al., (2016). Luteinizing hormone-releasing hormone peptide tethered nanoparticulate system for enhanced antitumoral efficacy of paclitaxel. *Nanomedicine, 11*(7), 797–816.

Hao, J., Fang, X., Zhou, Y., Wang, J., Guo, F., Li, F., & Peng, X., (2011). Development and optimization of solid lipid nanoparticle formulation for ophthalmic delivery of chloramphenicol using a box-behnken design. *Int. J. Nanomedicine, 6,* 683–692.

He, W., Guo, X., Feng, M., & Mao, N., (2013). *In vitro* and *in vivo* studies on ocular vitamin A palmitate cationic liposomal *in situ* gels. *International Journal of Pharmaceutics, 458,* 305–314.

International Federation on Ageing, (2013). *The High Cost of Low Vision: The Evidence on Ageing and the Loss of Sight*. LT Publication.

Janagam, D. R., Wu, L., & Lowe, T. L., (2017). Nanoparticles for drug delivery to the anterior segment of the eye. *Adv. Drug Deliv. Rev., 122,* 31–64.

Kabiri, M., Kamal, S. H., Pawar, S. V., Roy, P. R., Derakhshandeh, M., Kumar, U., Hatzikiriakos, S. G., et al., (2018). A stimulus-responsive, *in situ*-forming, nanoparticle-laden hydrogel for ocular drug delivery. *Drug Deliv. Transl. Res., 8*(3), 484–495.

Kakkar, S., & Kaur, I. P., (2011). Spanlastics: A novel nanovesicular carrier system for ocular delivery. *Int. J. Pharm., 413*(1), 202–210.

Kaskoos, R. A., (2014). Investigation of moxifloxacin loaded chitosan-dextran nanoparticles for topical instillation into eye: *In-vitro* and *ex-vivo* evaluation. *Int. J. Pharm. Investig., 4*(4), 164–173.

Kaur, I. P., & Kakkar, S., (2014). Nanotherapy for posterior eye diseases. *J. Control Release, 193,* 100–112.

Khan, N., Ameeduzzafar, Khanna, K., Bhatnagar, A., Ahmad, F. J., & Ali, A., (2018). Chitosan coated PLGA nanoparticles amplify the ocular hypotensive effect of forskolin: Statistical design, characterization, and *in vivo* studies. *Int. J. Biol. Macromol., 116,* 648–663.

Kim, H., Choi, J. S, Kim, K. S., Yang, J. A., Joo, C K., & Hahn, S. K., (2012). Flt1 peptide-hyaluronate conjugate micelle-like nanoparticles encapsulating genistein for the treatment of ocular neovascularization. *Acta Biomater., 8*(11), 3932–3940.

Kumar, R., & Sinha, V. R., (2014). Preparation and optimization of voriconazole micro emulsion for ocular delivery. *Colloids Surf B Biointerfaces, 117*(Supplement C), 82–88.

Lakhani, P., Patil, A., Taskar, P., Ashour, E., & Majumdar, S., (2018). Curcumin-loaded nanostructured lipid carriers for ocular drug delivery: Design optimization and characterization. *Journal of Drug Delivery Science and Technology*, doi: 10.1016/j.jddst.2018.07.010.

Li, J., Guo, X., Liu, Z., Okeke, C. I., Li, N., Zhao, H., Aggrey, M. O., et al., (2014). Preparation and evaluation of charged solid lipid nanoparticles of tetrandrine for ocular drug delivery system: Pharmacokinetics, cytotoxicity and cellular uptake studies. *Drug Dev. Ind. Pharm., 40*(7), 980–987.

Li, J., Liu, D., Tan, G., Zhao, Z., Yang, X., & Pan, W., (2016). A comparative study on the efficiency of chitosan-N-acetylcysteine, chitosan oligosaccharides, or carboxymethyl chitosan surface modified nanostructured lipid carrier for ophthalmic delivery of curcumin. *Carbohydr Polym., 146,* 435–444.

Li, J., Tan, G., Cheng, B., Liu, D., & Pan, W., (2017). Transport mechanism of chitosan-N-acetylcysteine, chitosan oligosaccharides, or carboxymethyl chitosan decorated coumarin-6 loaded nanostructured lipid carriers across the rabbit ocular. *Eur. J. Pharm. Biopharm., 120,* 89–97.

Li, M., Xin, M., Guo, C., Lin, G., & Wu, X., (2017). New nanomicelle curcumin formulation for ocular delivery: Improved stability, solubility, and ocular anti-inflammatory treatment. *Drug Dev. Ind. Pharm., 43*(11), 1846–1857.

Lim, C., Kim, D. W., Sim, T., Hoang, N. H., Lee, J. W., Lee, E. S., Youn, Y. S., & Oh, K. T., (2016). Preparation and characterization of a lutein loading nanoemulsion system for ophthalmic eye drops. *Journal of Drug Delivery Science and Technology, 36,* 168–174.

Liu, D., Li, J., Cheng, B., et al., (2017). *Ex vivo* and *in vivo* evaluation of the effect of coating a coumarin-6-labeled nanostructured lipid carrier with chitosan-N-acetylcysteine on rabbit ocular distribution. *Mol. Pharm., 14*(8), 2639–2648.

Liu, D., Li, J., Cheng, B., Wu, Q., & Pan, H., (2017). *Ex vivo* and *in vivo* evaluation of the effect of coating a coumarin-6-Labeled nanostructured lipid carrier with chitosan-N-acetylcysteine on rabbit ocular distribution. *Mol. Pharm., 14*(8), 2639–2648.

Liu, D., Li, J., Pan, H., He, F., Liu, Z., Wu, Q., Bai, C., Yu, S., & Yang, X., (2016). Potential advantages of a novel chitosan-N-acetylcysteine surface modified nanostructured lipid carrier on the performance of ophthalmic delivery of curcumin. *Sci. Rep., 6,* 28796.

Liu, R., Liu, Z., Zhang, C., & Zhang, B., (2012). Nanostructured lipid carriers as novel ophthalmic delivery system for mangiferin: Improving *in vivo* ocular bioavailability. *J. Pharm. Sci., 101*(10), 3833–3844.

Liu, R., Sun, L., Fang, S., Wang, S., Chen, J., Xiao, X., & Liu, C., (2016). Thermosensitive *in situ* nanogel as ophthalmic delivery system of curcumin: Development, characterization, *in vitro* permeation and *in vivo* pharmacokinetic studies. *Pharm. Dev. Technol., 21*(5), 576–582.

Liu, Z., Zhang, X., Wu, H., Li, J., Shu, L., Liu, R., Li, L., & Li, N., (2011). Preparation and evaluation of solid lipid nanoparticles of baicalin for ocular drug delivery system *in vitro* and *in vivo. Drug Development and Industrial Pharmacy,37*(4),475–481.

Lou, J., Hu, W., Tian, R., Zhang, H., Jia, Y., Zhang, J., & Zhang, L., (2014). Optimization and evaluation of a thermoresponsive ophthalmic *in situ* gel containing curcumin-loaded albumin nanoparticles. *Int. J. Nanomedicine, 9,* 2517–2525.

Madni, A., Rahem, M. A., Tahir, N., et al., (2017). Non-invasive strategies for targeting the posterior segment of eye. *Int. J. Pharm., 530*(1/2), 326–345.

McGrath, C., Rudman, D. L., Trentham, B., et al., (2017). Reshaping understandings of disability associated with age-related vision loss (ARVL): Incorporating critical disability perspectives into research and practice. *Disabil. Rehabil., 39*(19), 1990–1998.

Meyer, H., Stöver, T., Fouchet, F., et al., (2012). Lipidic nanocapsule drug delivery: Neuronal protection for cochlear implant optimization. *Int. J. Nanomedicine, 7,* 2449–2464.

Motwani, S. K., Chopra, S., Talegaonkar, S., Kohli, K., Ahmad, F. J., & Khar, R. K., (2008). Chitosan-sodium alginate nanoparticles as submicroscopic reservoirs for ocular delivery: Formulation, optimization and *in vitro* characterization. *Eur. J. Pharm. Biopharm., 68*(3), 513–525.

Pandit, J., Sultana, Y., & Aqil, M., (2017). Chitosan-coated PLGA nanoparticles of bevacizumab as novel drug delivery to target retina: Optimization, characterization, and *in vitro* toxicity evaluation. *Artif. Cells Nanomed. Biotechnol., 45*(7), 1397–1407.

Peptu, C. A., Popa, M., Savin, C., et al., (2015). Modern drug delivery systems for targeting the posterior segment of the eye. *Curr. Pharm. Des., 21*(42), 6055–6069.

Preeti U. P., Kumar, M., & Pathak, K., (2016). Norfloxacin loaded pH triggered nanoparticulate *in-situ* gel for extraocular bacterial infections: Optimization, ocular irritancy and corneal toxicity. *Iran J. Pharm. Res., 15*(1), 3–22.

Prosperi-Porta, G., Kedzior, S., Muirhead, B., et al., (2016). Phenylboronic-acid-based polymeric micelles for mucoadhesive anterior segment ocular drug delivery. *Biomacromolecules, 17*(4), 1449–1457.

Robinson, M., & Zhang, X., (2011). The world medicines situation. *Traditional Medicines: Global Situation, Issues and Challenges* (pp. 1–12). Geneva: World Health Organization.

Song, K., Xin, M., Yu, H., Zheng, Z., Li, J., Li, M., Guo, H., Tan, Y., & Wu, X., (2018). Novel ultra-small micelles based on rebaudioside A: A potential nanoplatform for ocular drug delivery. *Int. J. Pharm., 552*(1/2), 265–276.

Souto, E. B., & Doktorovová, S., (2009). Chapter six-solid lipid nanoparticle formulations: Pharmacokinetic and biopharmaceutical aspects in drug delivery. In: Düzgünes, N., (ed.), *Methods in Enzymology* (pp. 105–129). Amsterdam (AMS): Academic Press.

Tekade, R. K., Youngren-Ortiz, S. R., Yang, H., et al., (2014). Designing hybrid on conase nanocarriers for mesothelioma therapy: A Taguchi orthogonal array and multivariate component driven analysis. *Mol. Pharm., 11*(10), 3671–3683.

Thrimawithana, T. R., Young, S., Bunt, C. R., et al., (2011). Drug delivery to the posterior segment of the eye. *Drug Discov. Today, 16*(5/6), 270–277.

Vadlapudi, A. D., Cholkar, K., Vadlapatla, R. K., et al., (2014). Aqueous nanomicellar formulation for topical delivery of biotinylated lipid prodrug of acyclovir: Formulation development and ocular biocompatibility. *J. Ocul. Pharmacol. Ther., 30*(1), 49–58.

Vandamme, T. F., (2002). Microemulsions as ocular drug delivery systems: Recent developments and future challenges. *Prog. Retin. Eye Res., 21*(1), 15–34.

Wang, F., Chen, L., Jiang, S., He, J., Zhang, X., Peng, J., Xu, Q., & Li, R., (2014). Optimization of methazolamide-loaded solid lipid nanoparticles for ophthalmic delivery using Box-Behnken design. *J. Liposome Res., 24*(3), 171–181.

Wang, J., Zhao, F., Liu, R., Chen, J., Zhang, Q., Lao, R., Wang, Z., Jin, X., & Liu, C., (2017). Novel cationic lipid nanoparticles as an ophthalmic delivery system for multi component drugs: Development, characterization, *in vitro* permeation, *in vivo* pharmacokinetic and molecular dynamics studies. *Int. J. Nanomedicine, 12*, 8115–8127.

Weng, Y., Liu, J., Jin, S., et al., (2017). Nanotechnology-based strategies for treatment of ocular disease. *Acta Pharmaceutica, Sinica B, 7*(3), 281–291.

Yu, Y., Feng, R., Yu, S., Li, J., Wang, Y., Song, Y., Yang, X., Pan, W., & Li, S., (2018). Nanostructured lipid carrier-based pH and temperature dual-responsive hydrogel composed of carboxymethyl chitosan and poloxamer for drug delivery. *Int. J. Biol. Macromol., 114*, 462–469.

Zeng, W., Li, Q., Wan, T., Liu, C., Pan, W., Wu, Z., Zhang, G., Pan, J., Qin, M., Lin, Y., Wu, C., & Xu, Y., (2016). Hyaluronic acid-coated niosomes facilitate tacrolimusocular delivery: Mucoadhesion, precorneal retention, aqueous humor pharmacokinetics, and transcorneal permeability. *Colloids Surf B Biointerfaces, 141*, 28–35.

Zhang, J., Liang, X., Li, X., Guan, Z., Liao, Z., Luo, Y., & Luo, Y., (2016). Ocular delivery of cyanidin-3-glycoside in liposomes and its prevention of selenite-induced oxidative stress. *Drug Development and Industrial Pharmacy,42*(4),546–553.

CHAPTER 10

Rosmarinic Acid: A Boon in the Management of Cardiovascular Disease

MD. ADIL SHAHARYAR,[1,2] MAHFOOZUR RAHMAN,[3] KUMAR ANAND,[2] CHOWDHURY MOBASWAR HOSSAIN,[1] IMRAN KAZMI,[4] and SANMOY KARMAKAR[2]

[1]*Bengal School of Technology, Chinsurah, Hooghly, West Bengal, India, Tel.: +91-9748902723, E-mail: adil503@yahoo.co.in (M. A. Shaharyar)*

[2]*Department of Pharmaceutical Technology, Jadavpur University, Kolkata, West Bengal, India, Tel.: +91-8017136385, E-mail: sanmoykarmakar@gmail.com (S. Karmakar)*

[3]*Department of Pharmaceutical Sciences, Faculty of Health Sciences, Sam Higginbottom Institute of Agriculture, Technology, and Sciences, Allahabad, Uttar Pradesh, India, Tel.: +91-8627985598, E-mail: mahfoozkaifi@gmail.com*

[4]*Glocal School of Pharmacy, Glocal University, Mirzapur Pole, Saharanpur, Uttar Pradesh, India*

ABSTRACT

Cardiovascular disease has been a source of morbidity and mortality in the world. The American Heart Association states that though the mortality has decreased yet the burden and impact are still threatening. Molecules from the plants have been a boon for mankind. These gifted molecules from nature have been a source of cure for various diseases, the cardiovascular disease being one of them. Many molecules have been investigated and rosmarinic acid obtained from various plants being one of them. Rosmarinic acid, till now, has received less attention in terms of its cardiovascular potential from the scientific community. This book chapter deals with the cardiovascular disease-modifying activities of rosmarinic acid and sheds light for carrying out research in this domain. This book chapter has covered the attenuation or inhibition of AMI, arrhythmia, hypertension (HTN), etc., by Rosmarinic acid. For studying the effect of rosmarinic acid on cardiovascular disease, various protocols have been mentioned. After this discussion Rosmarinic, acid turns out to be a strong candidate having promising results in the management of cardiovascular diseases (CVDs).

10.1 INTRODUCTION

Heart and its ailments find a special place in the contemporary scientific circle. Cardiovascular disease is a menace to the society. According to the American Heart Association, the mortality rate has declined but the impact and burden of the disease remain unchanged. The mortality rate in 2006 from cardiovascular disease was 262.5 per 100,000 (International Classification of disease 10, 100–199). The value was a higher for white males. For white males 306.6 per 100,000 and for black males 422.8 per 100,000. In the case of females, it was lower 215.5 and 298.2 per 100,000 for white and black females respectively. A 2006 report of AHA foregrounded the fact that 2300 Americans die per day of cardiovascular disease. One of every six deaths in the US is due to CHD. Every 6 deaths in the US are due to CHD. Each year around 95,000 people experience a new or recurrent stroke. According to a survey conducted by the National Health and Nutrition Examination (NHANES) 2003–2006 points out that 33.6% of US adults $\geq$ 20 years of age have hypertension (HTN). The data of cardiovascular disease affecting people presents a disturbing picture, which needs immediate attention (Jones et al., 2010).

Plant extracts have always been useful and exploited by mankind for the treatment of various diseases since ancient civilization. Rosmarinic acid is one such molecule extracted from various plants having a cardiovascular effect.

10.1.1 SOURCE

Rosmarinic acid oil found in *Perilla frutescens* (Lee et al., 2013) from which glucoside of rosmarinic acid (rosmarinic acid-3-O-glucoside) is obtained (Makino et al., 2001). Rosemary (Al Sereiti et al., 1999) (*Rosmarinus officinalis Linn.*), Sage which is a spice herb Mint (Ellis et al., 1970), Thyme (Dapkevicius et al., 2002), Basil (rosmarinic acid and related phenolics in hairy root cultures of *Ocimum basilicum*) and the Ayurvedic medicine Holy Basil (Hakkim et al., 2007), *Melissa officinalis* (*Labiatae*) at 2.2–5.5%,

Orthosiphon stamineus (Malahubban et al., 2013), *Clerodendranthus spicatus* (*Thunberg*) (Zheng et al., 2012), *Verbascumxantho phoeniceum* (*Scrophulariaceae*) (Georgiev et al., 2012), and *Heliotropium foertherianum* (*Boraginaceae*) (Braidy et al., 2013).

10.1.2 BIOSYNTHESIS OF ROSMARINIC ACID

The phenylpropanopid pathway uses 4-coumaroyl CoA. Thus, 4-coumaroyl CoA acts as a hydroxycinnamoyl donor. The hydroxy cinnamoyl acceptor is synthesized from the Shikimic acid pathway.

From chemical and biological point of view, rosmarinic acid is synthesized from an ester of caffeic acid (CAA) with 3,4-dihydroxyphenyllactic acid and 4-coumaroyl-4'-hydroxyphenyllactate respectively. Rosmarinate is synthesized with the help of rosmarinate synthase which utilizes caffeoyl-CoA and 3,4-dihydroxyphenyllactic acid to produce the same (Petersen et al., 1988) (Figure 10.1).

The pathway has many enzymes taking part which probably came from the pathway that involves synthesis of chlorogenic and caffeoylshikimic acid (Petersen et al., 2009).

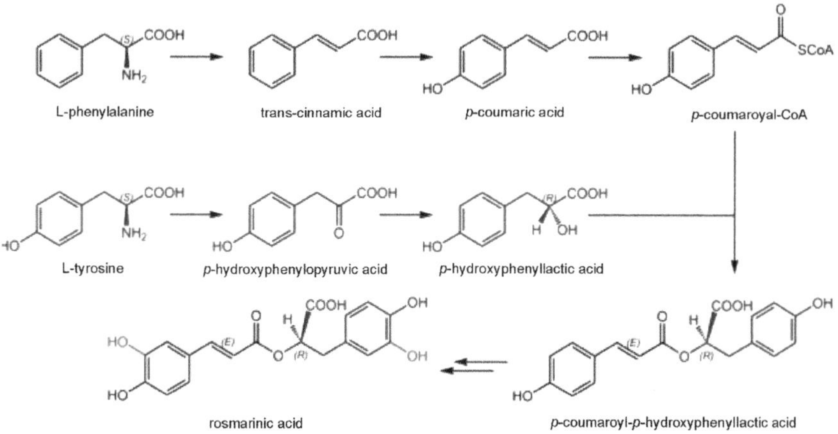

FIGURE 10.1   Biosynthesis of rosmarinic acid.
(*Source:* Reprinted from Wu et al., 2015. © Elsevier.)

10.1.3 CHEMICAL NATURE OF ROSMARINIC ACID

Two eminent Italian scientists namely M. L. Scarpatti and G. Oriente are credited with the isolation of rosmarinic acid from the plant Rosemary (*Rosmarinus officinalis*). *The* Iupacname of the rosmarinic acid is (2R)-3- (3,4-dihy-droxyphenyl)-2-[(E)-3-(3,4-dihydroxyphenyl)prop-2-enoyl]oxypropanoic acid (pubchem.ncbi.nlm.nih.gov) (Figure 10.2).

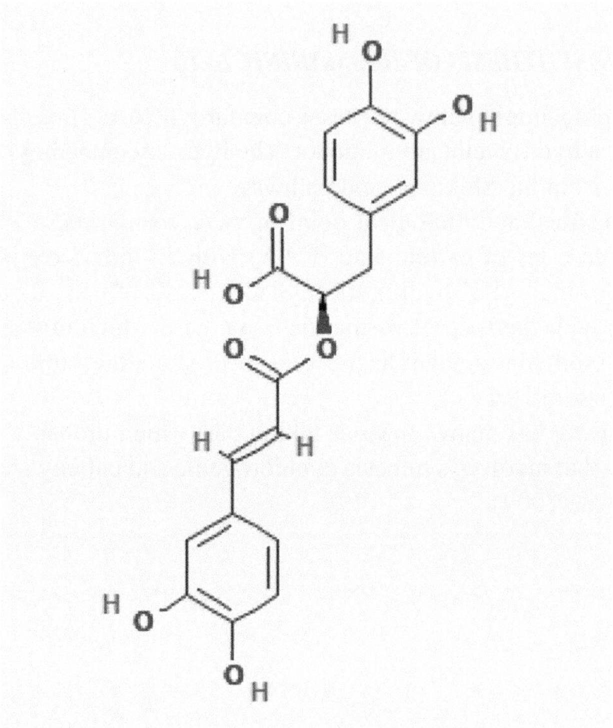

FIGURE 10.2   Rosmarinic acid.

Source: PubChem URL: https://pubchem.ncbi.nlm.nih.gov.

It is a powder with red-orange color having slight solubility in water and soluble in almost all the organic solvent (Petersen et al., 2003).

10.2   VARIABILITY OF ROSMARINIC ACID CONTENT IN DIFFERENT SPECIES OF PLANT BELONGING TO FAMILY LABIATAE

Labiatae family of the plant kingdom has been tremendously exploited as traditional medicine for conditions like depression, strengthening of fragile blood vessels, memory enhancement, weakness, circulation improvement, exhaustion (Wang et al., 2004), infection, inflammation (Vieira, 2010), gastritis, and indigestion (Hajimehdipoor et al., 2010). Researchers have shown that rosmarinic acid possesses anti-oxidant (Zheng et al., 2001), anti-inflammatory (Al-Sereiti et al., 1999), anti-allergic (Ito et al., 1998), anti-depression (Takeda et al., 2002), anti-hyperglycemic (Kumar et al., 2010) and antimicrobial (Nascimento, 2009; Jain, 2010; Zomorodian et al., 2011).

An investigation was conducted to find out the best source of rosmarinic acid in plants belonging to family Labiatae which predominantly grows in Iran. HPLC was used to ascertain the RA contents in 29 plants, using the mobile phase as 0.085% *O*-phosphoric acid in water: 0.085% *O*-phosphoric acid in methanol: 0.085% *O*-phosphoric acid in 2-propanol in gradient mode for 20 min (Table 10.1).

TABLE 10.1   Rosmarinic Acid Content Analysis from Gradient Time Perspective

Water Containing o-Phosphoric Acid (%)	Methanol Containing o-Phosphoric Acid (%)	Isopropyl Alcohol Containing o-Phosphoric Acid (%)	Time (mins)
10	10	80	0
15	15	70	10
20	20	60	15
20	20	60	20

Source: Shekarchi et al. (2012).

The separation was best with the above HPLC protocol. C_8 and C_{18} columns were compared and the best separation efficacy was obtained by C_{18} column. HPLC chromatogram of *Mentha spicata* sample and UV spectrum of RA in 11.16 min obtained from PDA detector. Different genus of the labiata family was analyzed and rosmarinic acid contents were found greatest in *Mentha* species. From Table 10.2, it is observed all *Mentha* species contain RA in fairly good concentration (19.3–58.5 mg g^{-1}) and *M. spicata* revealed the highest rosmarinic acid content (Shekarchi et al., 2012).

10.3   PHARMACOKINETIC ASPECTS OF ROSMARINIC ACID

The pharmacokinetic parameters of rosmarinic acid, tissue distribution studies, excretion, and metabolism as well as its metabolism in serum are not clear. In a Pharmacokinetic study miltiorrhiza depside salts in a dose of 60 mg/kg S were administered to Sprague Dawley rats were administered and elimination half-life of RA was found to be 0.75 h while Pharmacokinetic parameters after IV were found to be AUC (0-tn) (mg. h/l) 6.6 ± 1.8, Mean residence time (0-) (h) 0.32 ± 0.07, $t_{1/2}$ (h) 0.12 ± 0.04, Clearance (l/h/kg) 1.02 ± 0.32 26 (Li et al., 2007).

TABLE 10.2 Different Concentration of Rosmarinic Acid from Different Plants Belonging to Labiatae Family

Plant Scientific Name	Region of Collection in IRAN	Concentration of Rosmarinic Acid in mg gm^{-1}
Lavendula angustifolia	Tehran, Abali road	1.7 ± 0.2
Mellisa officinalis	Mazandaran, Salmanshahr	36.5 ± 0.8
Mentha aquatica	Golestan, Gorgan	24.6 ± 0.2
Mentha crispa	Golestan, Gorgan	19.3 ± 0.2
Mentha longifolia	Golestan, Gorgan	26.6 ± 0.3
Mentha piperita	Golestan, Gorgan	28.2 ± 0.3
Mentha pulegium	Golestan, Gorgan	23.4 ± 0.3
Mentha spicata	Golestan, Gorgan	58.5 ± 1.4
Oreganum vulgare	Mazandaran, Salmanshahr	25.0 ± 0.1
Perovskia artemisoides	Khorasan	31.3 ± 0.2
Rosmarinus officinalis	Tehran, Abali road	7.2 ± 0.1
Salvia hypoleuka	Tehran, Damavand	4.3 ± 0.03
Salvia limbata	Semnan, Ahovan	7.5 ± 0.1
Salvia macrosiphon	Tehran, Delichaee	6.4 ± 0.1
Salvia officinalis	Mazandaran, Salmanshahr	39.3 ± 0.9
Salvia virgata	Mazandaran, Ghaemshahr	16.4 ± 0.9

Source: Shekarchi et al. (2012).

Absorption, conjugation, and methylation of RA from Perilla Extract took place and a small proportion of RA was found to be degraded into various components, such as conjugated forms of CAA, FA (ferulic acid) and COA (m-coumaric acid). Excretion of these metabolites was found in the urine. Pharmacokinetics (PKs) studies on rosmarinic acid was applied to the evaluation of RA, in rats following intravenous and oral administrations demonstrated more rapid distribution and was eliminated more rapidly from the systemic circulation with a $t_{1/2}$,λZ of (56.45 ± 0.67) min after intravenous administration as described in Table 10.1. After being administered orally,

RA was absorbed and eliminated more rapidly, with a T_{max1} of 10 min, a T_{max2} of 45 min, and a $t_{1/2}, \lambda Z$ of (63.68 ± 13.11) min (Baba et al., 2005).

On intravenous administration of S. miltiorrhiza depside salts in a dose of 60 mg/kg in Sprague-Dawley rats, concentration-time curves were obtained which reflected a two-compartment model. The elimination half-lives and AUC_{0-6h} for rosmarinic acid were 0.75 h and 6.6 h, respectively (Li et al., 2007).

Intestinal absorption of rosmarinic acid was investigated through oral route where portal vein peaked at 10 mins having C (max) 1.36 micro mol/L.

AUC of the intact rosmarinic acid in portal vein was calculated from the serum concentration-time profile and was found to be 60.4 micromol min L^{-1} (Konishi et al., 2005).

Further, a study involving absorption, metabolism, degradation, and urinary excretion of rosmarinic acid, administered via oral route in rats was conducted. The concentration of rosmarinic acid reached its peak in the plasma in 0.5 h.

The majority of rosmarinic acid degraded into conjugated and/or methylated forms of CAA, FA and m-coumaric acid before being excreted slowly in the urine (Baba et al., 2004).

10.4 PHARMACOLOGICAL ASPECTS OF ROSMARINIC ACID

RA was found to have four phenolic hydrogen that are responsible for controlling free radical oxidation. Further, it contains other two catechol containing 1,2-dihydroxybenzene rings which gives polarity to it (Shahidi et al., 1992).

10.4.1 ROSMARINIC ACID AS AN ANTI-INFLAMMATORY ANTI-BACTERIAL AGENT

For long natural compounds have been investigated in the treatment of inflammations specially those having potential either to reduce or eliminate the synthesis of leukotriene. These natural compounds ideally should have no adverse effects.

Rosmarinic acid has been found to inhibit the activation of the complementary system both *in vitro* and *in vivo* using both classical and alternate pathway (Englberger, 1988; Peake et al., 1991). In an *in vivo* study, rosmarinic acid has been found to inhibit cobra venom factor (CVF)-induced paw edema in rats (Rampart, 1986; Bult et al., 1985).

Experimental Investigation reveals that rosmarinic acid actively binds covalently with the activated complement component C3b surface, thereby inhibiting the complement system (Sahu et al., 1999). NSAID and gluco-corticoids (GCs) are the modulators that inhibit the complement activation system through cyclo-oxygenase pathway while rosmarinic acid prevents inflammation through prostanoid pathway and does not meddle in the COX pathway leading to reduction in side effects (Kuhnt et al., 1995).

Natural compounds such as chlorogenic acid, rabdosiin, and rosmarinic acid have CAA which exerts anti-allergic activities that encompasses free radical oxygen scavenging and inhibition of release of β-hexosaminidase and hyaluronidase. Rabdosiin showed the highest hyaluronidase-inhibitory activity. Among the compounds that were tested for radical scavenging activities, involving oxygen species were superoxide anion radicals and hydroxyl radicals. These radical oxygen species were also inhibited by rabdosiin. More than 90% of β-hexosaminidase release from cultured cells was inhibited by both rabdosiin and CAA at a concentration of 2 mM (Sanchez-Campillo et al., 2009).

Remarkable anti-bacterial activity of rosmarinic acid was noted against *Escherichia coli, Bacillus subtilis,* and *Micrococcus luteus.*

Thus, the anti-bacterial and anti-inflammatory activity of rosmarinic acid makes it a good candidate in the treatment of skin infections of the epidermis and oral mucosa (Kuhnt et al., 1995).

10.4.2   ROSMARINIC ACID AS A PHOTO PROTECTIVE AGENT

The UV radiation present in the solar spectrum generates ROS (reactive oxygen species) that imbalances the homeostasis of the skin by causing damage of DNA in the cell. The photoprotective activity of rosmarinic acid is exerted by the free radical scavenging activity. Rosmarinic acid erects its own defense wall by the stimulation of melanin synthesis and modulation of tyrosinase activity (Sanchez-Campillo et al., 2009).

After screening of phyto compounds or extracts, those with anti-oxidant and anti-inflammatory properties may also be used to protect the skin from getting damaged by UV radiations (Vostálová et al., 2010).

10.4.3   ROSMARINIC ACID AS AN ANTI-CANCER AGENT

After performing some mutagenic assays, it was found that there was no increment in the frequency of micronuclei as compared to the negative controls, when different concentrations of rosmarinic acid were administered to animals in an experimental protocol (Furtado et al., 2008)

Oral carcinogenesis was induced by 7,12-dimethylbenz anthracene (DMBA) to investigate the inhibitory anti-cancer activities of rosmarinic acid. For this study, the biomarkers involved in lipid peroxidation (LPO), Inhibitory effects of rosmarinic acid against DMBA-induced oral carcinogenesis by evaluating both the expression patterns of immunity (p53 and bcl-2) and biochemical markers (LPO, antioxidants, and detoxification enzymes) (Anusuya et al., 2011). Phytochemicals like carnosol, ursolic acid, carnosic acid obtained from rosemary have anti-oxidant and chemoprotective properties. These act by inhibiting the P-glycoprotein and can cause food-drug interaction (Nabekura et al., 2010)

10.4.4 ROSMARINIC ACID AS AN ANTI-DEPRESSIVE AGENT

Anti-depressive activity was observed in rosmarinic acid that was obtained from the leaves of *Perilla frutescens* Britton var. acuta Kudo (*Perillae Herba*). CAA is the major metabolite of rosmarinic acid and both the chemical moiety has been found to reduce the time of immobility of mice in the forced swimming test. Histamine has been found to possess depression causing effect and rosmarinic acid inhibits its release from mast cells thus exerts anti-depressive activity at a single dose while CAA inhibits the synthesis and release of nitric oxide (NO) which is a vasodilator through a 1-adrenoreceptor.

It is speculated that brain adrenoreceptors may be the reason behind stress and depression. Forced swimming in mice causes an increase of histamine as well as its turnover in the brain while antagonism of H1 and H3 receptor using different antagonists markedly reduced the period of immobility. From different types of assay systems it was established that anti-depressants such as amitriptyline, mianserin, and doxepin are potent competitive H1 receptor antagonists. Further studies are required to establish the mechanism involving anti-depressant activities of rosmarinic acid and CAA in the brain (Takeda et al., 2002)

As evident from the chemical structure, rosmarinic acid is a major polyphenolic compound and is one of the components of *Perillae Herba* (a leaf of Perilla frutescens) having anti-depressant properties as found in animal models (Takeda et al., 2002).

In one of the cellular studies, cell proliferation was induced using rosmarinic acid and is believed to be one of the probable pathways of exerting anti-depressant effect (Makino et al., 2001).

10.4.5   *ROSMARINIC ACID AS AN INHIBITOR OF ANGIOGENESIS*

Angiogenesis stems from the Greek word 'Angeion' which means vessel, i.e., formation of new blood vessel from the existing one. It continues to form (new blood vessels) through the life cycle of both healthy and diseased person. It inhibits multiple steps involved in angiogenesis like proliferation, migration, adhesion, and tube formation of human umbilical vein endothelial cells (HUVEC). It also reduced the level of various biomarkers like IL-8 release of endothelial cells, intracellular ROS level, H_2O_2-dependent VEGF expression (Huang et al., 2006).

10.5   ROLE OF ROSMARINIC ACID IN CARDIOVASCULAR DISEASE

Role of rosmarinic acid has not been properly brought to notice. It has been widely investigated in various cardiovascular diseases (CVDs) as discussed below.

10.5.1   *ROSMARINIC ACID AS A HYPOLIPIDEMIC AND ANTI-ATHEROSCLEROTIC AGENT*

Polyphenols obtained from dietary sources are potent and highly useful in inhibiting the lipid membranes alteration caused due to oxidative stress. Among the various polyphenols found in nature, rosmarinic acid founds special mention and is widely studied. A study involving rosmarinic acid confirms its LPO inhibiting activity.

An investigation by atomic force microscopy of transferred lipid/RA monolayers showed that at nanoscale level, a concentration of 1 mol% was insufficient in altering the structure of the membrane and further no sign of changes in the permeability and fluidity of the membrane was noted. 1,2-dilinoleoyl-sn-glycero-3-phosphocholine (DLPC) vesicles loaded with rosmarinic acid was prepared which showed that up to 1 mol% of Rosmarinic acid, when inserted spontaneously within the membrane, inhibited LPO without causing any alteration in the membrane (Fadel et al., 2011).

Low-density lipoprotein (LDL) that gets modified due to oxidation possesses an atherogenic property which can be prevented by using anti-oxidants that act by LDL inhibition. Rosmarinic acid was found to inhibit LDL oxidation in a dose-dependent manner (Fuhrman et al., 2000)

10.5.2   SIGNIFICANCE OF ROSMARINIC ACID IN METABOLIC SYNDROME (METS)

Cardiac abnormalities and HTN prevention potential of rosmarinic acid was investigated in fructose-fed rats (FFR). A high fructose-fed model of insulin resistance was chosen and RA was found to be insulin-sensitizing as well as anti-oxidant. Rosmarinic acid administered to FFR rats efficiently improved insulin sensitivity, reduced lipid levels, oxidative damage, and the concentration of p22phox subunit of nicotinamide adenine dinucleotide phosphate reduced oxidase, and prevented cardiac hypertrophy. A decrease in blood pressure (BP) by rosmarinic acid was achieved by causing a decrease in endothelin-1 and angiotensin-converting enzyme activity and increase of NO levels. Histology studies showed significant lowering of myocardial damage in fructose-fed rats when rosmarnic acid was administered thus, exhibiting vasoactive and cardioprotective activity and lowering cardiovascular risk-associated with IR (Karthik et al., 2011).

10.5.3   ROSMARINIC ACID IN CARDIOMYOPATHY

The study used melaton to induce rat cardiopathology. Rosmarinic acid-like luteolin and echinochrome could not provide cardioprotective activities and increased survival probability (Tsibul'skiĭ et al., 2011).

At the mechanism level, another study was carried out to probe the inhibitory action of rosmarinic acid on adriamycin (ADR)-induced apoptosis in H9c2 cardiac muscle cells causing a decrease in the liabilities of H9c2 cells, with the development of apoptotic characters like nuclear morphological changes and activation of caspase protease enzyme. Rosmarinic acid was bestowed with the ability to inhibit these apoptotic characters by decreasing the intracellular ROS generation and also by regaining the potential of mitochondrial membrane. These exhaustive studies revealed the pharmacological abilities of rosmarinic acid to inhibit ADR-induced apoptosis. These results concludes that

Rosmarinic acid is a potential chemotherapeutic agent that can prevent cardiotoxicity in patients exposed to ADR (Kim et al., 2005).

A study involving the evaluation of the cardioprotective effect of *Prunella vulgaris* ethylacetate fraction (PVEF) and its component, i.e., rosmarinic acid was executed on isolated rat cardiomyocytes with the help of doxorubicin-induced oxidative stress. PVEF and rosmarinic acid showed cytoprotective effect in the concentration range of 0.005 to 0.05 mg/mL. The data showed that the action of PVEF correlated with the RA content. From the probable mechanistic point of view the extract containing rosmarinic acid possessed remarkable cardioprotective effects due to anti-oxidant property (high phenolic content) and inhibition of LPO of membrane (Psotová et al., 2005). Promising results were obtained in terms of chemoprotective effect of rosmarinic acid achieved by induction of toxicity in rat cardiomyocytes by anthracycline (Chlopcíková et al., 2004).

10.5.4 *ROSMARINIC ACID AS AN ANTI-HYPERTENSIVE AGENT*

For addressing HTN, there are many drugs which are floating in the market but still HTN is affecting millions all over the world. Medicinal plants are slowly superseding the synthetic ones. The leverage being in terms of high manufacturing cost of synthetic drugs, low cost of herbal-based medicine and very few adverse affects of these natural products. One of the ways to treat HTN is the use of ACE inhibitor. Lie et al. and Karthik et al. has shown that rosmarinic acid inhibits or modulates ACE thus affecting BP but unfortunately literature related to it is very less (Li, 2008; Karthik et al., 2011). It has been reported that rosmarinic acid has endothelium-dependent vasodilator effect (Ersoy et al., 2008). The vasodilator effect is attributed to the polyphenolic group present in rosmarinic acid which exert this effect through activation of NO, prostacyclin (PGI$_2$) and endothelium-dependent hyperpolarizing factor (EDHF) (Ersoy, 2008; Fernandes et al., 2005). One of the pathways of rosmarinic acid's working is by increasing the level of Ca^{+2} in endothelial cells as well as activation of PI3-kinase/Akt, finally causing NOS activation and subsequent hyperpolarization. Rosmarinic acid also exerts anti-oxidant effect by inhibiting the oxygen free radical and peroxynitrate production thus leading to the prevention of damaging of the tissues (Fernandes et al., 2005).

10.5.5 SIGNIFICANCE OF ROSMARINIC ACID IN ACUTE MYOCARDIAL INFARCTION (AMI) AND ARRHYTHMIA

Acute myocardial infarction (AMI) and arrhythmia are a menace to the society and a great cause of hospitalization and mortality respectively. The cellular calcium level is regulated by both Sarcoplasmic reticulum Ca^{2+} ATPase (SERCA2) and Ryanodine receptor (RyR2), respectively. The protocol was designed in such a way so as to investigate whether rosmarinic acid can safeguard cardiac functions against AMI and arrhythmia induced by Isoproterenol, modulated by both SERCA2 and RyR2 genotypically. For mechanism of rosmarinic acid in myocardial infarction refer to Figure 10.1 (Javidanpour et al., 2018).

To run this protocol male Sprague-Dawley rats were used for both *in vivo* and *ex vivo* studies. Rosmarinic acid was administered to these rats in a dose of 10, 15, and 30 mg/kg for 14 days, respectively. Isoproterenol in a dose of 100 mg/kg was administered subcutaneously in consecutive mode to induce AMI. *In vivo* study was carried out to evaluate various parameters like heart rate, BP, ECG parameters, antioxidative enzymes, plasma levels of cardiac biomarkers. Langendorff set up was used to measure cardiac functions in isolated heart. Left ventricle of the heart was explored for gene expressions ofSERCA2 and RyR2.

A significant fall in QRS voltage, BP, activities of antioxidant enzymes, gene expressions of SERCA2 and RyR2 and cardiac function was noted on administration of isoproterenol. The results reflected an increase in ST-elevation, heart rate, antioxidant enzymes, and cardiac biomarkers at a dose of 30 mg/kg. This study reveals cardioprotective potential of rosmarinic acid against AMI and arrhythmia, the management of arrhythmic and AMI is probably due to its potential to augment the expression of plasma antioxidant enzymes and genes involved in Ca^{2+} homeostasis. Basically, its anti-adrenergic action is the main reason for its protective role (Javidanpour et al., 2018).

10.5.6 SIGNIFICANCE OF ROSMARINIC IN ADVERSE CARDIAC REMODELING

Cardiac remodeling occurs when the heart adapts itself to the hostile stimuli which causes failure of the heart and is the chief reason for enhanced death after myocardial Infarction.

Protocol was designed to investigate whether Rosemary leaves had any effect on cardiac remodeling after MI. For running the protocol male Wistar rats were taken and divided into 6 groups. These groups were as follows:

- **Group I:** Sham group fed with standard chow (SR0, n = 23);
- **Group II:** Sham group-fed with standard chow along with 0.02% rosemary (R002) (SR002, n = 23);
- **Group III:** Sham group fed standard chow along with 0.2% rosemary (R02) (SR02, n = 22);
- **Group IV:** Induced to MI and fed with standard chow (IR0, n = 13);
- **Group V:** induced to MI and fed with standard chow supplemented with R002 (IR002, n = 8); and
- **Group VI:** induced to MI and fed with standard chow supplemented with R02 (IR02, n = 9).

The drug was administered to the animals for 3 months and after that systolic pressure was evaluated. Echocardiography and euthanasia was performed. Samples of Left ventricle were evaluated for cytokine levels, fibrosis, apoptosis, oxidative stress, and energy metabolism enzymes. The protocol constituting oral administration of Rosemary showed attenuation of cardiac remodeling by enhancing metabolism of energy as well as lowering the oxidative stress.

Hypertrophy after MI was found to be reduced along with improvement of diastolic function to the tune of 0.02% when supplementation of Rosemary was administered. Investigation has revealed that a dose of 0.02% and 0.2% of Rosemary in humans is equivalent to 11 mg and 110 mg, respectively (Murino et al., 2017).

10.5.7 SIGNIFICANCE OF ROSMARINIC IN CARDIAC FIBROSIS

Cardiac fibrosis is described as a transformation of cardiac fibroblast to myofibroblast through unnecessary differentiation accompanied by disturbed homeostasis between synthesis and degradation of the extra-cellular matrix (ECM) (Kong et al., 2014). The ECM is secreted by the converted CF's (cardiac fibroblasts) which gives support to the cardiomyo-cytes and non-structural components. When cardiomyoctes are subjected to chronic stimuli (Rienks et al., 2014) excessive ECM deposition takes place causing mechanical and electrical impulse disturbance and finally succumbing to heart failure and Arrhythmia (Khan et al., 2006). CF's are the main rogue behind causing cardiac fibrosis. So if the CF's are targeted cardic fibrosis can be prevented, decrease the chances of cardiac remodeling, and delay the occurrence of heart failure (Nagpal et al., 2016). To investigate Rosmarinic acid's anti-fibrotic effect male mice aged 8–10 weeks with bodyweight 25. 5 ± 2 gm were used. To anesthetize mice, 3% pentobarbital sodium at a dose of 50 mg per kg was administered intraperitoneally and arbitrarily assigned to the AB (aortic banding) surgery group or sham-operated control group. Severe aortic constriction was produced by surgery. The sham-operated group underwent the same process but no ligation of the Aortic was done. For post-operative pain relief Temgesic (qd) at a dose of 0.1 mg/kg was used subcutaneously. After one week, the following operation Doppler was used to confirm adequate ligation. The animals were administered rosmarinic acid in a dose of 100 mg per Kg intragastrically once daily or a vehicle of the same volume for 7 weeks (Govindaraj, 2016; Boonyarikpunchai et al., 2014). The animals were segregated into 4 groups namely sham + vehicle, sham + rosmarinic acid, AB + vehicle and AB+ rosmarinic acid. Each group comprised of 15 mice. After one week of surgery, mice were provided with rosmarinic acid in a dose of 100 mg/kg/d for 3 weeks so as to establish *In vivo* inflammatory action. After the completion of experimental protocol, mice were sacrificed for heart and tibia for HW/BW and HW/TL calculation. For the experiment, AMPKα and AMPKα2 KO mice were employed to study cardiac fibrosis (Ma et al., 2016). Transthoracic echocardiography was performed using the advance My Lab 30 CV ultrasound (Ma, 2017; Xu et al., 2017). Further, for studying invasive hemodynamic, cardiac catheterization was employed. Western blot quantitative real-time PCR and immunofluorescence staining was also used. The result sharply indicates that rosmarinic acid improved cardiac dysfunction and Cardiac Fibrosis. Cardiac fibrosis was found to be inhibited through AMPK activation and Smad3 inhibition (as shown in Figure 10.2).

10.6   CONCLUSION

Rosmarinic acid has been extracted from different plant species but its effect on cardiovascular disease has always been underestimated. This chapter gives an assimilated account of its cardiovascular disease-modifying potential. Rosmarinic acid showed cardioprotective effect due to its anti-oxidant property. It also possessed endothelium-dependent vasodilator effect which acted through NO, PGI_2, and EDHF pathway. It was also found to protect the cardiac functions against isoproterenol-induced AMI and arrhythmia along with the involvement of SERCA2 and RyR2 receptors. During the study, it also revealed its potential in cardiac remodeling attenuation. In the case of cardiac fibrosis, rosmarinic acid meticulously targeted Cf's and through AMPK activation and Smad3 inhibition cardiac fibrosis was inhibited. The results point out a bigger role that rosmarinic acid can play in modifying CVDs.

ACKNOWLEDGMENT

We express our sincere thanks to the DST-INSPIRE fellowship program, DST-SERB, UGC-UPE II, and AICTE-RPS schemes of Govt. of India for providing financial support which was utilized for the present study.

KEYWORDS

- **acute myocardial infarction**
- **aortic banding**
- **arrhythmia**
- **caffeic acid**
- **cardiovascular**
- **rosmarinic acid**

REFERENCES

Al-Sereiti, M. R., Abu-Amer, K. M., & Sen, P., (1999). Pharmacology of rosemary (*Rosmarinus officinalis* Linn.) and its therapeutic potentials. *Indian J. Exp., Biol., 37*(2), 124–130.

Anusuya, C., & Manoharan, S., (2011). Antitumor initiating potential of rosmarinic acid in 7,12-dimethylbenz anthracene-induced hamsterbuccal pouch carcinogenesis. *J. Environ. Pathol. Toxicol. Oncol., 30*(3), 199–211.

Baba, S., Osakabe, N., Natsume, M., et al., (2004). Orally administered rosmarinic acid is present as the conjugated and/or methylated forms in plasma, and is degraded and metabolized to conjugated forms of caffeic acid, ferulic acid and m-coumaric acid. *Life Sci., 75*(2), 165–178.

Baba, S., Osakabe, N., Natsume, M., et al., (2005). Absorption, metabolism, degradation, and urinary excretion of rosmarinic acid after intake of *Perilla frutescens* extract in humans. *European Journal of Nutrition, 44*(1), 1–9.

Boonyarikpunchai, W., Sukrong, S., & Towiwat, P., (2014). Antinociceptive and antiinflammatory effects of rosmarinic acid isolated from *Thunbergia laurifolia* Lindl. *Pharmacol. Biochem. Behav., 124*, 67–73.

Braidy, N., Matin, A., Rossi, F., et al., (2013). Neuroprotective effects of rosmarinic acid on ciguatoxin in primary human neurons. *Neurotox. Res., 25*(2), 226–234.

Bult, H., Herman, A. G., & Rampart, M., (1985). Modification of endotoxin-induced haemodynamic and haematological changes in the rabbit by methylprednisolone, F(ab')2 fragments and rosmarinic acid. *British Journal of Pharmacology, 84*(2), 317–327.

Chlopcíková, S., Psotová, J., Miketová, P., et al., (2004). Chemoprotective effect of plant phenolics against anthracycline-induced toxicity on rat cardiomyocytes. Part II caffeic, chlorogenic and rosmarinic acids. *Phytother. Res., 18*(5), 408–413.

Dapkevicius, A., Van, B. T. A., Lelyveld, G. P., et al., (2002). Isolation and structure elucidation of radical scavengers from thymus vulgaris leaves. *J. Nat. Prod., 65*(6), 892–896.

Ellis, B. E., & Towers, G. H., (1970). Biogenesis of rosmarinic acid in mentha. *Biochem. J., 118*(2), 291–297.

Englberger, W., Hadding, U., Etschenberg, E., et al., (1988). Rosmarinic acid: A new inhibitor of complement C3-convertase with anti-inflammatory activity. *International Journal of Immunopharmacology, 10*(6), 729–737.

Ersoy, S., Orhan, I., Turan, N. N., et al., (2008). Endothelium dependent induction of vasorelaxation by *Melissa officinalis* L. ssp. Officinal is in rat isolated thoracic aorta. *Phytomedicine, 15*(12), 1087–1092.

Fadel, O., El Kirat, K., & Morandat, S., (2011). The natural antioxidant rosmarinic acid spontaneously penetrates membranes to inhibit lipid peroxidation *in situ. Biochem. Biophys. Acta, 1808*(12), 2973–2980.

Fernandes, L., Fortes, Z. B., Casarini, D. E., et al., (2005). Role of PGI2 and effects of ACE inhibition on the bradykinin potentiation by angiotensin-(1-7) in resistance vessels of SHR. *Regul Pept., 127*(1–3), 183–189.

Fuhrman, B., Volkova, N., Rosenblat, M., et al., (2000). Lycopene synergistically inhibits LDL oxidation in combination with vitamin E glabridin, rosmarinic acid, carnosic acid, or garlic. *Antioxid. Redox Signal, 2*(3), 491–506.

Furtado, M. A., De Almeida, L. C. F., Furtado, R. A., et al., (2008). Antimutagenicity of rosmarinic acid in Swiss mice evaluated by the micronucleus assay. *Mutation Research/ Genetic Toxicology and Environmental Mutagenesis, 657*(2), 150–154.

Georgiev, M., Pastore, S., Lulli, D., et al., (2012). Verbascum xanthophoeniceum-derived phenylethanoid glycosides are potent inhibitors of inflammatory chemokines in dormant and interferon-gamma-stimulated human keratinocytes. *J. Ethnopharmacol., 144*(3), 754–760.

Govindaraj, J., & Sorimuthu, P. S., (2015). Rosmarinic acid modulates the antioxidant status and protects pancreatic tissues from glucolipotoxicity mediated oxidative stress in high-fat diet: Streptozotocin-induced diabetic rats. *Mol. Cell. Biochem., 404*(1/2), 143–159.

Hajimehdipoor, H., Shekarchi, M., Khanavi, M., et al., (2010). A validated high performance liquid chromatography method for the analysis of thymol and carvacrol in *Thymus vulgaris* L. volatile oil. *Pharmacogn. Mag., 6*(23), 154–158.

Hakkim, F. L., Shankar, C. G., & Girija, S., (2007). Chemical composition and antioxidant property of holy basil (*Ocimum sanctum* L.) leaves, stems, and inflorescence and there *in vitro* callus cultures. *J. Agric. Food Chem., 55*(22), 9109–9117.

https://pubchem.ncbi.nlm.nih.gov/compound/5281792 (accessed on 26 June 2020).

Huang, S. S., & Zheng, R. L., (2006). Rosmarinic acid inhibits angiogenesis and its mechanism of action *in vitro*. *Cancer Lett., 239*(2), 271–280.

Ito, H., Miyazaki, T., Ono, M., & Sakurai, H., (1998). Antiallergic activities of rabdosiin and its related compounds: Chemical and biochemical evaluations. *Bioorg. Med. Chem., 6*(7), 1051–1056.

Jain, R., Kosta, S., & Tiwari, A., (2010). Ayurveda and urinary tract infection. *J. Young Pharm., 2*(3), 337.

Javidanpour, S., Dianat, M., Badavi, M., et al., (2018). The inhibitory effect of rosmarinic acid on over expression of NCX1 and stretch-induced arrhythmias after acute myocardial infarction in rats. *Biomedicine and Pharmacotherapy, 102*, 884–893.

Jones, D. L., Adams, R. J., Brown, T. M., et al., (2010). *Heart Disease and Stroke Statistics-2010 Update A Report from the American Heart Association, 121*, e46–e215.

Karthik, D., Viswanathan, P., & Anuradha, C. V., (2011). Administration of rosmarinic acid reduces cardio pathology and blood pressure through inhibition of p22phox NADPH oxidase in fructose-fed hypertensive rats. *J. Cardiovasc. Pharmacol., 58*(5), 514–521.

Khan, R., & Sheppard, R., (2006). Fibrosis in heart disease: Understanding the role of transforming growth factor-beta in cardiomyopathy, valvular disease and arrhythmia. *Immunology, 118*(1), 10–24.

Kim, D. S., Kim, H. R., Woo, E. R., et al., (2005). Inhibitory effects of rosmarinic acid on adriamycin-induced apoptosis in H9c2 cardiac muscle cells by inhibiting reactive oxygen species and the activations of c-Jun N-terminal kinase and extracellular signal-regulated kinase. *Biochem. Pharmacol., 70*(7), 1066–1078.

Kong, P., Christia, P., & Frangogiannis, N. G., (2014). The pathogenesis of cardiac fibrosis. *Cell. Mol. Life. Sci., 71*(4), 549–574.

Konishi, Y., Hitomi, Y., Yoshida, M., et al., (2005). Pharmacokinetic study of caffeic and rosmarinic acids in rats after oral administration. *J. Agric. Food Chem., 53*(12), 4740–4746.

Kuhnt, M., Pröbstle, A., Rimpler, H., et al., (1995). Biological and pharmacological activities and further constituents of *Hyptisverticillata*. *Planta Med., 61*(3), 227–232.

Kumar, P. M., Sasmal, D., & Mazumder, P. M., (2010). The antihyperglycemic effect of aerial parts of *Salvia splendens* (scarlet sage) in streptozotocin-induced diabetic-rat. *Pharmacogn. Res., 2*(3), 190–194.

Lee, J., Hun, P. K., Myoung-Hee, L., et al., (2013). Identification, characterization, and quantification of phenolic compounds in the antioxidant activity-containing fraction from the seeds of Korean perilla (*Perilla frutescens*) cultivars. *Food Chemistry, 136*, 843–852.

Li, Q. L., Li, B. G., Zhang, Y., et al., (2008). Three angiotensin-converting enzyme inhibitors from *Rabdosiacoetsa*. *Phytomedicine, 15*(5), 386–388.

Li, X., Yu, C., Lu, Y., et al., (2007). Pharmacokinetics, tissue distribution, metabolism, and excretion of depside salts from *Salvia miltiorrhiza* in rats. *Drug Metabolism and Disposition, 35*(2), 234–239.

Ma, Z. G., Dai, J., Wei, W. Y., et al., (2016). Asiatic acid protects against cardiac hypertrophy through activating AMPKα signaling pathway. *International Journal of Biological Sciences, 12*(7), 861–871.

Ma, Z. G., Yuan, Y. P., & Xu, S. C., (2017). CTRP3 attenuates cardiac dysfunction, inflammation, oxidative stress, and cell death in diabetic cardiomyopathy in rats. *Diabetologia, 60*(6), 1126–1137.

Makino, T., Ito, M., Kiuchiu, F., et al., (2001). Inhibitory effect of decoction of *Perilla frutescens* on cultured murine mesangial cell proliferation and quantitative analysis of its active constituents. *Planta Medica, 67*(1), 24–28.

Malahubban, M., Alimon, M. R., Sazili, A. Q., et al., (2013). Phytochemical analysis of *Andrographis paniculata* and *Orthosiphon stamineus* leaf extracts for their antibacterial and antioxidant potential. *Trop. Biomed., 30*(3), 467–480.

Murino, R. B. P., Portugal, D. S. P., Gonc, Ë. A. D. F., et al., (2017). Rosemary supplementation (*Rosmarinus oficinallis* L.) attenuates cardiac remodeling after myocardial infarction in rats. *PLoS One, 12*(5), e0177521.

Nabekura, T., Yamaki, T., Hiroi, T., et al., (2010). Inhibition of anticancer drug efflux transporter P-glycoprotein by rosemary phytochemicals. *Pharmacological Research, 61*(3), 259–263.

Nagpal, V., Rai, R., Place, A. T., et al., (2016). MiR-125b is critical for fibroblast-to-myofibroblast transition and cardiac fibrosis. *Circulation, 133*(3), 291–301.

Nascimento, E. M., Rodrigues, F. F., Campos, A. R., et al., (2009). Phytochemical prospection, toxicity and antimicrobial activity of *Mentha arvensis* (Labiatae) from northeast of Brazil. *J. Young Pharm., 1*(3), 210–212.

Peake, P. W., Pussell, B. A., Martyn, P., et al., (1991). The inhibitory effect of rosmarinic acid on complement involves the C5 convertase. *International Journal of Immuno Pharmacology, 13*(7), 853–857.

Petersen, M., & Simmonds, M. S., (2003). Rosmarinic acid. *Phytochemistry, 62*(2), 121–125.

Petersen, M., Abdullah, Y., Benner, J., et al., (2009). Evolution of rosmarinic acid biosynthesis. *Phytochemistry, 70*(15/16), 1663–1679.

Petersen, M., Alfermann, A. W., & Naturforsch, Z., (1988). Two new enzymes of Rosmarinic acid biosynthesis from cell cultures of coleus blumei: Hydroxyphenylpyruvate reductase and rosmarinic acid synthase. *C: Biosci., 43c*, 501–504.

Psotová, J., Chlopcíková, S., Miketová, P., et al., (2005). Cytoprotectivity of *Prunella vulgaris* on doxorubicin-treated rat cardiomyocytes. *Fitoterapia, 76*(6), 556–561.

Rampart, M. R., Beetens, J. R., Bult, H., et al., (1986). Complement-dependent stimulation of prostacyclin biosynthesis: Inhibition by rosmarinic acid. *Biochemical Pharmacology, 35*(8), 1397–1400.

Rienks, M., Papageorgiou, A. P., Frangogiannis, N. G., et al., (2014). Myocardial extracellular matrix: An ever-changing and diverse entity. *Circ. Res., 114*(5), 872–888.

Sahu, A., Rawal, N., & Pangburn, M. K., (1999). Inhibition of complement by covalent attachment of rosmarinic acid to activated C3b. *Biochem. Pharmacol., 57*(12), 1439–1446.

Sanchez-Campillo, M., Gabaldon, J. A., Castillo, J., et al., (2009). Rosmarinic acid, a photo-protective agent against UV and other ionizing radiations. *Food Chem. Toxicol., 47*(2), 386–392.

Shahidi, F., & Wanasundara, P. K., (1992). Phenolic antioxidants. *Critical Reviews in Food Science and Nutrition, 32*(1), 67–103.

Shekarchi, M., Hajimehdipoor, H., Saeidnia, S., et al., (2012). Comparative study of rosmarinic acid content in some plants of Labiatae family. *Pharmacognosy Magazine, 8*(29), 37–41.

Takeda, H., Tsuji, M., Inazu, M., et al., (2002). Rosmarinic acid and caffeic acid produce antidepressive-like effect in the forced swimming test in mice. *European Journal of Pharmacology, 449*(3), 261–267.

Takeda, H., Tsuji, M., Matsumiya, T., et al., (2002). Identification of rosmarinic acid as a novel antidepressive substance in the leaves of *Perilla frutescens* Britton var. *acuta* Kudo (*Perillae* Herba). *Nihon Shinkei Seishin Yakurigaku Zasshi, 22*(1), 15–22.

Tsibul'skiĭ, A. V., Popov, A. M., Artiukov, A. A., Kostetskiĭ, É., et al., (2011). The comparative study of the medical action of lyuteolin, rosmarinic acid, and echinochrom A at experimental stress-induced cardio pathology. *Biomed. Khim., 57*, 314–325.

Vieira, A., (2010). A comparison of traditional anti-inflammation and anti-infection medicinal plants with current evidence from biomedical research: Results from a regional study. *Pharmacogn. Res., 2*(5), 293–295.

Vostálová, J., Zdařilová, A., & Svobodová, A., (2010). *Prunella vulgaris* extract and rosmarinic acid prevent UVB-induced DNA damage and oxidative stress in HaCaT keratinocytes. *Arch. Dermatol. Res., 302*(3), 171–181.

Wang, H., Provan, G. J., & Helliwell, K., (2004). Determination of rosmarinic acid and caffeic acid in aromatic herbs by HPLC. *Food Chem., 87*(2), 307–311.

Xu, S. C., Ma, Z. G., Wei, W. Y., et al., (2017). Beza fibrate attenuates pressure overload-induced cardiac hypertrophy and fibrosis. *Ppar. Res, 12*.

Zheng, Q., Sun, Z., Zhang, X., et al., (2012). Clerodendranoic acid, a new phenolic acid from *Clerodendranthus spicatus. Molecules, 17*(11), 13656–13661.

Zheng, W., & Wang, S. Y., (2001). Antioxidant activity and phenolic compounds in selected herbs. *J. Agric. Food Chem., 49*(11), 5165–5170.

Zomorodian, K., Saharkhiz, M. J., Rahimi, M. J., et al., (2011). Chemical composition and antimicrobial activities of the essential oils from three ecotypes of *Zataria multiflora. Pharmacogn. Mag., 7*(25), 53–59.

CHAPTER 11

Long-Term Toxicity and Regulations for Bioactive-Loaded Nanomedicines

IQBAL AHMAD,[1,2] SOBIYA ZAFAR,[2] SHAKEEB AHMAD,[2] SUMA SAAD,[2] S. M. KAWISH,[2] SANJAY AGARWAL,[1] and FARHAN JALEES AHMAD[2]

[1]*Formulation Research Lab., Advance Nanomeds, Plot No. 142/20A, NSEZ, Noida – 201305, Uttar Pradesh, India*

[2]*Nanomedicine Research Lab., Department of Pharmacy, School of Pharmaceutical Education and Research, Jamia Hamdard, New Delhi – 110025, India*

ABSTRACT

Incorporation of natural bioactive into nanomedicines, their applications, and evaluation have aggressively been put forward during the last couple of decades. The enormous ability of nanocarriers in enhancing the bioavailability, targeting, and efficacy of natural molecules have been well documented. Many findings also demonstrate the application of nanosystems in toxicity reduction and lessening of possible side effects of drugs effective targeting and thereby decrease the dose required. However, it should be noted that the conversion of molecules from natural to the nanoscale can display entirely new or significantly altered physicochemical as well as biological properties and may impose some newer risks to the patient. For instance, some drugs that are not crossing biological barriers may surpass them when transformed into nanoparticles, opening up new dimensions to therapeutic strategies specifically for brain delivery. In addition, they may also get into other cellular compartments and undesirably cause a cascade of adverse reactions including genotoxicity. This chapter outlines the suitability of various bioactive loaded nanocarriers in therapeutics, their toxicity, and regulatory considerations.

11.1   INTRODUCTION

Natural products have continued to be the major driver of primary healthcare throughout human history with about 80% prevalence found in developing countries and up to 30% in developed countries. This equates to approximately 5.1 billion world population depends on natural products for medicinal applications (Picking, 2017). Bioactive, obtained from natural products, including antioxidants, probiotics, polyunsaturated fatty acids (PUFAs), and proteins have demonstrated great potential as therapeutic agents for the treatment of several medical conditions including cancer, central nervous system-related disorders, arthritis, inflammation, infections, and several others. However, the stability, solubility, and hence the bioavailability severely limits the successful clinical translation of the herbal bioactive for therapeutic applications. Although most of the natural compounds exhibit low toxicity, high-dose-induced side effects are a major reason limiting patient compliance (Watkins et al., 2015). Nanocarrier based delivery of bioactive has been a major advancement in the efforts to increase the therapeutic effectiveness of herbal bioactive.

Nanotechnology is the science and technology of manipulating matter of size <100 nm to produce devices with new molecular properties, organizations, and functions, that cannot be achieved at large scales. Nanotechnology is a rapidly evolving field and can be considered as the start of a new technological revolution with immense potential in healthcare, environment, smarter electronics, and advanced agriculture and energy (Hoet et al., 2009). Nanotechnology in the food sector is focused on the production of nanofood ingredients and additives developing delivery systems for the bioactive molecules and food packaging. The major applications of nanotechnology in the area of food and additives include-improving nutraceuticals stability, augmenting bioavailability of poorly soluble functional food ingredients, enhancing shelf life, and modifying the flavor and texture of food products (Chaudhry et al., 2008).

Nanomedicine is a branch of nanotechnology that encompasses specific medical intervention through which the human biological system can be monitored and controlled at the molecular level. Nanomaterials (NMs) such as metallic nanoparticles, ceramic, or carbon-based nanoparticles can be developed using simple molecules or they can be organized structures such as liposomes and nanoemulsion, or as dendrimers and polymers (Satalkar et al., 2016). Numerous benefits offered by nanomedicines include but not limited to, enhanced solubility of poorly soluble bioactive and thereby improved bioavailability, protection from degradation of bioactive, reduction in toxicity, decreased drug's immunogenicity and selective targetability (Sastry et al., 2010; Viacava et al., 2017). The United States-Food and Drug Administration (US-FDA) and the European Medicines Agency (EMA) have approved several nanomedicine-based products for therapeutic applications. Functionalization of nanoparticles with specific ligands, antigen, aptamer, peptide, etc., enhances the accumulation of nanoparticles in ischemic tissue, tumor, and organ inflamed area. Stimuli sensitiveness to pH, temperature, light, enzymes can mediate triggered drug release to the target site. Nanoparticles can also bypass biological barriers including cell membranes and blood-brain barrier bringing about increased drug concentrations to the diseased site (Smolkova et al., 2017).

NMs have different physicochemical and biological properties as compared to their larger counterparts. These characteristics confer double identity to the nanoparticles as their utilization implies novel medical and/or industrial applications as well as the possible hazardous outcome for both human and environmental health. The physicochemical characteristics of the nanoparticles, including, particle size, shape, and surface chemistry influences the cellular uptake, biodistribution patterns, and clearance mechanisms (Hoet et al., 2009). Any modification to any of these features induces new functions and potential toxicity. Challenges in the optimization procedure, characterization, and screening methods, instability under biological environments, robust, and reproducible manufacturing and scale-up, batch-to-batch consistency and regulatory barriers further impedes the successful clinical translation of a range of nanoparticles (Agrahari and Hiremath, 2017). Bioactive targeting is still a major challenge. Nanoparticles can enter the cells via endocytosis and can potentially cause the systemic toxicity if their bio-distribution is not controlled or if they form toxic metabolites. Non-biodegradable nanoparticle accumulation in the body over time could further lead to unwanted toxicity and cell death. For the product to be commercially successful, the two primary and essential qualifications are the high therapeutic efficacy and safety. Majority of the nanomedicines, however, fail to accomplish these requirements which impede their successful commercialization. Furthermore, the safety concerns with the nanoparticles stem from their translocation potential to the tissues attributed to their small size and higher-than-physiologically-normal concentrations of the delivered bioactive in the tissues. Oxidative stress is the major mechanism underlying NMs induced toxicity which further mediates inflammatory cell responses, immunotoxicity, and genotoxicity. Epigenetic alteration is another issue of

NMs induced toxicity to be taken into consideration (Smolkova et al., 2017; Stoccoro et al., 2013).

The long-term toxicity of nanoparticles is crucial to determine, especially if these systems are to be used for the treatment of chronic human diseases. When setting up a long-term toxicity (or safety) test for a nanomaterial, the route of administration and the vehicle used should correspond to the expected usage in humans. Species selection is another important consideration and the immune responses to the biological molecules should be comparable to that in humans. The test design and test outcomes necessitate supervision with great caution (Hoet et al., 2009).

Facilitating human safety is the prime concern with any delivery system. Nanotechnology is revolutionizing the field of medicine and drug delivery, but the unpredictable nature and the underlying nanotoxicity has the potential for harm. This necessitates the development of a regulation plan for nanotechnology that will serve the dual purpose of fostering innovation and keeping the public safe. Fiedler and Reynolds have correctly stated, "the law of unintended consequences operates with a vengeance where technology is concerned" (Fiedler and Reynolds, 1993).

11.2 TOXICITY WITH NATURAL BIOACTIVES

Consuming plants for potential health benefits for the prevention and treatment of several disorders has been a common practice since ancient times. Developments in phytochemical and pharmacological sciences have successfully enabled to interpret the composition as well as biological effectiveness of natural bioactive (Kamboj, 2000). The past few decades have witnessed the exponential increase in the use of phytochemical based dietary supplements and herbal remedies. The sudden surge in the use of dietary supplements has been particularly observed in cancer patients who consume these in conjunction with traditional cancer treatment, without informing their physicians. Epidemiological studies indicate that the phytochemicals are considered safe and might be a more natural alternative to conventional medication, however, only limited data are available for the safety and efficacy of most phytochemicals for disease interventions (Bode and Dong, 2015). Flavonoids are the constituents of fruits, vegetables, plant-derived beverages and are also present in a huge number of herbal-containing dietary supplements. They have shown to be potent antioxidants, however, a dark side still remains. Dietary phenolics act as prooxidants in systems containing redox-active metals. Series of chemical reactions are involved to mediate the prooxidant effects of the dietary phenolics. Transition metals such as copper (Cu) and iron (Fe) catalyze the redox cycling of phenolic compounds, in the presence of O_2, resulting in the formation of reactive oxygen species (ROS) and phenoxyl radicals which cause damage to DNA, lipids, and other biological molecules. Epigallocatechin gallate (EGCG), a green tea catechin, induce hydrogen peroxide (H_2O_2) generation in the presence of transition metal ions, subsequently causing oxidative damage to isolated and cellular DNA. The *in vitro* studies have further demonstrated the DNA oxidation induction ability of EGCG in promyeloblast cell line, HL60 cells, for acute promyelocytic leukemia. EGCG induced DNA oxidation was more pronounced in glutathione (GSH) depleted cells while no such activity was observed in H_2O_2-resistant HP100 cells that have 18 times higher catalase (CAT) activity than HL-60 cells. This implies that the H_2O_2 generation by EGCG is involved in DNA oxidation. This also relates to the prooxidant activity of EGCG on enhancing the dimethylhydrazine or nitrosamine colon carcinogenesis in rats. Another phenolic component of green tea, Pyrogallol produced significant hepatic damage in rats when administered at a dose of 100 mg/kg, intraperitoneally (I.P.). The increased level of serum enzymes aspartate aminotransferase (AST) and alanine aminotransferase (ALT) along with the increased level of malondialdehyde (MDA) suggests the formation of free radical and pro-oxidant effects as the key mediator of hepatic damage. Tea flavonoids, EGCG, propyl gallate and gallic acid (GAE) at a dose of 120 mg/kg, 170 mg/kg and 500 mg/kg, respectively, caused a 4-fold increase in plasma ALT levels, on the administration to the CD-1 mice indicating significant hepatic damage in rodent models (Galati and O'brien, 2004; Furukawa et al., 2003; Hirose et al., 2001). The catechol B ring containing flavonoids, such as quercetin, upon oxidation by peroxidase, forms semiquinone-and quinone-type metabolites that may act as electrophiles which bind to cellular macromolecules producing ROS through redox cycling. Peroxidase-mediated oxidation of phenol B ring containing flavonoids such as, apigenin (API), naringenin, resulted in the formation of phenoxyl radicals which catalyzed GSH or NADH co-oxidation and generated ROS. Another toxicity concern with flavonoid is the cytochrome P (CYPs)-flavonoid interaction. The CYP enzymes inhibiting or inducing the ability of flavonoids depends upon their structures, concentrations, or the experimental conditions. CYP activity is inhibited with flavonoids possessing hydroxyl groups while those lacking hydroxyl groups may induce the enzyme. Flavonoid-drug interactions may occur with the simultaneous administration of flavonoids and therapeutic agents. This can modulate the pharmacokinetics (PKs) of the active molecule with either increasing their toxicity or reducing their therapeutic effect, depending on the flavonoid structure. The flavanone present in grapefruit juice, Naringenin, when co-administered with calcium channel blockers (CCBs) like verapamil and nitrendipine, impairs the metabolism of CCBs mediated due to inhibition of intestinal CYP3A4 by naringenin. The naringenin can also produce lethal and teratogenic effects as observed in the amphibian embryo toxicity test. The dose of 10 mg/l exerted 100% malformations causing the death of 30% of the abnormal embryos. The major abnormalities observed were decreased body size, axial curves, microcephaly, abdominal edema, underdeveloped gills, and delayed development (Galati and O'brien, 2004). Likewise, Curcumin can inhibit the activity of the drug-metabolizing enzymes CYP450, glutathione-S-transferase, and UDP-glucuronosyltransferase, leading to increased plasma concentration of concomitantly administered drug and hence its toxicity (Burgos-Morón et al., 2010).

Another important polyphenol, Curcumin, obtained from the plant *Curcuma longa*, has demonstrated substantial safety and efficacy in the prevention and treatment of several human ailments. Curcumin has anti-inflammatory, anti-microbial, anticancer, thrombosuppressive, hepatoprotective, hypoglycemic, antiarthritic, and antioxidant activities. It is therefore not surprising to note that curcumin is widely available as a dietary supplement and is a popular subject in the ongoing clinical trials (Russo et al., 2010). However, there is accumulating evidence that has raised concern on the safety and effectiveness of curcumin. Several reports have demonstrated that curcumin may cause a dose and time-dependent induction of chromosome aberrations and DNA damage in both *in vitro* and *in vivo* conditions. The National Toxicology Program (USA), in 1993, published an extensive report on the toxicity and carcinogenicity of the organic extract of turmeric oleoresin containing 79–85% curcumin. The long term toxicity studies carried out for 3 months and 2 years on the rodents fed with diets containing varied concentrations of turmeric oleoresin demonstrated possible toxic and carcinogenic effects of turmeric oleoresin. In the rats, increased incidences of ulcers, hyperplasia, and inflammation of the forestomach, cecum, and colon was observed. The female mice developed thyroid gland follicular cell hyperplasia. Carcinogenic activity evident with increased incidences of clitoral gland adenomas, hepatocellular adenomas in female mice, and carcinomas of the small intestine was also observed in all the species tested. The probable mechanism involved in the carcinogenesis process is the generation of ROS, such as, superoxide anion and hydrogen peroxide. The ROS generation involves a series of chemical reaction, called Michael addition, wherein, 2 α,β-unsaturated ketones in the chemical structure of curcumin reacts covalently with exposed thiol groups of cysteine residues of the proteins. Curcumin at low concentrations works as an antioxidant, however, at higher concentrations, increases the cellular levels of ROS. Curcumin was also found to be an active iron chelator which induced a state of overt iron deficiency anemia in mice fed with an iron-deficient diet (Burgos-Morón et al., 2010; Program, 1993).

Resveratrol, a compound found in grapes, mulberries, and peanuts, has demonstrated antioxidant, anti-inflammatory, antiproliferative, and pro-apoptotic properties. The dose-limiting toxicity studies were carried out for determining any potential toxicity associated with resveratrol. A dose of 3000 mg/Kg body weight (BW) for 28 days caused nephrotoxicity in rats, evident with an enhanced level of serum BUN and creatinine levels, increased kidney weights, and gross renal pathology changes, also caused anemia due to reduced erythropoietin synthesis in the kidneys. The dose of 1000 or 300 mg/kg BW/day did not result in nephrotoxic findings (Crowell et al., 2004). Some active constituents of cruciferous vegetables can also produce toxic effects. Akagi et al. reported that the oral administration of 0.1% phenethyl isothiocyanate (PEITC) and benzyl isothiocyanate (BITC) in the rat diet-induced continuous urinary epithelial cell proliferation and simple and papillary or nodular (PN) hyperplasias, resulting in bladder carcinogenesis in rats (Akagi et al., 2003). The intracellular ROS generated from the N=C=S group of the isothiocyanates (ITCs) produces the cytotoxic and genotoxic effects and subsequent oxidative DNA damage (Russo et al., 2010).

Many findings have suggested that most of the natural compounds are still far from reaching the clinical stage due to low solubility, poor oral bioavailability, low stability, as well as possible toxicity at effective dosage. To overcome these challenges, nanotechnology-based approaches have been applied and found to have shown some desirable output which includes potentiation of the activity, reducing the side effects as well also reducing the required dose (Wachtel-Galor and Benzie, 2011). Moreover, bioactive incorporated nanomedicines have also been used to target individual organs through both passive and active mechanisms (Allen and Cullis, 2004; Kostarelos, 2003; Majumder, 2017).

11.3   TOXICITY WITH BIOACTIVE NANOMATERIALS (NMS)

Nanoparticulate systems including polymeric nanoparticles, lipidic nanoparticles, metallic nanoparticles, carbon nanotubes (CNTs), dendrimers, nanofibers, quantum dots, etc., are manufactured around the world due to the advantages offered by them in disease diagnosis and drug delivery for the management and amelioration of so many diseases (Borel and Sabliov, 2014). Fabrication of a bioactive loaded nanoparticulate system helps to achieve a water-soluble and stable drug delivery system owing to the enhanced surface area. But at the same time, the enhanced surface area also makes the NMs more reactive in the biological system (Kahru and Savolainen, 2010; Oberdörster et al., 2005). Nanoscale size reduction allows the particles to enter the distal biological sections which were not possible for the larger particles (Vega-Villa et al., 2008). The general mechanism of NMs induced toxicity is illustrated in Figure 11.1. The nanosize of the particle can form electronic states in the NPs which undergo electron transfer reactions resulting in the generation of ROS and free radicals which in turn induce oxidative stress and disturb the biological electron transfer reactions. The free radicals can mediate the mutilation of the biomolecules via lipid peroxidation (LPO), protein destabilization, and damage to the DNA helix. The oxidative stress enhances the inflammatory process via the upregulation of NF-KB, kinase, and activator protein (Ahmad et al., 2016). Figure 11.1 shows the possible mechanism of NMs induced toxicity.

Drug delivery systems such as microemulsions, self-micro emulsifying drug-delivery systems, nanoemulsions, solid lipid nanoparticles (SLNs), liposomes, etc., are advantageous in terms of selective tissue targeting and bioavailability enhancement of drugs (Pariser et al., 2011). But due to the presence of lipid in their structure, these carriers are susceptible to the phagocytic uptake. This interaction of NMs with phagocytes has some immunogenic potential. In addition to this, NMs when interact with lymphocytes and other cells may develop immune responses (swelling, immunomodulation, allergy) (Singh and Nalwa, 2007).

11.3.1 ROUTES OF NANOCARRIERS EXPOSURE AND POSSIBLE SYSTEMIC AND ORGANS TOXICITY

NMs induced toxicity is worrisome and cognizance has been taken by the scientific community in the past few years. To extract the maximum therapeutic effect of a drug with the help of a nanocarrier, one needs to pay attention towards the toxicity evaluation of such nanocarriers. The toxicity assessment strategies among the scientists have also been evolved in last few years. For the toxicity evaluation, mainly pharmacokinetic parameters such as absorption (Leite-Silva et al., 2013), distribution (Balogh et al., 2007; Goel et al., 2009), biochemistry involved in metabolism and clearance are supposed to be observed. Apart from these, predictive strategies for the assessment of NMs induced toxicity are also trending among the scientists (Fischer and Chan, 2007).

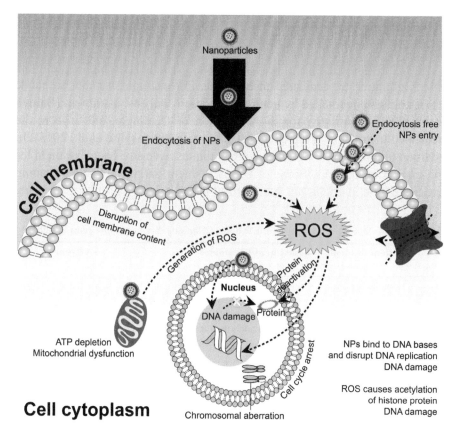

FIGURE 11.1 The possible mechanisms of nanoparticles (NPs) induced toxicity; NPs directly generates reactive oxygen species (ROS) by oxidants and free radicals on the NPs surface. NPs also activate inflammatory cells (macrophages); ROS generation results in activation of a proinflammatory transcription factor NF-κβ. Reduced clearance of NPs leads to increased interaction of NP with epithelium. NPs when reaching the nucleus oxidation and acetylation of histone protein occur resulting in DNA modification; NPs alter the mitochondrial functions, generates ROS which in turn may lead to cell injury and apoptosis.

NMs induced toxicity has also been estimated in animal models based on the phenotypic changes of cells/tissues (Guo et al., 2013; Sayes et al., 2007) programmed cell death, i.e., apoptosis (Sarhan and Hussein, 2014; Coccini et al., 2013) infiltration and inflammation of vital organs (brain, heart, lung, spleen, and kidney). For example, NMs tend to deposit in Kupffer cells and hepatic sinusoids and may alter the hepatic metabolism and detoxication process.

The distribution extent of NMs is a function of their physicochemical properties (particle size, surface charge, chemistry of coating material) and is responsible for the toxic effects of NMs *in vivo*. Extent of distribution is usually estimated after excising the tissues or organs followed by the physical detection of NMs. The estimation of metallic NMs is comparatively easier and done by dedicated instruments. For example, a nanochip made up of gold can be tracked by neutron activation analysis instrument (Balogh et al., 2007). Similarly, for the estimation of Cadmium and Silicon, the dedicated instrument is optical emission spectrometry (Guo et al., 2013). In addition, fluorescent or radiolabeled techniques have also been exploited for the estimation of Nms. Some of the assessment parameters for evaluating toxicity of nanoparticles are summarized in Table 11.1.

TABLE 11.1 Various Approaches for Evaluating Nanotoxicity in Major Organ Systems

Sl. No.	System Studied	Assessment Parameter	References
1.	Hepatic system	Quantitative analysis of functional changes was assessed by serum enzymology of aspartate aminotransferase, c-glutamyl transferase, and alkaline phosphatase, alanine aminotransferase.	Pan et al., 2012; Yamagishi et al., 2013; Cho et al., 2009
2.	Renal system	Cell nuclear antigen measurement was used for the cell proliferation study. Detection of pathological changes is determined by using various markers like fibrotic and mesenchymal markers which transform the growth factor-β1, interferon-6, type I collagen, fibronectin, and vimentin.	Coccini et al., 2013; Gross et al., 2015; Pan et al., 2012
3.	Gastrointestinal system	Gastrointestinal microvilli, epithelial atrophy, and the mast cell count in the stomach were analyzed by the histological assay.	Lin et al., 2014; Han et al., 2012; Wang et al., 2013
4.	Pulmonary system	Lactate dehydrogenase (LDH) assay for biochemical examination was performed on Bronchoalveolar lavage (BAL) fluid for determining pneumonocyte injury.	Paranjpe and Müller-Goymann, 2014; Zhang et al., 2002

TABLE 11.1 *(Continued)*

5.	Cardiovascular system	The cardiac injury was assessed by using serum markers such as creatine kinase-MB, troponin-T, and myoglobin. Venous tolerance was indicated by edema, purple lump, blood clot, and eye witness. Analysis of oxidative stress was done by using biomarkers such as LPO, ROS, and Antioxidant enzymes such as GPx, catalase, and SOD	Zhang et al., 2015; Laverman et al., 2001; Fornaguera et al., 2015
6.	Nervous system	After i.v administration, brain uptake was determined by calculating the ratio between the concentration in brain and in blood plasma, for impairment in brain, glutamate uptake was analyzed and for determining acute toxicity, histology of brain was performed.	Win-Shwe and Fujimaki, 2011; Liu et al., 2014; Blasi et al., 2013
7.	Immune and reproductive system	Assessment of toxicity was done by assessing variation in immune cytokine, molecules, and immune organs as well as in hematological systems. Female reproductive organ functioning was evaluated, histopathology was performed. Some reports for NPs suggest the effect the offspring development due to crossing of placenta blood barrier in rats. For the male reproductive system, toxicity was evaluated by changes in sperm parameters, sexual hormones, i.e., testosterone, and testicular tissue structure.	Li et al., 2016; Layali et al., 2016; Ren et al., 2016

An immunohistochemistry study was performed as a part of a toxicological study for determining any inflammation of hepatic cells and liver fibrosis (Pan et al., 2012). Degradation of renal glomerulus a parameter for renal toxicity was identified by histopathological study (Coccini et al., 2013). For determining the degree of injury of the glomerular filtration membrane (Petrica et al., 2015) various parameters, such as glomerular filtration rate, urine protein, total proteins, albumin, hematuria, and creatinine ratio were analyzed (Gandhi et al., 2013).

Oral route of administration is the most widely used mode of administration but the drawback is bioavailability due to the first-pass metabolism. Polymeric based or lipid-based nano-sized carriers (Pridgen et al., 2014) increases the bioavailability by intercepting the acidic and enzymatic inactivation and degradation and facilitates the GIT transportation.

Analysis of short term (Ma-Hock et al., 2009) and long term toxicity (Bermudez et al., 2004) for pulmonary system by collecting the bronchoalveolar lavage (BAL) fluid for biochemical assessment like lactate dehydrogenase (LDH) assay (Paranjpe and Müller-Goymann, 2014). The total number of neutrophils obtained from BAL indicates the inflammation level (Zhang et al., 2002).

The amount of drug crossing through the blood-brain barrier can be analyzed by radiography methods such as PET and CT systems (Frigell et al., 2013). Acute toxicity can be determined by brain histology examination (LM and TEM) and fluorescence imaging (Blasi et al., 2013). The nerve injury can be assessed by electrophysiological and behavioral studies. Animal models for the behavioral study show clinical symptoms such as convulsions, diarrhea, lethargy, salivation, nausea, etc., (Pradhan et al., 2014).

11.3.2 REPRODUCTIVE TOXICITY

Teratogenicity induced by NMs is the main toxicity related to the reproductive system. Phytomedicines loaded nanoparticulate systems and excipients must be screened to avoid such functional abnormalities. It has been observed experimentally that NMs can slow down the embryo developmental processes. It has been suggested through various modern-day experimental studies that nanoparticles can have an effect on the developmental process which in turn influences the reproductive functions apart from other physiological functions. The toxicity estimation in the reproductive system takes a longer time as the reproductive system is somewhat different from the other systems which is differentiated into male and female. For the male reproductive system, the testicular histological structure, sexual hormones (e.g., testosterone), parameters of epididymal sperm, and the nanoparticles concentration harbored in the serum and testis need to be evaluated (Li et al., 2016; Layali et al., 2016). For the female reproductive system toxicity study in different sexual hormone (e.g., follicle-stimulating hormone, LH (luteinizing hormone and estradiol) levels need to be measured in the serum (Saunders et al., 2015) along with the functions of major organs like ovary, uterus, and vaginal tract. For a detailed investigation, the histopathological study should be performed, especially for organs like uterus, placenta, testes, etc. This investigation should be performed for both parental as well as offspring (Mozaffari et al., 2015).

11.3.3 IMMUNOTOXICITY

Immunogenic activity and related toxicity are mainly due to the surface properties of NMs (Dobrovolskaia et al., 2016). The entire immune system is intricated, hence the extent of toxicity produced by NMs is not easy to determine. In that case, changes in the hematological system, inflammatory markers (cytokines) and immune organs, etc., are supposed to be observed. For example, estimation of NMs induced immunotoxicity can be done by observing the generation and discharge of tumor necrosis factor (TNF) and Interleukins (Wang et al., 2016; Baron et al., 2016). In addition, one of the main immune organs, the spleen is usually examined for any histological changes and for this purpose, staining of the spleen with the help of hematoxylin and eosin dye has to be done (Wang et al., 2016).

11.3.4 GENOTOXICITY

There has been a growing concern about the potentially hazardous effects of NMs on the health of human beings. For that purpose, a great deal of effort was made to investigate the potentially hazardous effects of NMs, including genotoxicity. NMs with genotoxic effects can affect various small cellular components such as DNA or RNA through a different mechanism of actions. The nanoscale size and higher surface area when they focus on low solubility particles, their ability to generate ROS is the main area of concern for the Genotoxicity (Wang et al., 2016).

Furthermore, reduced particle size and higher surface area collectively generate more ROS as compared to larger particles (Brown et al., 2000) and hence may produce more genotoxicity. Type of target in the phases of the cell cycle, mutagen, DNA replication, and methods of DNA repairment collectively develop a genotoxic effect. For example, NMs may alter the strands of DNA in G1-phase, may negatively affect the formation of spindle fibers in phase G2. In addition, NMs on getting the right to permeate through the nuclear membrane may also affect the chromatin during interphase or mitosis. Examples of NMs induced ROS are; singlet oxygen, superoxide, hydrogen peroxide, hydroxyl radicals (Fubini and Hubbard, 2003).

Leukocytes (mainly neutrophil) rush during inflammation may generate ROS which in turn damages the DNA and ultimately may produce secondary genotoxicity. Mammalian cells and bacteria are mainly used to identify the genetic mutation but the later is comparatively less suitable as the cell membrane composition of bacteria differs from the mammalian cell membrane. For the assessment of secondary genotoxicity, *in vivo* models with similar end-points are selected (Driscoll et al., 1997).

11.4   RISK ASSESSMENT AND RISK MINIMIZATION IN NANOMEDICINE

The cutting edge nanotechnological advancement in the field of medicine has many advantages as it helps in early disease diagnosis, personalized or customized treatment, and better disease amelioration at lower cost. However, the potential risk assessment and risk minimization associated with the nano-technology-based drug and delivery system are quintessentially important. The term "risk" can be defined as the potential "hazard" that can be produced on "exposure" to certain NMs. The risk assessment includes hazard identification, hazard characterization, and exposure assessment, and risk characterization.

The prime objective of risk assessment and nanosafety studies is to produce a nanomedicine with minimum risk of toxicity. In that context, the utmost important thing is to find and authenticate some alternate and new approaches. For this purpose, European initiatives such as "Safety-by-design" have been taken to interpret the acute *in vitro* toxicity results for the prediction of long term toxicity in animal models (Accomasso et al., 2018).

Before starting an *in vitro* toxicity study of a NM, *in silico* study is recommended which includes quantitative nanostructure-activity relation-ships (QNAR), categorization, or grouping of NMs and read-across. As the name suggests, QNAR is a relationship developed between a chemical structure with certain physicochemical properties and a specifically deter-mined biological activity. Categorization of NM can be done on the basis of commercial viability/production volume, materials used (such as Polymer, Lipid, Metal, Carbon, etc.), morphology (shape and size), mechanism of action, etc., (Lynch et al., 2014). Categorization of NM based on chemical properties is particularly important as their structural similarity likely to produce toxicity with similar pattern. Read-across technique helps in predicting the end-point of a test nanomaterial by using information of same end-point previously obtained from other NMs.

High throughput screening (HTS) and high content screening (HCS) are the automated tools used for the estimation of *in vitro* toxicity related to NMs. HTS is mainly a type of automated assay and usually focuses on a separate biological mechanism or biochemical alteration. HTS-based screening of test NMs do not observe the whole phenotypical changes in cell. HCS is also an automated screening tool and mainly uses fluorescence and microscopic images for the toxicity analysis. Contrary to HTS, it is used to estimate multiple changes in the phenotype of similar cell population (Godwin et al., 2015) The HTS based *in vitro* assays are comparatively simple, less time consuming and less expensive than complicated animal model experiments. However, it cannot be used solely for the *in vitro* toxicity study due to the poor *in vitro-in vivo* correlation (IVIC); as a small cell cannot be a representative of an animal with complex body structure.

Small animals such as mice, rats, workhorse, zebrafish, etc., are the gold standard animals for the *in vivo* toxicity screening of NMs. In such animals, it is also important to understand the fate of NM at the cellular level, tissue level, and organ level. Hence, a right approach for the toxicity testing of NMs should include *in silico, in vitro,* and *in vivo* study for the sufficient IVIC and proper risk assessment.

When a NM comes in contact of biological media, they tend to undergo transformation such as aggregation or chemical degradation (dissolution, corrosion, and oxidation) and this transformation ultimately may produce toxicity. Hence, physicochemical characterization of developed NMs is required to scrutinize for the risk minimization (Bian et al., 2011). Coating of FDA approved biocompatible polymers (PEG or PVP) on such NMs may help improving their stability in biological media.

Early risk assessment and risk minimization strategies are prerequisite for the successful development of a nanomedicine and regulation from governing bodies on hazardous NMs must be welcome for the welfare of human community, ecosystem, and environment (Duncan and Gaspar, 2011).

11.5   REGULATION OF NANOMEDICINES

Emerging technologies create an atypical, often complex, and fundamentally political problem for global governance due to the persistent uncertainty that surrounds their potential risks. The regulation of any new technology is crucial to establish its safety and effectiveness. Nanomedicine has demonstrated significant potential in providing better health outcomes and is rapidly shifting from bench to bedside, closer to the realm of practical applicability. The global nanomedicine market is likely to reach $344.0 billion by 2024 (Agrahari and Hiremath, 2017). The rapid shift and the huge market share in the near future necessitate the examination of the adequacy of the current methods and regulatory guidelines for the assessment of the delivery, fate, safety, and efficacy of nanomedicines. Considering the peculiar adverse human health and environmental effects, investment is needed for the systematic toxicological evaluation of the NMs during the product development process. Toxicological research to address the potential hazards of nanoparticles has now caught the eye of the regulatory bodies and hence the government agencies have begun funding the field of toxicological research. Thus, it is of paramount significance to understand the fundamental and regulatory aspects of nanomedicine (Zhao and Castranova, 2011).

However, the large number of nanomedicines has been approved for biomedical applications, but the lack of specific protocols and the standard operating procedures for their development and characterization has hampered the realization of their full potential in clinical practice. A closer collaboration is still required between the regulatory agencies but significant steps have been taken in the last 5 years. According to the regulator's perspective, the specifications for the nanomedicine are described according to the therapeutic moiety in the product (Sainz et al., 2015). The standardization and characterization of the physicochemical properties including particle size, surface charge, and morphology of the nanoparticles is crucial for the successful development of nanomedical product. Modification in the physicochemical properties can significantly alter the biological properties and biodistribution patterns of the developed nanosystem. New and robust quality control assays methods should also be developed for monitoring the performance, drug release, protein binding, metabolism assessment, and cellular uptake and hence the therapeutic effectiveness of nanoparticles (Muthu and Feng, 2009; Dobrovolskaia and McNeil, 2013; Sainz et al., 2015).

A close collaboration between scientists, regulators, industry, patient representatives, and patient advocacy institutions, is being developed through research policy and alliances, to accelerate the development of new technologies and improved strategies for appropriate translational requirements and clinical development of nanomedicine (Agrahari and Hiremath, 2017). The various efforts by the industry and regulatory agencies to promote the clinical translation of nanomedicine are discussed in the subsequent sections-

11.5.1 FOOD AND DRUG ADMINISTRATION (FDA) PERSPECTIVES

The regulation of Nanotechnology product in the United States is carried out by the FDA, which coordinates the legislative supervision by the Office of

Science and Health Coordination through the Office of Commissioners. The working group suggests the scientific proposals and regulations for development, evaluation, and promotion of new pharmaceutical products (Demetzos, 2016). FDA has approved several nanomedicine products including liposomes, nanocrystals, albumin-based nanoparticles, polymeric nanoparticles. The important decision-making centers within FDA include Center for Drug Evaluation and Research (CDER), Center for Biological Evaluations and Research (CBER), Center for Device and Radiological Health (CDRH) and Center for Veterinary (CVM). The office for control and compliance is the office of regulatory affairs (ORA). According to CDER, the controls for the nanomedicinal products should be similar to the controls of new medicine safety, as described by FDA (Zolnik and Sadrieh, 2009).

Several initiatives have been put forward by the FDA to regulate the nanotechnology-based products. FDA, in the year 2001, along with other federal agencies, launched the National Nanotechnology Initiative (NNI) program to coordinate the research and development efforts on nanotechnology at the federal level (D'Silva and Van Calster, 2009). Nanoscale science, engineering, and technology (NSET) Subcommittee consisting of the managing board and representatives from each Federal agency, govern, and coordinate the actions of NNI (Preble, 2010). NNI defines nanotechnology as "the understanding and control of matter at dimensions of roughly 1 to 100 nm and involves imaging, measuring, modeling, and manipulating matter at this length scale" and Nanosimilars are "the copies of the off-patent nanotechnological therapeutic products consisting of a bioactive molecule and the nanocarrier which can be considered as the innovative excipient." The NNI mainly aims to foster the translation of novel technologies into commercial products, to broaden and maintain the educational resources, skilled manpower, and the supporting infrastructure for bringing the advancements in technology. Research and Development Act (NRDA) was developed in 2005 to authorize funding (of approximately $849 million) to 10 federal agencies for nanotechnology research for a period of four years. Federal funding for this initiative increased to $1.5 billion dollars in the fiscal year 2009 (Preble, 2010; Demetzos, 2016; Bawa, 2013).

The FDA also established a nanotechnology task force (NTF) in 2006 that addressed the knowledge or policy gaps to facilitate the continued development of the innovative, safe, and effective use of NMs in the FDA-regulated products. The FDA Task Force Report issued by NTF in 2007 concluded that the existing regulations were sufficiently comprehensive to ascertain the safety of nanoproducts because these products would endure premarket testing and approval either as new drugs under the New Drug Application (NDA) process, or in the case of medical devices, under the Class III Premarket Approval (PMA) process. The Task Force's research encouraged the development of appropriate analytical methods and that a case-by-case approach should be adopted to evaluate if sufficient evidence exists for the product to satisfy the applicable statutory and regulatory standards (Pita et al., 2018; Harris, 2009; Food and Force, 2007).

FDA involves actively in the activities of International forums such as the International Organization for Standardization (ISO) and the Organization for Economic Co-operation and Development (OECD). ISO has further published several standards related to nanotechnology. Some of which may include ISO 19007:2018-*In vitro* MTS assay for measuring the cytotoxic effects of nanoparticles, ISO 10808:2010 – Characterization of nanoparticles in inhalation exposure chambers for inhalation toxicity testing, ISO 209701:2010-Endotoxin test on nanomaterial samples for *in vitro* systems – Limulus amebocyte lysate (LAL) test. FDA has also issued several guidance documents on the subject matter of nanotechnology application in FDA-regulated products, these include, Final Guidance for Industry-Considering Whether an FDA-Regulated Product Involves the Application of Nanotechnology, Final Guidance for Industry-Safety of NMs in Cosmetic Products, Final Guidance for Industry-Assessing the Effects of Significant Manufacturing Process Changes, Including Emerging Technologies, on the Safety and Regulatory Status of Food Ingredients and Food Contact Substances, Including Food Ingredients that are Color Additives and Final Guidance for Industry-Use of NMs in Food for Animals (Food and Administration, 2011, 2014).

11.5.2 EUROPEAN MEDICINES AGENCY (EMA) PERSPECTIVE

In the European Union, the EMA regulates provisions for biotechnological and nanotechnological products. The EMA comprises of six committees, including, Committee for Medicinal Products for Human Use (CHMP), Committee for Medicinal Products for Veterinary Use (CVMP), Committee on Herbal Medicinal Products (HMPC), Committee for Orphan Medicinal Products (COMP), Pediatric Committee (PDCO) and Committee for Advanced Therapies (CAT). The committees consider the risk/benefit ratio for the therapeutic product to ascertain its safety and efficacy as per the European regulations and legislation (Demetzos, 2016). The product development includes the preclinical studies in animals for determining any associated toxicity, the clinical studies for evaluating the effectiveness and defining the appropriate dose and also the post-approval studies for monitoring the safety and efficacy, when the product is already in the market.

Nanomedicines, as defined by The European Science Foundation (ESF), is "the science and technology of diagnosing, treating, and preventing disease and the traumatic injury, of relieving pain, and preserving and improving the human health, using molecular tools and molecular knowledge of the human body" (D'Silva and Van Calster, 2009). The nanobiotechnological compositions, as per EU, falls under three preexisting Directive frameworks. The first Directive 90/385/EEC includes products that are medical devices and are both "active" and "implantable," of which nanomedicines can be a part as they can be implanted. The second, Directive 93/42/EEC, defines as "any instrument, apparatus, appliance, software, material or other article, whether used alone or in combination, including the software intended by its manufacturer to be used specifically for diagnostic and/or therapeutic purposes and necessary for its proper application, intended by the manufacturer to be used for human beings." The third is the Directive 98/79EC-*in vitro* diagnostic medical devices (Preble, 2010).

The European Technology Platform on Nanomedicine (ETP) has been developed comprising of a group of 53 European stakeholders, including industrial and academic experts to write a vision document describing the extrapolation of needs and possibilities until 2020 for the nanotechnology-based healthcare. The focus areas were based on the Strategic Research Agenda wherein the disease that have a great impact on the patients and have a high prevalence in the society were identified and the expected beneficial impact of the nanomedicine on the identified disease in the near future, was addressed. The focus of ETP includes three specific areas of nanomedicine: (a) *in vitro* diagnostics (nanodiagnostics for medical imaging), (b) targeted drug delivery and release (multi-reservoir drug delivery and microchips), and (c) regenerative medicine (nerve regeneration for spinal and limb repair) (Tomellini et al., 2005).

Reflection papers have been drafted to address the specific technical and regulatory principles for the nanoformulations. These include data requirements for intravenous iron-based nanocolloidal products developed with reference to an innovator medicinal product (Ema/Chmp/Swp/100094/2011); data requirements for intravenous liposomal products developed with reference to an innovator liposomal product (Ema/Chmp/Swp/100094/2011 2013); general issues for consideration regarding parenteral administration of coated nanomedicine products (EMA/325027/2013); development of block copolymer micelle medicinal products (Ema/Chmp/13099/2013) (Agency, 2015; Use, 2013, 2017). The EU-NCL (Nanomedicine Characterization Laboratory) was set up as a cooperative arrangement between six European Laboratories and the NCI-NCL of the US to provide access to the public and private developers for characterizing the quality and safety of nanomedicines which are planning to enter into clinical trials or seeking application for marketing authorization. For the strategic research and development, the ITF and the EU Innovation Offices Network provides support to the sponsors to discuss and plan the Regulatory and Scientific advice at the individual, national or EU level (Pita et al., 2018).

11.5.3   REGULATION OF HERBAL NANOMEDICINE PRODUCTS IN INDIA

India, though being in the third rank in the production of nanotechnology-related research articles, but lacks any nanospecific regulation in place, at present. However, now the various scientific agencies with different stakeholders such as government, academia, research organizations, industry, and international collaborative network, have initiated support for creating capacity and directing applications to the nanotechnology developments in the healthcare sector.

Department of Science and Technology (DST), Government of India that is the nodal department for nanotechnology development in India created a working group for the regulation of nanotechnology. Nanomission, a programme of DST has announced the establishment of a National Regulatory Authority Framework Roadmap for Nanotechnology and also framed draft guidelines and best practices for safe handling of NMs. Associated Chambers of Commerce and Industry in India (ASSOCHAM), the Confederation of Indian Industry (CII), and Federation of Indian Chambers of Commerce and Industry (FICCI) are the three major industry associations involved in the promotion of nanotechnology in India. A nanotechnology initiative was put forward by the CII in 2002 to generate a supportive environment for the industry through knowledge exchange missions, workshops, market research, awareness programmes, and other range of services. Council for Scientific and Industrial Research (CSIR) also started a project, "Nano-SHE that is NMs: Application and Impact on Safety, Health, and Environment" for toxicological evaluation of the nanostructured materials. India has also collaborated with International Organizations to foster the development and clinical translation of nanomedicines. A close collaboration between India and Europe was set up in the name of Euro-India net under the six framework programme (FP6) to encourage the collaborations between scientists in the area of nanotechnology. UNESCO and India have also signed a memorandum of understanding to establish a regional center for education and training in biotechnology or nanobiotechnology (Bhatia and Chugh, 2017; Ali and Sinha, 2014).

11.6 CONCLUSION

Natural bioactives are being increasingly used for the prevention and treatment of several human disorders. The low solubility, poor bioavailability, and the toxicity associated with the herbal medicines limit their potential benefits. Development of nanomedicines has paved a way to overcome the challenges with the delivery of natural molecules. However, reducing to nanoscale modifies the physicochemical and the biological properties which may additionally impose newer risks to the patient. This warrants the assessment of toxicity associated with the nanoparticles. Harmonization of the regulatory requirements is crucial for successful clinical translation of nanomedicine.

KEYWORDS

- alanine aminotransferase
- calcium channel blockers
- epigallocatechin gallate
- glutathione
- high content screening
- *in vitro-in vivo* correlation

REFERENCES

Accomasso, L., Cristallini, C., & Giachino, C., (2018). Risk assessment and risk minimization in nanomedicine: A need for predictive, alternative, and 3Rs strategies. *Frontiers in Pharmacology, 9,* 228.

Agency, E. M., (2015). Reflection paper on the data requirements for intravenous iron-based nano-colloidal products developed with reference to an innovator medicinal product. In: *EMA/CHMP/SWP/620008/2012*.

Agrahari, V., & Hiremath, P., (2017). Challenges associated and approaches for successful translation of nano medicines into commercial products. In: *Future Medicine*.

Ahmad, M. Z., Abdel-Wahab, B. A., Alam, A., Zafar, S., Ahmad, J., Ahmad, F. J., Midoux, P., et al., (2016). Toxicity of inorganic nanoparticles used in targeted drug delivery and other biomedical application: An updated account on concern of biomedical nanotoxicology. *Journal of Nanoscience and Nanotechnology, 16,* 7873–7897.

Akagi, K., Sano, M., Ogawa, K., Hirose, M., Goshima, H., & Shirai, T., (2003). Involvement of toxicity as an early event in urinary bladder carcinogenesis induced by phenethyl isothiocyanate, benzyl isothiocyanate, and analogues in F344 rats. *Toxicologic Pathology, 31,* 388–396.

Ali, A., & Sinha, K., (2014). Prospects of nanotechnology development in the health sector in India. *Int. J. Health Sci., 2,* 109–125.

Allen, T. M., & Cullis, P. R., (2004). Drug delivery systems: Entering the mainstream. *Science, 303,* 1818–1822.

Balogh, L., Nigavekar, S. S., Nair, B. M., Lesniak, W., Zhang, C., Sung, L. Y., Kariapper, M. S., et al., (2007). Significant effect of size on the *in vivo* biodistribution of gold composite nanodevices in mouse tumor models. *Nanomedicine: Nanotechnology, Biology and Medicine, 3,* 281–296.

Baron, L., Gombault, A., Fanny, M., Villeret, B., Savigny, F., Guillou, N., Panek, C., et al., (2016). The NLRP3 inflammasome is activated by nanoparticles through ATP, ADP and adenosine. *Cell Death and Disease, 6,* e1629.

Bawa, R., (2013). *41 FDA and Nanotech: Baby Steps Lead to Regulatory Uncertainty.*

Bermudez, E., Mangum, J. B., Wong, B. A., Asgharian, B., Hext, P. M., Warheit, D. B., & Everitt, J. I., (2004). Pulmonary responses of mice, rats, and hamsters to subchronic inhalation of ultrafine titanium dioxide particles. *Toxicological Sciences, 77,* 347–357.

Bhatia, P., & Chugh, A., (2017). A multilevel governance framework for regulation of nanomedicine in India. *Nanotechnology Reviews, 6,* 373–382.

Bian, S. W., Mudunkotuwa, I. A., Rupasinghe, T., & Grassian, V. H., (2011). Aggregation and dissolution of 4 nm ZnO nanoparticles in aqueous environments: Influence of pH, ionic strength, size, and adsorption of humic acid. *Langmuir, 27,* 6059–6068.

Blasi, P., Schoubben, A., Traina, G., Manfroni, G., Barberini, L., Alberti, P. F., Cirotto, C., & Ricci, M., (2013). Lipid nanoparticles for brain targeting III. Long-term stability and *in vivo* toxicity. *International Journal of Pharmaceutics, 454,* 316–323.

Bode, A. M., & Dong, Z., (2015). Toxic phytochemicals and their potential risks for human cancer. *Cancer Prevention Research, 8,* 1–8.

Borel, T., & Sabliov, C., (2014). Nanodelivery of bioactive components for food applications: Types of delivery systems, properties, and their effect on ADME profiles and toxicity of nanoparticles. *Annual Review of Food Science and Technology, 5,* 197–213.

Brown, D. M., Stone, V., Findlay, P., MacNee, W., & Donaldson, K., (2000). Increased inflammation and intracellular calcium caused by ultrafine carbon black is independent of transition metals or other soluble components. *Occupational and Environmental Medicine, 57,* 685–691.

Burgos-Morón, E., Calderón-Montaño, J. M., Salvador, J., Robles, A., & López-Lázaro, M., (2010). The dark side of curcumin. *International Journal of Cancer, 126,* 1771–1775.

Chaudhry, Q., Scotter, M., Blackburn, J., Ross, B., Boxall, A., Castle, L., Aitken, R., & Watkins, R., (2008). Applications and implications of nanotechnologies for the food sector. *Food Additives and Contaminants*, *25,* 241–258.

Cho, W. S., Cho, M., Jeong, J., Choi, M., Cho, H. Y., Han, B. S., Kim, S. H., et al., (2009). Acute toxicity and pharmacokinetics of 13 nm-sized PEG-coated gold nanoparticles. *Toxicology and Applied Pharmacology*, *236,* 16–24.

Coccini, T., Barni, S., Manzo, L., & Roda, E., (2013). Apoptosis induction and histological changes in rat kidney following Cd-doped silica nanoparticle exposure: Evidence of persisting effects. *Toxicology Mechanisms and Methods*, *23,* 566–575.

Crowell, J. A., Korytko, P. J., Morrissey, R. L., Booth, T. D., & Levine, B. S., (2004). Resveratrol-associated renal toxicity. *Toxicological Sciences*, *82,* 614–619.

D'Silva, J., & Van, C. G., (2009). Taking temperature: A review of European Union regulation in nanomedicine. *European Journal of Health Law*, *16,* 249–269.

Demetzos, C., (2016). Regulatory framework for nanomedicines. In: *Pharmaceutical Nanotechnology.* (Springer).

Dobrovolskaia, M. A., & McNeil, S. E., (2013). Understanding the correlation between *in vitro* and *in vivo* immunotoxicity tests for nanomedicines. *Journal of Controlled Release*, *172,* 456–466.

Dobrovolskaia, M. A., Shurin, M., & Shvedova, A. A., (2016). Current understanding of interactions between nanoparticles and the immune system. *Toxicology and Applied Pharmacology*, *299,* 78–89.

Driscoll, K. E., Deyo, L. C., Carter, J. M., Howard, B. W., Hassenbein, D. G., & Bertram, T. A., (1997). Effects of particle exposure and particle-elicited inflammatory cells on mutation in rat alveolar epithelial cells. *Carcinogenesis*, *18,* 423–430.

Duncan, R., & Gaspar, R., (2011). Nanomedicine(s) under the microscope. *Molecular Pharmaceutics*, *8,* 2101–2141.

Fiedler, F. A., & Reynolds, G. H., (1993). Legal problems of nanotechnology: An overview. *S. Cal. Interdisc. LJ.*, *3,* 593.

Fischer, H. C., & Chan, W. C., (2007). Nanotoxicity: The growing need for *in vivo* study. *Current Opinion in Biotechnology*, *18,* 565–571.

Food and Drug Administration, (2007). *Nanotechnology: A Report of the US Food and Drug Administration Nanotechnology Task Force* (Food and Drug Administration).

Food and Drug Administration, (2011). *Guidance for Industry, Considering Whether an FDA-Regulated Product Involves the Application of Nanotechnology.*

Food and Drug Administration, (2014). *Guidance for Industry Safety of Nanomaterials in Cosmetic Products.* Center for Food Safety and Applied Nutrition, US Department of Health and Human Services, Rockville, MD. http://www.fda.gov/downloads/Cosmetics/GuidanceRegulation/GuidanceDocuments/UCM.300932 (accessed on 26 June 2020).

Fornaguera, C., Calderó, G., Mitjans, M., Vinardell, M. P., Solans, C., & Vauthier, C., (2015). Interactions of PLGA nanoparticles with blood components: Protein adsorption, coagulation, activation of the complement system and hemolysis studies. *Nanoscale*, *7,* 6045–6058.

Frigell, J., García, I., Gómez-Vallejo, V., Llop, J., & Penadés, S., (2013). 68Ga-labeled gold glyconanoparticles for exploring blood-brain barrier permeability: Preparation, biodistribution studies, and improved brain uptake via neuropeptide conjugation. *Journal of the American Chemical Society*, *136,* 449–457.

Fubini, B., & Hubbard, A., (2003). Reactive oxygen species (ROS) and reactive nitrogen species (RNS) generation by silica in inflammation and fibrosis. *Free Radical Biology and Medicine, 34,* 1507–1516.

Furukawa, A., Oikawa, S., Murata, M., Hiraku, Y., & Kawanishi, S., (2003). (−)-Epigallocatechin gallate causes oxidative damage to isolated and cellular DNA. *Biochemical Pharmacology, 66,* 1769–1778.

Galati, G., & O'brien, P., (2004). Serial review: Flavonoids and isoflavones (phytoestrogens): Absorption, metabolism, and bioactivity. *Free Radical Biol. Med., 37,* 287–303.

Gandhi, S., Srinivasan, B., & Akarte, A. S., (2013). An experimental assessment of toxic potential of nanoparticle preparation of heavy metals in streptozotocin induced diabetes. *Experimental and Toxicologic Pathology, 65,* 1127–1135.

Godwin, H., Nameth, C., Avery, D., Bergeson, L. L., Bernard, D., Beryt, E., Boyes, W., et al., (2015). *Nanomaterial Categorization for Assessing Risk Potential to Facilitate Regulatory Decision-Making.* ACS Publications.

Goel, R., Shah, N., Visaria, R., Paciotti, G. F., & Bischof, J. C., (2009). Biodistribution of TNF-α-coated gold nanoparticles in an *in vivo* model system. *Nanomedicine, 4,* 401–410.

Gross, E., Toste, F. D., & Somorjai, G. A., (2015). Polymer-encapsulated metallic nanoparticles as a bridge between homogeneous and heterogeneous catalysis. *Catalysis Letters, 145,* 126–138.

Guo, M., Xu, X., Yan, X., Wang, S., Gao, S., & Zhu, S., (2013). *In vivo* biodistribution and synergistic toxicity of silica nanoparticles and cadmium chloride in mice. *Journal of Hazardous Materials, 260,* 780–788.

Han, X. Y., Du, W. L., Huang, Q. C., Xu, Z. R., & Wang, Y. Z., (2012). Changes in small intestinal morphology and digestive enzyme activity with oral administration of copper-loaded chitosan nanoparticles in rats. *Biological Trace Element Research, 145,* 355–360.

Harris, S., (2009). The regulation of nanomedicine: Will the existing regulatory scheme of the FDA suffice. *Rich. JL and Tech., 16,* 1.

Hirose, M., Hoshiya, T., Mizoguchi, Y., Nakamura, A., Akagi, K., & Shirai, T., (2001). Green tea catechins enhance tumor development in the colon without effects in the lung or thyroid after pretreatment with 1, 2-dimethylhydrazine or 2, 2'-dihydroxy-di-n-propylnitrosamine in male F344 rats. *Cancer Letters, 168,* 23–29.

Hoet, P., Legiest, B., Geys, J., & Nemery, B., (2009). Do nanomedicines require novel safety assessments to ensure their safety for long-term human use? *Drug Safety, 32,* 625–636.

Kahru, A., & Savolainen, K., (2010). Potential hazard of nanoparticles: From properties to biological and environmental effects. *Toxicology, 2,* 89–91.

Kamboj, V. P., (2000). Herbal medicine. *Current Science, 78,* 35–39.

Kostarelos, K., (2003). Rational design and engineering of delivery systems for therapeutics: Biomedical exercises in colloid and surface science. *Advances in Colloid and Interface Science, 106,* 147–168.

Laverman, P., Dams, E. T. M., Storm, G., Hafmans, T. G., Croes, H. J., Oyen, W. J., Corstens, F. H., & Boerman, O. C., (2001). Microscopic localization of PEG-liposomes in a rat model of focal infection. *Journal of Controlled Release, 75,* 347–355.

Layali, E., Tahmasbpour, E., & Jorsaraei, S., (2016). The effects of silver nanoparticles on oxidative stress and sperm parameters quality in male rats. *Journal of Babol University of Medical Sciences, 18,* 48–55.

Leite-Silva, V. R., Le Lamer, M., Sanchez, W. Y., Liu, D. C., Sanchez, W. H., Morrow, I., Martin, D., et al., (2013). The effect of formulation on the penetration of coated and uncoated zinc oxide nanoparticles into the viable epidermis of human skin *in vivo*. *European Journal of Pharmaceutics and Biopharmaceutics*, *84,* 297–308.

Li, X., Yang, X., Yuwen, L., Yang, W., Weng, L., Teng, Z., & Wang, L., (2016). Evaluation of toxic effects of CdTe quantum dots on the reproductive system in adult male mice. *Biomaterials*, *96,* 24–32.

Lin, S., Wang, X., Ji, Z., Chang, C. H., Dong, Y., Meng, H., Liao, Y. P., et al., (2014). Aspect ratio plays a role in the hazard potential of CeO_2 nanoparticles in mouse lung and zebra fish gastrointestinal tract. *ACS Nano, 8,* 4450–4464.

Liu, D., Lin, B., Shao, W., Zhu, Z., Ji, T., & Yang, C., (2014). *In vitro* and *in vivo* studies on the transport of PEGylated silica nanoparticles across the blood-brain barrier. *ACS Applied Materials and Interfaces*, *6,* 2131–2136.

Lynch, I., Weiss, C., & Valsami-Jones, E., (2014). A strategy for grouping of nanomaterials based on key physico-chemical descriptors as a basis for safer-by-design NMs. *Nano Today*, *9,* 266–270.

Ma-Hock, L., Burkhardt, S., Strauss, V., Gamer, A. O., Wiench, K., Van, R. B., & Landsiedel, R., (2009). Development of a short-term inhalation test in the rat using nano-titanium dioxide as a model substance. *Inhalation Toxicology, 21,* 102–118.

Majumder, P., (2017). Nanoparticle-assisted herbal synergism an effective therapeutic approach for the targeted treatment of breast cancer: A novel prospective. glob. *J. Nanomed.*, *2,* 555595.

Mozaffari, Z., Parivar, K., Roodbari, N. H., & Irani, S., (2015). Histopathological evaluation of the toxic effects of zinc oxide (ZnO) nanoparticles on testicular tissue of NMRI adult mice. *Adv. Stud. Biol.*, *7,* 275–291.

Muthu, M. S., & Feng, S. S., (2009). Pharmaceutical stability aspects of nanomedicines. *Nanomedicine, 4,* 857–860.

Oberdörster, G., Oberdörster, E., & Oberdörster, J., (2005). Nanotoxicology: An emerging discipline evolving from studies of ultrafine particles. *Environmental Health Perspectives*, *113,* 823.

Pan, T. L., Wang, P. W., Al-Suwayeh, S. A., Huang, Y. J., & Fang, J. Y., (2012). Toxicological effects of cationic nanobubbles on the liver and kidneys: Biomarkers for predicting the risk. *Food and Chemical Toxicology*, *50,* 3892–3901.

Paranjpe, M., & Müller-Goymann, C. C., (2014). Nanoparticle-mediated pulmonary drug delivery: A review. *International Journal of Molecular Sciences*, *15,* 5852–5873.

Pariser, A. R., Xu, K., Milto, J., & Cote, T. R., (2011). Regulatory considerations for developing drugs for rare diseases: Orphan designations and early phase clinical trials. *Discovery Medicine*, *11,* 367–375.

Petrica, L., Vlad, A., Gluhovschi, G., Zamfir, A., Popescu, C., Gadalean, F., Dumitrascu, V., et al., (2015). Glycated peptides are associated with proximal tubule dysfunction in type 2 diabetes mellitus. *International Journal of Clinical and Experimental Medicine*, *8,* 2516.

Picking, D., (2017). The global regulatory framework for medicinal plants. In: *Pharmacognosy.* (Elsevier).

Pita, R., Ehmann, F., & Thürmer, R., (2018). Regulation of biomedical applications of functionalized nanomaterials in the European Union. In: *Biomedical Applications of Functionalized Nanomaterials.* (Elsevier).

Pradhan, S., Patra, P., Mitra, S., Dey, K. K., Jain, S., Sarkar, S., Roy, S., et al., (2014). Manganese nanoparticles: Impact on non-nodulated plant as a potent enhancer in nitrogen metabolism and toxicity study both *in vivo* and *in vitro*. *Journal of Agricultural and Food Chemistry*, *62*, 8777–8785.

Preble, E. S., (2010). Preemptive legislation in the European Union and the united states on the topic of nanomedicine: Examining the questions raised by smart medical technology. *Ind. Health L. Rev.*, *7*, 397.

Pridgen, E. M., Alexis, F., & Farokhzad, O. C., (2014). Polymeric nanoparticle technologies for oral drug delivery. *Clinical Gastroenterology and Hepatology*, *12*, 1605–1610.

Program, N. T., (1993). NTP toxicology and carcinogenesis studies of turmeric oleoresin (CAS No. 8024-37-1)(major component 79%-85% curcumin, CAS No. 458-37-7) in F344/N rats and B6C3F1 mice (feed studies). *National Toxicology Program Technical Report Series*, *427*, 1.

Ren, L., Zhang, J., Zou, Y., Zhang, L., Wei, J., Shi, Z., Li, Y., Guo, C., Sun, Z., & Zhou, X., (2016). Silica nanoparticles induce reversible damage of spermatogenic cells via RIPK1 signal pathways in C57 mice. *International Journal of Nanomedicine*, *11*, 2251.

Russo, M., Spagnuolo, C., Tedesco, I., & Russo, G. L., (2010). Phytochemicals in cancer prevention and therapy: Truth or dare? *Toxins*, *2*, 517–551.

Sainz, V., Conniot, J., Matos, A. I., Peres, C., Zupanðið, E., Moura, L., Silva, L. C., et al., (2015). Regulatory aspects on nanomedicines. *Biochemical and Biophysical Research Communications*, *468*, 504–510.

Sarhan, O. M. M., & Hussein, R. M., (2014). Effects of intraperitoneally injected silver nanoparticles on histological structures and blood parameters in the albino rat. *International Journal of Nanomedicine*, *9*, 1505.

Sastry, K., Rashmi, H., & Rao, N., (2010). Nanotechnology patents as R & D indicators for disease management strategies in agriculture. *Journal of Intellectual Property Rights*, *15*, 197–205.

Satalkar, P., Elger, B. S., & Shaw, D. M., (2016). Defining nano, nanotechnology, and nanomedicine: Why should it matter? *Science and Engineering Ethics*, *22*, 1255–1276.

Saunders, M., Hutchison, G., & Carreira, S. C., (2015). Reproductive toxicity of nanomaterials. *Therapy*, *40*, 44.

Sayes, C. M., Marchione, A. A., Reed, K. L., & Warheit, D. B., (2007). Comparative pulmonary toxicity assessments of C60 water suspensions in rats: Few differences in fullerene toxicity *in vivo* in contrast to *in vitro* profiles. *Nano Letters.*, *7*, 2399–2406.

Singh, S., & Nalwa, H. S., (2007). Nanotechnology and health safety-toxicity and risk assessments of nanostructured materials on human health. *Journal of Nanoscience and Nanotechnology*, *7*, 3048–3070.

Smolkova, B., Dusinska, M., & Gabelova, A., (2017). Nanomedicine and epigenome. Possible health risks. *Food and Chemical Toxicology*, *109*, 780–796.

Stoccoro, A., Karlsson, H. L., Coppedè, F., & Migliore, L., (2013). Epigenetic effects of nano-sized materials. *Toxicology*, *313*, 3–14.

Tomellini, R., Faure, U., & Panzer, O., (2005). European technology platform on nanomedicine. nanotechnology for health. Vision paper and basis for a strategic research agenda for nanomedicine. *European Technology Platform Nanomedicine*, 1–35.

Use, C. F. M. P. F. H., (2013). Joint MHLW/EMA reflection paper on the development of block copolymer micelle medicinal products. In.: *EMA/CHMP/13099*.

Vega-Villa, K. R., Takemoto, J. K., Yáñez, J. A., Remsberg, C. M., Forrest, M. L., & Davies, N. M., (2008). Clinical toxicities of nanocarrier systems. *Advanced Drug Delivery Reviews*, *60*, 929–938.

Viacava, G. E., Vázquez, F. J., Ayala-Zavala, J. F., & Ansorena, M. R., (2017). Sustainability challenges involved in use of nanotechnology in the agro food Sector. *Sustainability Challenges in the Agro-Food Sector, 343.*

Wachtel-Galor, S., & Benzie, I. F., (2011). *Herbal Medicine: Biomolecular and Clinical Aspects.*

Wang, X., Tian, J., Yong, K. T., Zhu, X., Lin, M. C. M., Jiang, W., Li, J., et al., (2016). Immunotoxicity assessment of CdSe/ZnS quantum dots in macrophages, lymphocytes, and BALB/c mice. *Journal of Nanobiotechnology, 14,* 10.

Wang, Y., Chen, Z., Ba, T., Pu, J., Chen, T., Song, Y., Gu, Y., et al., (2013). Susceptibility of young and adult rats to the oral toxicity of titanium dioxide nanoparticles. *Small, 9,* 1742–1752.

Watkins, R., Wu, L., Zhang, C., Davis, R. M., & Xu, B., (2015). Natural product-based nanomedicine: Recent advances and issues. *International Journal of Nanomedicine, 10,* 6055.

Win-Shwe, T. T., & Fujimaki, H., (2011). Nanoparticles and neurotoxicity. *International Journal of Molecular Sciences, 12,* 6267–6280.

Yamagishi, Y., Watari, A., Hayata, Y., Li, X., Kondoh, M., Tsutsumi, Y., & Yagi, K., (2013). Hepatotoxicity of sub-nanosized platinum particles in mice. *Die Pharmazie: An International Journal of Pharmaceutical Sciences, 68,* 178–182.

Zhang, D. D., Hartsky, M. A., & Warheit, D. B., (2002). Time course of quartz and TiO_2 particle-induced pulmonary inflammation and neutrophil apoptotic responses in rats. *Experimental Lung Research, 28,* 641–670.

Zhang, W., Wang, G., See, E., Shaw, J. P., Baguley, B. C., Liu, J., Amirapu, S., & Wu, Z., (2015). Post-insertion of poloxamer 188 strengthened liposomal membrane and reduced drug irritancy and *in vivo* precipitation, superior to PEGylation. *Journal of Controlled Release, 203,* 161–169.

Zhao, J., & Castranova, V., (2011). Toxicology of nanomaterials used in nanomedicine. *Journal of Toxicology and Environmental Health, Part B14,* 593–632.

Zolnik, B. S., & Sadrieh, N., (2009). Regulatory perspective on the importance of ADME assessment of nanoscale material containing drugs. *Advanced Drug Delivery Reviews, 61,* 422–427.

CHAPTER 12

Resveratrol-Loaded Phytomedicines for Management of Cancer

SHAKIR SALEEM, RUQAIYAH KHAN, and SANDEEP ARORA

Department of Pharmacology, Chitkara College of Pharmacy, Chitkara University, NH-64, Jansla, Rajpura, Punjab – 140401, India, E-mails: shakirsaleem@gmail.com; shakir.saleem@chitkara.edu.in (*S. Saleem*)

ABSTRACT

Cancer has recently become one of the prominent reasons for human mortality. Since ages, humans have used natural products to prevent illnesses and this hints us that bioactive compounds are one of the best alternative sources which can be employed in the prevention and treatment of various kinds of diseases including cancer. Resveratrol, chemically known as 3,4,'5-trihydroxytrans-stilbene, is a non-flavonoid polyphenol phytoalexin that naturally occurs in various species of plants, including peanuts, grapes, pines, and berries. It has been used since ages in Chinese and Japanese traditional medicine to treat inflammation, headaches, cancers, and amenorrhea. There are several reports of nanoformulations loaded with resveratrol has potential anticancer activity including but not limited to cancer of stomach, prostate, ovaries, alimentary canal, and breast. The nanoformulation of resveratrol has also enhanced its bioavailability in humans. The stability can be adjusted using several natural polymers, such as gelatin, PEG, and PLGA, alone or in combination with synthetic polymers, like chitosan (CS) and casein. Further studies are required to establish it as a potent clinical anticancer agent.

12.1   INTRODUCTION

Cancer is one of the most commonly diagnosed diseases, and its related morbidity and mortality constitute a very significant health problem worldwide. Since decades, great efforts are in process to discover an effective cure but cancer persists as one of the prominent reasons for human mortality. It has been estimated that by 2025, more than 2 million new cases of cancer will be diagnosed, and more than 600,000 cancer-related mortality is expected in the United States (Ko et al., 2017). There have been a multitude of unique advances in the diagnosis and surveillance of cancer, nevertheless, the overall survival rate for cancer has not bettered yet. Improved clinical outcomes have been achieved through various individualized care medicines, including but not limited to targeted therapies (Okimoto et al., 2014). But, some of the recent advances in cancer treatment ended up giving rise to acquired resistance to many chemotherapeutic agents (Krepler et al., 2016).

The development of cancer is a multistep phenomenon involving multifactorial processes where clear and discrete molecular and cellular alterations can be seen. These cellular changes are distinct and have closely connected phases of initiation, promotion, and progression of cancer (Hong et al., 1997; Sethi et al., 2012; Chai et al., 2015). Development of resistance is the prime concern of the current cancer therapies, which includes chemotherapy, targeted agents, radiation, surgery, and immunosuppression (Sethi et al., 2009). The alternate way to encounter grave situations involving severe cancer is to detect and diagnose early in the benign stage, this can help in managing cancer in a better way giving more chances of survival. But the even the diagnosis of cancer is not guaranteed with the latest trends in diagnostics (Janakiram et al., 2016). The discovery of a lead molecule with fervent anticancer activity and minimal side effects is the primary objective in the fight against cancer.

12.2   PHYTOMEDICINE AND ITS HISTORY

Since ancient times, natural products have been used to prevent several chronic diseases, including cancer (Shanmugam et al., 2011; Aggarwal et al., 2009; Yang et al., 2013; Tang et al., 2014; Kannaiyan et al., 2011; Hsieh et al., 2015; Bishayee et al., 2016; Shrimali et al., 2013). Bioactive compounds are one of the best alternative sources which can be employed in the prevention and treatment of various kinds of diseases including cancer (Shanmuugam et al., 2012, 2016, 2017, 2018; Prasannan et al., 2012). Phytochemicals like phytoestrogens have been found to interfere with several cellular-signaling pathways simultaneously, with no or minimal toxicity to normal cells (Newman et al., 2016; Aggarwal et al., 2004). The application of substances to prevent or delay the development of carcinogenesis has been termed chemoprevention (Hong et al., 1997), and there is a burgeoning interest in the use of natural compounds as possible chemopreventive and therapeutic agents for human populations.

Resveratrol has been frequently reported as a potent anti-cancer agent and this is why it has gained prominence recently (Aggarwal et al., 2004; Bishayee et al., 2009, 2010; Sinha et al., 2016). Resveratrol, chemically known as 3,4,'5-trihydroxy-trans-stilbene, is a non-flavonoid polyphenol phytoalexin that naturally occurs in various species of plants, including peanuts, grapes, pines, and berries. It helps the plant to develop immunity against the infection from different pathogens (Cucciolla et al., 2007). Surprisingly, it has been used since ages in Chinese and Japanese traditional medicine to treat inflammation, headaches, cancers, and amenorrhea.

12.3   RESVERATROL AND ITS ANALOGS

The stressful conditions like climatic vicissitude, ozone exposure, sunlight, heavy metal, and infection to a pathogen like *Botrytis cinerea* leads to the activation of stilbene synthase enzyme in plants which in turns produces resveratrol ($C_{14}H_{12}O_3$). It has two isoforms: trans-resveratrol (more stable) and cis-resveratrol (Athar et al., 2007).

The trans-isoform is the major isoform of resveratrol and is also extensively studied for several pharmacological actions. Trans-isoform is transformed into cis isoform on exposure to heat and ultraviolet radiation. Resveratrol has been classed as a phytoestrogen as its structure is like that of the synthetic estrogen diethylstilbestrol. Its biological sources are very common as, resveratrol is easily available in common food items and augments health in ways similar to viniferins, pterostilbene, and piceid (Jeandet et al., 2002). Moreover, few semi-synthetic resveratrol analogs were found to have specific pharmacological benefits like chemopreventive actions (Cai et al., 2004), antioxidant effects (Colin et al., 2008) and anti-aging properties (Moran et al., 2009). It had also been reported that resveratrol can reverse the resistance to some drugs in different types and sizes of a tumor by over-sensitizing them to chemotherapeutic agents (Mondal et al., 2016; Lee et al., 2016). Many pharmacological effects have been elucidated by the trans-resveratrol and its glucoside including cardio-protective, anti-oxidative, anti-inflammatory, estrogenic, and anti-estrogenic, and anti-tumor activities (Stagos et al., 2012; Carter et al., 2014). Additionally, the antimicrobial action (Stagos et al., 2012) of trans-resveratrol was reported to be useful in the management of cognitive impairments like dementia (Mazzanti et al., 2016; Molino et al., 2016).

Resveratrol has broad-spectrum antimicrobial activity and has a wide-spectrum pharmacological activity like antioxidant and cardioprotective functions. But it has been trending recently because of its outstanding anti-cancer as well as chemopreventive potential (Gupta et al., 2011). It has been demonstrated that resveratrol can modulate many intracellular targets of cancer, which influence many vital processes like cell growth, inflammation, apoptosis, angiogenesis, cellular, and lymphatic invasion, and metastasis. Resveratrol boosts the pro-apoptotic effects of cytokines (namely TRAIL), chemotherapeutic agents, and gamma radiation (Athar et al., 2013).

12.4 *IN VITRO* PHARMACOLOGICAL PROPERTIES AND ANTI-CANCER EFFECTS OF RESVERATROL

Resveratrol is reported to possess multidimensional properties which produce salubrious effects like anti-inflammatory, anti-oxidative, and anti-aging qualities (Wadsworth et al., 1999; Ray et al., 1999; Baur et al., 2006). It has also been found in red wine, and hence it is often hypothesized that resveratrol is the prime element behind French Paradox, the minimized risk of cardiovascular disorders in French people despite the high intake of satu-rated fats; which has been linked with high red wine consumption (Renaud et al., 1992). Jang et al. in 1997 reported that resveratrol inhibits carcinogenesis in a mouse-skin cancer model, and thereafter a resveratrol related publication became superfluous. A multitude of research papers have reported the anti-cancer potential of resveratrol in human cell lines, including but not limited to, myeloid, and lymphoid cancer cells, breast, skin, cervix, ovary, stomach, prostate, colon, liver, pancreas, and thyroid cancer cells (Aggarwal et al., 2004; Minamoto et al., 1999; Khansari et al., 2009; Barzilai et al., 2004). Resveratrol has a grand role in preventing cancer and affects different stages of cancer ranging from initiation and promotion to progression by interfering and modulating the diverse signal-transduction pathways that monitor cell growth, cell division, inflammation, apoptosis, metastasis, and angiogenesis.

Many *in vitro* studies have examined the anti-proliferative and proapoptotic activity of resveratrol in human prostate cancer cells, and its mechanism of action. It was found that the growth of LNCaP cells (hormone-sensitive cells), DU-145 (androgen-independent) cells, and PC-3 (hormone-independent line possessing dysfunctional androgen receptors) cells were arrested in a concentration-dependent manner. Resveratrol also antagonized the formation of free radicals in macrophages and reduced the oxidative stress within premalignant cells, and it decreased the production of NO in PC-3 and DU-145 cells, reducing growth and metastasis of prostate cancer (Ratan et al., 2002).

Resveratrol-induced apoptosis in LNCaP and DU145 prostate cancer cell lines through different PKC-mediated and MAPK dependent pathways (Shih et al., 2004). Furthermore, resveratrol-mediated apoptosis is reported to be associated with p53 activation and occurs by the death receptor Fas/CD95/APO-1 in several human cancer cells (Athar et al., 2009). It is also assumed that resveratrol exerts its chemopreventive action partially by interfering with the expression or function of the androgen receptor (Ratan et al., 2002). Resveratrol has a very interesting mechanism of chemoprevention, i.e., by sensitization effect as reported by many *in vitro* and *in vivo* research studies, resveratrol can overcome chemoresistance in tumor cells by regulating apoptotic pathways, downregulating drug transporters, downmodulating proteins involved in the proliferation of tumor cell, and by inhibiting NF-κB and STAT-3 pathway (Gupta et al., 2011).

12.4.1 ANTI-TUMOR INITIATION ACTIVITY

Initiation of neoplasia occurs via alteration or mutation of genes spontaneously due to exposure to a carcinogenic agent, and finally resulting in mutagenesis (Minamoto et al., 1999). Reactive oxygen species (ROS) react with the genetic material, DNA, and chromatin proteins, causing several types of DNA damage (Barzilai et al., 2004; Fruehauf et al., 2007). In fact, the chemical carcinogens must undergo phase-I biotransformation, especially via cytochrome P450 enzyme to damage DNA in cells and transforms them into reactive electrophiles. Additionally, the formation of carcinogen-DNA adducts gives rise to chemical-induced carcinogenesis (Windmill et al., 1997). This is irreversible initiation stage but can be stopped by inhibiting the activity and expression of certain cytochrome P450 enzymes and enhancing the activity of phase-II detoxification enzymes, which transform carcinogens into less toxic and soluble products (Galati et al., 2000; Guengerich et al., 2000) (see Table 12.1).

TABLE 12.1 Enlists the Anti-Tumor Activity of Resveratrol in Several Cell Lines and Proposes the Mechanism of Action Followed

Activity	Cell Line	Mechanism of Action
Anti-tumor	Human Leukemia HL-60 cells	Suppressed free radical formation induced by 12-O-tetradecanoylphorbol-13-acetate (Windmill et al., 1997).
		Scavenger of hydroxyls and superoxides, as well as radicals induced by metals/enzymes (Leonard et al., 2003).
		Protects against lipid peroxidation within cell membranes and damage to DNA resulting from ROS (Leonard et al., 2003).
	Human breast epithelial Michigan cancer foundation (MCF)-10A cells	Inhibit 2,3,7,8-tetrachlorodibenzo-p-dioxin (TCDD)–induced expression of cytochrome P450 1A1 (CYP1A1) and 1B1 (CYP1B1), as well as their catalytic actions (Chen et al., 2004).
	Human breast cancer MCF-7 and liver cancer HepG2 cells	Abrogate the CYP1A activity induced by environmental aryl hydrocarbon benzo[a] pyrene (B[a]P) and catalyzed by directly suppressing the CYP1A1/1A2 enzyme activity and the signal-transduction pathway that up-regulates the expression of carcinogen-activating enzymes (Ciolino et al., 1999).
		Inhibition of TCDD-induced recruitment of AhR and ARNT to the CYP1A1/1A2 and CYP1A1/1B1 promoter and decreased their expression (Beedanagari et al., 2009).
	Gastric cancer AGS cells	Reduced TCDD-induced, AhR-mediated CYP1A1 expression (Peng et al., 2009).
	Human leukemia K562 cells	Increases both the activity and expression of NAD (P)H: quinone oxidoreductase-1 (NQO1), a carcinogen-detoxifying phase-II enzyme (Hsieh et al., 2006).

12.4.2 ANTI-TUMOR-PROMOTION ACTIVITY

Tumor promotion involves clonally enlarging initiated cells to create a continuously proliferating, premalignant lesion. Tumor promoters are generally found to alter the expression of the gene, subsequently leading to increased cellular proliferation and decreased cell death (Klaunig et al., 2004). Studies conducted *in vitro* have revealed that resveratrol exerts anti-proliferative activity by inducing apoptosis in cells. Of these, resveratrol modifies the balance of cyclins as well as cyclin-dependent kinases, resulting in cell cycle inhibition at G0/G1 phase. For example, a link has been found between the inhibition of cyclin D1/CDK4 by resveratrol and cell cycle arrest in the G0/G1 phase within different cancer cells (Wolter et al., 2001; Benitez et al., 2007; Bai et al., 2010; Gatouillat et al., 2010). Resveratrol was also shown to elevate the levels of cyclin A and E, with cell cycle seizure in the G2/M and S phases (Ferry-Dumazet et al., 2002; Filippi-Chiela et al., 2011). Similar reports have specified that resveratrol causes the arrest of cell cycles and also causes the activation of the p53-dependent pathway (Liao et al., 2010; Rashid et al., 2011; Hsieh et al., 2011) (see Table 12.2).

TABLE 12.2 Describes the Mechanism of Action for Anti-Tumor Activity of Resveratrol in Different Types of Cancer Cell Lines

Activity	Cell Line	Mechanism of Action
Anti-tumor Promotion	Human skin cancer A431 cells	Downregulating the expression of cyclin D1, cyclin D2, and cyclin E.
		Inhibiting the activities and/or expression of CDK2, CDK4, and CDK6.
		Upregulating the expression of p21 (Gartel et al., 2002).
	Breast cancer MCF-7 and human prostate cancer DU-145 cells	Modulating CDK4 and cyclin D1 expression (Kim et al., 2003a).
	A549 cells	S phase arrest, reduced retinoblastoma protein (Rb) phosphorylation, and induced p21 and p53 protein expression (Kim et al., 2003b).
	HL-60 cells	Modulating diverse signal transduction pathways via regulation of the levels of Fas and Fas-ligand and inducing apoptosis (Clement et al., 1998; Delmas et al., 2003).
	Leukemic THP-1 cell line	Induces Fas-independent apoptosis (Tsan et al., 2000).
	Leukemia CEM-C7H2 cells	Induces Fas-independent apoptosis (Bernhard et al., 2000).

TABLE 12.2   *(Continued)*

Activity	Cell Line	Mechanism of Action
	Human breast cancer MDA-MB-231 cells	Resveratrol increased the cytoplasmic concentration of calcium in cancer cells and activate p53 causing the proapoptotic gene's transcription (Van Ginkel et al., 2015).
	Ovarian, (Kueck et al., 2007) breast, (Li et al., 2006) uterine, (Sexton et al., 2006) prostate, (Aziz et al., 2006) and multiple myeloma cells (Bhardwaj et al., 2007)	Abrogating Akt phosphorylation.

12.4.3   ANTI-TUMOR-PROGRESSION ACTIVITY

Progression of tumor implies the growth in size and increase in a number of cells in the tumor. This progression implicates various processes such as that lead to tumor metastasis. It has been seen that several genes are mutated or deleted physiologically that sustain the development of aggressive tumors. The invasion of healthy cells and metastasis of cancerous cells include the destruction of the extracellular matrix (ECM) and the basement membrane, by proteolytic enzymes, such as matrix metalloproteinases (MMPs). Out of all these enzymes, MMP-2 and MMP-9 are highly expressed within different types of malignant tumors modifying the cellular invasion and its metastatic properties (Nelson et al., 2000). Tissue inhibitor metalloproteinase proteins (TIMPs), on the other hand, are a protein group comprising TIMP-1, -2, -3, and -4 acting as natural MMP inhibitors (Jinga et al., 2006). Invasive tumors require new blood vessels which are fulfilled via angiogenesis. During the process of angiogenesis, endothelial cells can be activated by several growth factors, like fibroblast growth factor (FGF) and VEGF. Obstructing the development of newly formed blood vessels causes the supply of nutrients and oxygen to be reduced and, as a result, the size of the tumor and metastasis may also be reduced (see Table 12.3).

12.5   PRE-CLINICAL STUDIES

Resveratrol has also been reported to possess a significant anti-cancer property in various pre-clinical animal models (see Table 12.4). Table 12.4 summarizes the major outcomes of several research studies.

TABLE 12.3 The Anti-Tumor Progression Potential of Resveratrol and its Mode of Action

Activity	Cell Line	Mechanism of Action
Anti-tumor progression	Liver cancer HepG2 cells	Up-regulated TIMP-1 protein expression and down-regulated MMP-9 activity (Weng et al., 2010).
	Liver cancer Hep3B cells	Activities of MMP-2 and MMP-9 were decreased, along with a rise in the protein expression level of TIMP-2 (Weng et al., 2010).
	Breast cancer MDA-MB231 cells	Inhibition of the epidermal growth factor (EGF)-induced elevation of cell migration, and of the expression of MMP-9 (Lee et al., 2011).
	Human ovarian cancer cells	Abrogating the activation of the PI3K/Akt and MAPK signaling pathways (Cao et al., 2004).
	A549 lung cancer cells	Inhibited TGF--induced EMT by augmenting the expression of E-cadherin and attenuating the expression of vimentin and fibronectin, as well as the EMT-inducing transcription factors Slug and Snail (Wang et al., 2013).
	Pancreatic cancer PANC-1 cells	By regulating factors related to EMT (vimentin, E-cadherin, N-cadherin, MMP-2, and MMP-9) and modulating the activation of PI3K/Akt/NF-kB pathways (Lee et al., 2013).

TABLE 12.4 Enlists the Outcomes of *In Vivo* Study Involving Resveratrol

Cancer Model	Animal Model	Outcome
Skin	DMBA/TPA model in female CD-1 mice	Incidence decreases. Number of tumors per mouse decreases (Jang et al., 1997).
	Mouse xenograft models of A431 cells	Xenograft volume decreases. Free radical scavenging Incidence decreases. Number of tumors per mouse decreases (Hao et al., 2013).
	DMBA/TPA model in CD-1 mice	Skin tumor incidence decreases. Apoptosis increases; p53 increases; Bax increases; cytochrome C increases; APAF increases; Bcl2 decreases (Soleas et al., 2002).
	UVB-mediated photocarcinogenesis in female SKH-1 mice	Decrease hyperplasia; p53 increases.

TABLE 12.4 *(Continued)*

Cancer Model	Animal Model	Outcome
		Cox2 decreases; ODC decreases; surviving decreases mRNA and protein (Afaq et al., 2003).
Breast	Spontaneous mammary tumor in female FVB/N HER-2/neu mice	Onset of tumorigenesis decreases.
		Tumor volume decreases.
		Multiplicity decreases.
		Apoptosis increases (Provinciali et al., 2005).
	DMBA-induced mammary carcinogenesis in female Sprague-Dawley rats	Suppressed tumor growth Cell proliferation decreases, Apoptosis increases (Whitsett et al., 2006)
	Female HER-2/neu transgenic mice model	Delays the development and reduces the metastatic growth of spontaneous mammary tumors.
		Apoptosis increases, decreases HER-2/neu mRNA and protein (Provinciali et al., 2005).
Prostate	Athymic nude mice	Tumor volume decreases.
	xenograft models of PC-3 cells	Cell proliferation decreases.
		Apoptosis increases.
		Number of blood vessels decreases (Ganapathy et al., 2010).
	Male nude mice	Tumor growth decreases.
	xenograft models with Du145-EV-Luc	Progression, local invasion decreases.
	or Du145-MTA1	Spontaneous metastasis decreases.
	shRNA-Luc in anterior prostate	Angiogenesis decreases.
		Apoptosis increases (Li et al., 2013).
Lung	Female C57BL/6 mice]	Tumor volume/weight decreases.
	xenograft models of LLC tumors	Metastasis to lung decreases (Kimura et al., 2001).
	C57BL/6 mice implanted with Lewis's lung carcinoma lung tumor model	Angiogenesis decreases. Apoptosis increases (Lee et al., 2006).
Liver	Male Donryu rats	Tumor weight decreases.
	xenograft models of AH109A cells	Metastasis decreases (Miura et al., 2007).

TABLE 12.4 *(Continued)*

Cancer Model	Animal Model	Outcome
	DENA-initiated and PB-promoted hepatocyte nodule formation in female	Tumor growth decreases.
		Apoptosis increases.
	Sprague-Dawley rats	Cell proliferation decreases.
		Bcl2 decreases; Bax increases (Bishayee et al., 2009).
	Male Wistar rats implanted with AH-130 hepatoma cells	Tumor weight decreases.
		Apoptosis increases.
		Increases cells at G2/M (Kowalczyk et al., 2013).

12.6 RESVERATROL-LOADED POLYMERIC NANOTHERAPEUTICS FOR CANCER TREATMENT

In recent years, a number of approaches have been developed to encounter the molecular-level changes in the pathophysiology of carcinogenesis. The latest approach includes nano-diagnostic and nanotherapeutic modalities, like lipid nanoparticles, nanohybrids, and polymeric nanoparticles (Gharpure et al., 2015; Pacardo et al., 2015; Stylianopoulos et al., 2015). These nanocarrier modalities as drug delivery vehicles have elucidated promising results in preclinical and initial clinical trials (Eetezadi et al., 2015; Fernandes et al., 2015; Johnstone et al., 2016). Nanocarrier drug delivery systems have excellent salient features, including but not limited to improved stability, enhanced solubility, and increased surface area: volume ratio. Moreover, these carriers add extra edge as their surface properties are modifiable and can be adjusted to achieve manageable pharmacological and physicochemical characteristics, hence reducing impediments in attaining effective cancer chemotherapy (Kumari et al., 2016). In addition, an improved therapeutic index and moderated toxicity to normal healthy cells are also attained through nanotherapeutic carriers (Kumari et al., 2016). It is remarkable that active and passive targeting could be used to deliver drugs to specific sites. These characteristic features of nanocarriers are imperative for typical biologically active compounds like polyphenols for their rendition into novel therapeutic modalities. Irrespective of the assuring progress in basic cancer biology in preclinical studies, polyphenols possess inappropriate pharmacological properties like low bioavailability due to inept systemic access, and therefore high doses are required for elucidation of optimum therapeutic effect (Siddiqui et al., 2012). Although the biological effectiveness of polyphenols has been established through *in vitro* studies, similar results could not be reproduced in the *in vivo* studies and it was due to their instability in the physiological conditions of temperature, pH, and enzyme system. It was then proposed that the development of polyphenol loaded nanotherapeutics could resolve this issue by addressing the instability and systemic access of the active ingredient, resveratrol. Sooner a series of studies were carried out to evaluate the biologically active polyphenol combination with nano-sized carriers. The outcome from these studies revealed many solutions to overcome the shortcomings of conventional anticancer therapy and develop a clinically efficient anticancer treatment.

Some of the research studies have recorded intense toxicity of curcumin-loaded poloxamer nanocarriers in HeLa (Sahu et al., 2011) and ovarian cancer cells (Saxena et al., 2013). Moreover, resveratrol and doxorubicin (DOX) containing poloxamer nano-formulations exhibited a synergistic effect on ovarian cancer in mice (Carlson et al., 2014). Kim et al. (2015) reported that a combination of resveratrol-quercetin elucidated similar effect in ovarian tumors (Kim et al., 2015). In addition, resveratrol was encapsulated into PEG-polycaprolactone conjugate was used to encapsulate resveratrol and the surface modification of the resulting micelles was carried out using a polipoprotein and used to treat glioblastoma (Wang et al., 2015) as well as breast cancer. Finally, other studies mentioned that epigallocatechin gallate (EGCG) was delivered in colon cancer using PEG-polylactic acid (PLA) (Haratifar et al., 2014) and in pancreatic cancer using casein micelles as carriers (Sun et al., 2014) (see Table 12.5).

In another set of studies we found that resveratrol was nanoencapsulated in bovine serum albumin (Guo et al., 2015), gelatin (Karthikeyan et al., 2015), PLGA (Kumar et al., 2016), and PLGA-PEG derivatives (Sanna et al., 2013), and reported a significant elevation in the anticancer activity of resveratrol against prostate, ovarian, breasts, and lung cancer (Guo et al., 2015; Karthikeyan et al., 2015; Kumar et al., 2016; Sanna et al., 2013). Transferrin was used to modify the surface of resveratrol loaded PLGA-PEG nanoparticles for active targeting of glioma cancer cells *in vivo* (Guo et al., 2013).

Nanoparticles loaded with EGCG, resveratrol, quercetin, and 5-fluorouracil can be designed with enhanced stability and *in vitro* anticancer activity can be elucidated in various types of cancer including cancer of the stomach, prostate, ovaries, alimentary canal, and breast. The stability can be adjusted using several natural polymers, such as gelatin, PEG, and PLGA, alone or in combination with synthetic polymers, like chitosan (CS), and casein. Polyphenol-loaded polymeric conjugates for the treatment of cancer are summarized in Table 12.5.

TABLE 12.5 Enumerates Different Types of Nanoparticles Prepared Using Resveratrol and Synergistic Agents

Sl. No.	Type of Nano Formulation	Components of Nanoparticles	Method	Resveratrol + Synergistic Agent	Model Used
1.	Nanovesicles	Poloxamers F127	Thin-layer evaporation	Resveratrol + curcumin + Doxorubicin	Ovarian cancer SKOV-3 Healthy mice (Carlson et al., 2014)
2.		Poloxamers F127	Thin-layer evaporation	Resveratrol + quercetin + Doxorubicin	Ovarian cancer SKOV-3 Healthy mice (Cote et al., 2015)
3.		Apolipoprotein-E3	Recombinant DNA	Resveratrol	Glioblastoma A-172 (Kim et al., 2015)
4.		Polycaprolactone-PEG-Succinate	Thin-layer evaporation	Resveratrol	Breast cancer MCF-7 (Wang et al., 2015)
5.	Nanoparticles	PLGA-PEG	Nanoprecipitation	Resveratrol	Prostate cancer DU-145, LNCaP (Guo et al., 2015)
6.		Bovine Serum Albumin	Nanoprecipitation	Resveratrol	Lung cancer NCI-H460 (Karthikeyan et al., 2015)
7.		Bovine Serum Albumin	Nanoprecipitation	Resveratrol	Ovarian Cancer SKOV-3 (Kumar et al., 2016)
8.		PLGA	Emulsion method	Resveratrol	Breast cancer MCF-7 (Sanna et al., 2013)
9.		Maleimide-PEG-Polylactic acid	Self-assembly	Resveratrol	Glioblastoma CT26, U87 CT26 Xenograft mice (Guo et al., 2013)
10.	Polymeric conjugates	PEG	Condensation method	Resveratrol + Bicalutamide	Cervical cancer HeLa (Wang et al., 2016)
11.		PEG	Condensation method	Resveratrol + Bicalutamide	Breast cancer MCF-7 (Wang et al., 2016)
12.	Carbon-based nanohybrids	Graphene oxide	Reduction method	Resveratrol	Ovarian cancer A2780 (Gurunathan et al., 2015)

Curcumin-gemcitabine combination was encapsulated in PEG conjugates by a condensation reaction in the presence of carbodiimide for the treatment of pancreatic cancer (Li et al., 2009). PEG conjugates containing only curcumin have been formulated for prostate cancer (Safavy et al., 2007) and glioma cancer (Dey et al., 2015). Using the same conjugation technique, Wang et al. reported synergistic cytotoxicity by resveratrol-bicalutamide-PEG conjugates in breast and cervical cancer cells (Wang et al., 2016) and in hepatic cancer cells using quercetin-paclitaxel-carboxymethyl CS conjugates (Wang et al., 2014).

There is a multitude of polymeric conjugates which include nanoparticles loaded with resveratrol, quercetin, and curcumin in combination with standard anticancer drugs like paclitaxel, gemcitabine, or bortezomib for the treatment of hepatic, pancreatic, prostate, glioma, and breast cancer.

12.7 CONCLUSIONS AND FUTURE PERSPECTIVES

From the remarkable reports of resveratrol involved in preclinical and clinical anticancer studies, it can be deduced that resveratrol can attenuate carcinogenesis at various stages. As validated by experimental *in vivo* and *in vitro* studies, which are further supported by some clinical trial studies it can be stated that resveratrol has substantial potential as an anti-cancer agent and is involved in both prevention and therapy of a wide range of cancerous conditions. Resveratrol has many molecular targets and it acts on different protective and common pathways that are generally distorted in cancerous tumors. This suggests that resveratrol is a suitable anticancer agent and produces the pharmacological effect in conjunction with diverse chemotherapeutics and targeted therapies. The ability of resveratrol to prevent carcinogenesis includes the placation of oxidative stress, inflammation, and inhibition of cancer cell proliferation, and the activation of tightly regulated cell-death mechanisms.

Since resveratrol has complex involvement in the cellular processes, more studies must be carried out to understand better ways resveratrol could be exploited to prevent the carcinogenesis. Moreover, resveratrol has poor bioavailability in human subjects, and it has been a serious concern in transforming the outcomes of basic research to formulating therapeutic agents. Though clinical trials have revealed positive and beneficial outcomes, there are many conflicts which still need to be addressed. To enhance the bioavailability of resveratrol and to make it a potential anticancer agent, research that is more active should be directed toward the novel drug delivery system of resveratrol, its formulations, and its metabolism. Moreover, the possible interactions of resveratrol with other compounds also must be ruled out.

KEYWORDS

- **anticancer**
- **cancer**
- **chemoprevention**
- **fibroblast growth factor**
- **nanoformulation**
- **phytomedicine**
- **resveratrol**

REFERENCES

Afaq, F., Adhami, V. M., & Ahmad, N., (2003). Prevention of short-term ultraviolet Bradiation-mediated damages by resveratrol in SKH-1 hairless mice. *Toxicol. Appl. Pharmacol., 186*, 28–37.

Aggarwal, B. B., Bhardwaj, A., Aggarwal, R. S., Seeram, N. P., Shishodia, S., & Takada, Y., (2004). Role of resveratrol in prevention and therapy of cancer: Preclinical and clinical studies. *Anticancer Res., 24*, 2783–2840.

Aggarwal, B. B., Van, K. M. E., Iyer, L. H., Harikumar, K. B., & Sung, B., (2009). Molecular targets of nutraceuticals derived from dietary spices: Potential role in suppression of inflammation and tumorigenesis. *Exp. Biol. Med., 234*, 825–849.

Aggarwal, B. B., Vijayalekshmi, R. V., & Sung, B., (2009). Targeting inflammatory pathways for prevention and therapy of cancer: Short-term friend, long-term foe. *Clin. Cancer Res., 15*, 425–430.

Athar, M., Back, J. H., Kopelovich, L., Bickers, D. R., & Kim, A. L., (2009). Multiple molecular targets of resveratrol: Anticarcinogenic mechanisms. *Archives of Biochemistry and Biophysics, 486*(2), 95–102.

Athar, M., Back, J. H., Tang, X., Kim, K. H., Kopelovich, L., Bickers, D. R., & Kim, A. L., (2007). Resveratrol: A review of preclinical studies for human cancer prevention. *Toxicol. App. Pharmacol., 224*(3), 274–283.

Attia, S. M., (2012). Influence of resveratrol on oxidative damage in genomic DNA and apoptosis induced by cisplatin. *Mutat. Res., 741*, 22–31.

Aziz, M. H., Nihal, M., Fu, V. X., Jarrard, D. F., & Ahmad, N., (2006). Resveratrol-caused apoptosis of human prostate carcinoma LNCaP cells is mediated via modulation of phosphatidylinositol 30-kinase/Akt pathway and Bcl-2 family proteins. *Mol. Cancer Ther., 5*, 1335–1341.

Bai, Y., Mao, Q. Q., Qin, J., Zheng, X. Y., Wang, Y. B., Yang, K., Shen, H. F., & Xie, L. P., (2010). Resveratrol induces apoptosis and cell cycle arrest of human T24 bladder cancer cells *in vitro* and inhibits tumor growth *in vivo*. *Cancer Sci., 101*, 488–493.

Barzilai, A., & Yamamoto, K., (2004). DNA damage responses to oxidative stress. *DNA Repair, 3*, 1109–1115.

Baur, J. A., Pearson, K. J., Price, N. L., Jamieson, H. A., Lerin, C., Kalra, A., Prabhu, V. V., Allard, J. S., Lopez-Lluch, G., Lewis, K., et al., (2006). Resveratrol improves health and survival of mice on a high-calorie diet. *Nature, 444*, 337–342.

Beedanagari, S. R., Bebenek, I., Bui, P., & Hankinson, O., (2009). Resveratrol inhibits dioxin-induced expression of human CYP1A1 and CYP1B1 by inhibiting recruitment of the aryl hydrocarbon receptor complex and RNA polymerase II to the regulatory regions of the corresponding genes. *Toxicol. Sci., 110*, 61–67.

Benitez, D. A., Pozo-Guisado, E., Alvarez-Barrientos, A., Fernandez-Salguero, P. M., & Castellon, E. A., (2007). Mechanisms involved in resveratrol-induced apoptosis and cell cycle arrest in prostate cancer-derived cell lines. *J. Androl., 28*, 282–293.

Bernhard, D., Tinhofer, I., Tonko, M., Hubl, H., Ausserlechner, M. J., Greil, R., Kofler, R., & Csordas, A., (2000). Resveratrol causes arrest in the S-phase prior to Fas-independent apoptosis in CEM-C7H2 acute leukemia cells. *Cell Death Differ., 7*, 834–842.

Bhardwaj, A., Sethi, G., Vadhan-Raj, S., Bueso-Ramos, C., Takada, Y., Gaur, U., Nair, A. S., et al., (2007). Resveratrol inhibits proliferation, induces apoptosis, and overcomes chemo resistance through down-regulation of STAT3 and nuclear factor-kB-regulated antiapoptotic and cell survival gene products in human multiple myeloma cells. *Blood, 109*, 2293–2302.

Bishayee, A., & Dhir, N., (2009). Resveratrol-mediated chemoprevention of diethylnitrosamine-initiated hepatocarcinogenesis: Inhibition of cell proliferation and induction of apoptosis. *Chem. Biol. Interact., 179*, 131–144.

Bishayee, A., & Sethi, G., (2016). Bioactive natural products in cancer prevention and therapy: Progress and promise. *Semin. Cancer Biol., 40, 41*, 1–3.

Bishayee, A., (2009). Cancer prevention and treatment with resveratrol: From rodent studies to clinical trials. *Cancer Prev. Res., 2*, 409–418.

Bishayee, A., Politis, T., & Darvesh, A. S., (2010). Resveratrol in the chemoprevention and treatment of hepatocellular carcinoma. *Cancer Treat. Rev., 36*, 43–53.

Cai, Y. J., Wei, Q. Y., Fang, J. G., Yang, L., Liu, Z. L., Wyche, J. H., & Han, Z., (2004). The 3, 4-dihydroxyl groups are important for trans-resveratrol analogs to exhibit enhanced antioxidant and apoptotic activities. *Anticancer Res., 24*, 999–1002.

Cao, Z., Fang, J., Xia, C., Shi, X., & Jiang, B. H., (2004). trans-3,4,50-Trihydroxystibene inhibits hypoxia-inducible factor 1and vascular endothelial growth factor expression in human ovarian cancer cells. *Clin. Cancer Res., 10*, 5253–5263.

Carlson, L. J., Cote, B., Alani, A. W., & Rao, D. A., (2014). Polymeric micellar codelivery of resveratrol and curcumin to mitigate *in vitro* doxorubicin induced cardiotoxicity. *J. Pharm. Sci., 103*, 2315–2322.

Carter, L. G., D'Orazio, J. A., & Pearson, K. J., (2014). Resveratrol and cancer: Focus on *in vivo* evidence. *Endocr. Relat. Cancer, 21*, R209–R225.

Chai, E. Z., Siveen, K. S., Shanmugam, M. K., Arfuso, F., & Sethi, G., (2015). Analysis of the intricate relationship between chronic inflammation and cancer. *Biochem. J., 468*, 1–15.

Chen, Z. H., Hurh, Y. J., Na, H. K., Kim, J. H., Chun, Y. J., Kim, D. H., Kang, K. S., et al., (2004). Resveratrol inhibits TCDD-induced expression of CYP1A1 and CYP1B1 and catechol estrogen-mediated oxidative DNA damage in cultured human mammary epithelial cells. *Carcinogenesis, 25*, 2005–2013.

Ciolino, H. P., & Yeh, G. C., (1999). Inhibition of aryl hydrocarbon-induced cytochrome P-450 1A1 enzyme activity and CYP1A1 expression by resveratrol. *Mol. Pharmacol., 56*, 760–767.

Clement, M. V., Hirpara, J. L., Chawdhury, S. H., & Pervaiz, S., (1998). Chemo preventive agent resveratrol, a natural product derived from grapes, triggers CD95 signaling-dependent apoptosis in human tumor cells. *Blood, 92*, 996–1002.

Colin, D., Lancon, A., Delmas, D., Lizard, G., Abrossinow, J., Kahn, E., Jannin, B., & Latruffe, N., (2008). Antiproliferative activities of resveratrol and related compounds in human hepatocyte derived HepG2 cells are associated with biochemical cell disturbance revealed by fluorescence analyses. *Biochimie., 90*, 1674–1684.

Cote, B., Carlson, L. J., Rao, D. A., & Alani, A. W. G., (2015). Combinatorial resveratrol and quercetin polymeric micelles mitigate doxorubicin induced cardiotoxicity *in vitro* and *in vivo. J. Control Release, 213*, 128–133.

Cucciolla, V., Borriello, A., Oliva, A., Galletti, P., Zappia, V., & Della, R. F., (2007). Resveratrol: From basic science to the clinic. *Cell Cycle, 6*, 2495–2510.

Delmas, D., Rebe, C., Lacour, S., Filomenko, R., Athias, A., Gambert, P., Cherkaoui-Malki, M., Jannin, B., Dubrez-Daloz, L., Latruffe, N., et al., (2003). Resveratrol-induced apoptosis is associated with Fas redistribution in the rafts and the formation of a death-inducing signaling complex in colon cancer cells. *J. Boil. Chem., 278*, 41482–41490.

Dey, S., Ambattu, L. A., Hari, P. R., Rekha, M. R., & Sreenivasan, K., (2015). Glutathione-bearing fluorescent polymer-curcumin conjugate enables simultaneous drug delivery and label-free cellular imaging. *Polym. UK, 75*, 25–33.

Eetezadi, S., Ekdawi, S. N., & Allen, C., (2015). The challenges facing block copolymer micelles for cancer therapy, *in vivo* barriers, and clinical translation. *Adv. Drug Deliv. Rev., 91*, 7–22.

Fernandes, E., Ferreira, J. A., Andreia, P., Luís, L., Barroso, S., Sarmento, B., & Santos, L. L., (2015). New trends in guided nanotherapies for digestive cancers, a systematic review. *J. Control Release, 209*, 288–307.

Ferry-Dumazet, H., Garnier, O., Mamani-Matsuda, M., Vercauteren, J., Belloc, F., Billiard, C., Dupouy, M., Thiolat, D., Kolb, J. P., Marit, G., et al., (2002). Resveratrol inhibits the growth and induces the apoptosis of both normal and leukemic hematopoietic cells. *Carcinogenesis, 23*, 1327–1333.

Filippi-Chiela, E. C., Villodre, E. S., Zamin, L. L., & Lenz, G., (2011). Autophagy interplay with apoptosis and cell cycle regulation in the growth inhibiting effect of resveratrol in glioma cells. *PLoS One, 6*, e20849.

Fruehauf, J. P., & Meyskens, F. L. Jr., (2007). Reactive oxygen species: A breath of life or death? *Clin. Cancer Res., 13*, 789–794.

Galati, G., Teng, S., Moridani, M. Y., Chan, T. S., & O'Brien, P. J., (2000). Cancer chemoprevention and apoptosis mechanisms induced by dietary polyphenolics. *Drug Metab. Drug Interact, 17*, 311–349.

Ganapathy, S., Chen, Q., Singh, K. P., Shankar, S., & Srivastava, R. K., (2010). Resveratrol enhances antitumor activity of TRAIL in prostate cancer xenografts through activation of FOXO transcription factor. *PLoS One, 5*, e15627.

Gartel, A. L., & Tyner, A. L., (2002). The role of the cyclin-dependent kinase inhibitor p21 in apoptosis. *Mol. Cancer Ther., 1*, 639–649.

Gatouillat, G., Balasse, E., Joseph-Pietras, D., Morjani, H., & Madoulet, C., (2010). Resveratrol induces cell-cycle disruption and apoptosis in chemoresistant B16 melanoma. *J. Cell. Biochem., 110*, 893–902.

Gharpure, K. M., Wu, S. Y., Li, C., Lopez-Berestein, G., & Sood, A. K., (2015). Nanotechnology, future of oncotherapy. *Clin. Cancer Res., 21*, 3121–3130.

Guengerich, F. P., (2000). Metabolism of chemical carcinogens. *Carcinogenesis, 21*, 345–351.

Guo, L., Peng, Y., Li, Y., Jingping, Y., Guangmei, Z., Jie, C., Jing, W., & Lihua, S., (2015). Cell death pathway induced by resveratrol-bovine serum albumin nanoparticles in a human ovarian cell line. *Oncol. Lett., 9*, 1359–1363.

Guo, W., Li, A., Jia, Z., Yuan, Y., Dai, H., & Li, H., (2013). Transferrin modified PEG-PLA resveratrol conjugates, *in vitro* and *in vivo* studies for glioma. *Eur. J. Pharmacol., 718*, 41–47.

Gupta, S. C., Kannappan, R., Reuter, S., Kim, J. H., & Aggarwal, B. B., (2011). Chemo sensitization of tumors by resveratrol. *Annals of the New York Academy of Sciences, 1215*(1), 150–160.

Gurunathan, S., Han, J. W., Kim, E. S., Park, J. H., & Kim, J. H., (2015). Reduction of graphene oxide by resveratrol, a novel and simple biological method for the synthesis of an effective anticancer nanotherapeutic molecule. *Int. J. Nanomed., 10*, 2951–2969.

Hao, Y., Huang, W., Liao, M., Zhu, Y., Liu, H., Hao, C., Liu, G., Zhang, G., Feng, H., Ning, X., et al., (2013). The inhibition of resveratrol to human skin squamous cell carcinoma A431 xenografts in nude mice. *Fitoterapia, 86*, 84–91.

Haratifar, S., Meckling, K. A., & Corredig, M., (2014). Antiproliferative activity of tea catechins associated with casein micelles, using HT29 colon cancer cells. *J. Dairy Sci., 97*, 672–678.

Hong, W. K., & Sporn, M. B., (1997). Recent advances in chemoprevention of cancer. *Science, 278*, 1073–1077.

Hsieh, T. C., Lu, X., Wang, Z., & Wu, J. M., (2006). Induction of quinone reductase NQO1 by resveratrol in human K562 cells involves the antioxidant response element ARE and is accompanied by nuclear translocation of transcription factor Nrf2. *Med. Chem., 2*, 275–285.

Hsieh, T. C., Wong, C., John, B. D., & Wu, J. M., (2011). Regulation of p53 and cell proliferation by resveratrol and its derivatives in breast cancer cells: An *in silico* and biochemical approach targeting integrinαvβ3. *Int. J. Cancer, 129*, 2732–2743.

Hsieh, Y. S., Yang, S. F., Sethi, G., & Hu, D. N., (2015). Natural bioactives in cancer treatment and prevention. *BioMed. Res. Int.,* 182835.

Janakiram, N. B., Mohammed, A., Madka, V., Kumar, G., & Rao, C. V., (2016). Prevention and treatment of cancers by immune modulating nutrients. *Mol. Nutr. Food Res., 60*, 1275–1294.

Jang, M., Cai, L., Udeani, G. O., Slowing, K. V., Thomas, C. F., Beecher, C. W., Fong, H. H., Farnsworth, N. R., Kinghorn, A. D., Mehta, R. G., et al., (1997). Cancer chemo preventive activity of resveratrol, a natural product derived from grapes. *Science, 275*, 218–220.

Jeandet, P., Douillet-Breuil, A. C., Bessis, R., Debord, S., Sbaghi, M., & Adrian, M., (2002). Phytoalexins from the vitaceae: Biosynthesis, phytoalexin gene expression in transgenic plants, antifungal activity, and metabolism. *J. Agric. Food Chem., 50*, 2731–2741.

Jinga, D. C., Blidaru, A., Condrea, I., Ardeleanu, C., Dragomir, C., Szegli, G., Stefanescu, M., & Matache, C., (2006). MMP-9 and MMP-2 gelatinases and TIMP-1 and TIMP-2 inhibitors in breast cancer: Correlations with prognostic factors. *J. Cell. Mol. Med., 10*, 499–510.

Johnstone, T. C., Suntharalingam, K., & Lippard, S. J., (2016). The next generation of platinum drugs, targeted PtII agents, nanoparticle delivery, and PtIV prodrugs. *Chem. Rev., 116*, 3436–3486.

Kannaiyan, R., Shanmugam, M. K., & Sethi, G., (2011). Molecular targets of celastrol derived from thunder of god vine: Potential role in the treatment of inflammatory disorders and cancer. *Cancer Lett., 303*, 9–20.

Karthikeyan, S., Hoti, S. L., & Prasad, N. R., (2015). Resveratrol loaded gelatin nanoparticles synergistically inhibits cell cycle progression and constitutive NF-kappa B activation and induces apoptosis in non-small cell lung cancer cells. *Biomed. Pharmacother., 70*, 274–282.

Khansari, N., Shakiba, Y., & Mahmoudi, M., (2009). Chronic inflammation and oxidative stress as a major cause of age-related diseases and cancer. *Recent Pat. Inflamm. Allergy Drug Discov., 3*, 73–80.

Kim, H. J., Chang, E. J., Bae, S. J., Shim, S. M., Park, H. D., Rhee, C. H., Park, J. H., & Choi, S. W., (2002). Cytotoxic and antimutagenic stilbenes from seeds of *Paeonia lactiflora*. *Arch. Pharm. Res., 25*, 293–299.

Kim, S. H., Adhikari, B. B., Cruz, S., Schramm, M. P., Vinson, J. A., & Narayanaswami, V., (2015). Targeted intracellular delivery of resveratrol to glioblastoma cells using apolipoprotein E-containing reconstituted HDL as a nanovehicle. *PLoS One, 10*, e013.

Kim, Y. A., Lee, W. H., Choi, T. H., Rhee, S. H., Park, K. Y., & Choi, Y. H., (2003b). Involvement of p21WAF1/CIP1, pRB, Bax and NF-kB in induction of growth arrest and apoptosis by resveratrol in human lung carcinoma A549 cells. *Int. J. Oncol., 23*, 1143–1149.

Kim, Y. A., Rhee, S. H., Park, K. Y., & Choi, Y. H., (2003a). Antiproliferative effect of resveratrol in human prostate carcinoma cells. *J. Med. Food, 6*, 273–280.

Kimura, Y., & Okuda, H., (2001). Resveratrol isolated from *Polygonum cuspidatum* root prevents tumor growth and metastasis to lung and tumor-induced neovascularization in Lewis lung carcinoma-bearing mice. *J. Nutr., 131*, 1844–1849.

Klaunig, J. E., & Kamendulis, L. M., (2004). The role of oxidative stress in carcinogenesis. *Annu. Rev. Pharmacol. Toxicol., 44*, 239–267.

Ko, J. H., Sethi, G., Um, J. Y., Shanmugam, M. K., Arfuso, F., Kumar, A. P., Bishayee, A., & Ahn, K. S., (2017). The role of resveratrol in cancer therapy. *Int. J. Mol. Sci., 18*, 2589–2625.

Kowalczyk, M. C., Junco, J. J., Kowalczyk, P., Tolstykh, O., Hanausek, M., Slaga, T. J., & Walaszek, Z., (2013). Effects of combined phytochemicals on skin tumorigenesis in SENCAR mice. *Int. J. Oncol., 43*, 911–918.

Krepler, C., Xiao, M., Sproesser, K., Brafford, P. A., Shannan, B., Beqiri, M., Liu, Q., Xu, W., Garman, B., Nathanson, K. L., et al., (2016). Personalized preclinical trials in BRAF inhibitor-resistant patient-derived xenograft models identify second-line combination therapies. *Clin. Cancer Res., 22*, 1592–1602.

Kueck, A., Opipari, A. W. Jr., Griffith, K. A., Tan, L., Choi, M., Huang, J., Wahl, H., & Liu, J. R., (2007). Resveratrol inhibits glucose metabolism in human ovarian cancer cells. *Gynecol. Oncol., 107*, 450–457.

Kumar, S., Lather, V., & Pandita, D., (2016). A facile green approach to prepare core-shell hybrid PLGA nanoparticles for resveratrol delivery. *Int. J. Biol. Macromol., 84*, 380–384.

Kumari, P., Ghosh, B., & Biswas, S., (2016). Nanocarriers for cancer-targeted drug delivery. *J. Drug Target, 24*, 179–191.

Lee, E. O., Lee, H. J., Hwang, H. S., Ahn, K. S., Chae, C., Kang, K. S., Lu, J., & Kim, S. H., (2006). Potent inhibition of Lewis lung cancer growth by heyneanol A from the roots of *Vitis amurensis* through apoptotic and anti-angiogenic activities. *Carcinogenesis, 27*, 2059–2069.

Lee, M. F., Pan, M. H., Chiou, Y. S., Cheng, A. C., & Huang, H., (2011). Resveratrol modulates MED28(Magicin/EG-1) expression and inhibits epidermal growth factor (EGF)-induced migration in MDA-MB-231 human breast cancer cells. *J. Agric. Food Chem., 59*, 11853–11861.

Lee, Y. J., Lee, G. J., Yi, S. S., Heo, S. H., Park, C. R., Nam, H. S., Cho, M. K., & Lee, S. H., (2016). Cisplatin and resveratrol induce apoptosis and autophagy following oxidative stress in malignant mesothelioma cells. *Food Chem. Toxicol., 97*, 96–107.

Leonard, S. S., Xia, C., Jiang, B. H., Stinefelt, B., Klandorf, H., Harris, G. K., & Shi, X., (2003). Resveratrol scavenges reactive oxygen species and effects radical-induced cellular responses. *Biochem. Biophys. Res. Commun., 309*, 1017–1026.

Li, J., Wang, Y., Yang, C., Wang, P., Oelschlager, D. K., Zheng, Y., Tian, D. A., Grizzle, W. E., Buchsbaum, D. J., & Wan, M., (2009). Polyethylene glycosylated curcumin conjugate inhibits pancreatic cancer cell growth through inactivation of Jab1. *Mol. Pharmacol., 76*, 81–90.

Li, K., Dias, S. J., Rimando, A. M., Dhar, S., Mizuno, C. S., Penman, A. D., Lewin, J. R., & Levenson, A. S., (2013). Pterostilbene acts through metastasis-associated protein 1 to inhibit tumor growth, progression, and metastasis in prostate cancer. *PLoS One, 8*, e57542.

Li, W., Ma, J., Ma, Q., Li, B., Han, L., Liu, J., Xu, Q., Duan, W., Yu, S., Wang, F., et al., (2013). Resveratrol inhibits the epithelial-mesenchymal transition of pancreatic cancer cells via suppression of the PI-3K/Akt/NF-kB pathway. *Curr. Med. Chem., 20*, 4185–4194.

Li, Y., Liu, J., Liu, X., Xing, K., Wang, Y., Li, F., & Yao, L., (2006). Resveratrol-induced cell inhibition of growth and apoptosis in MCF7 human breast cancer cells are associated with modulation of phosphorylated Akt and caspase-9. *Appl. Biochem. Biotechnol., 135*, 181–192.

Liao, P. C., Ng, L. T., Lin, L. T., Richardson, C. D., Wang, G. H., & Lin, C. C., (2010). Resveratrol arrests cell cycle and induces apoptosis in human hepatocellular carcinoma Huh-7 cells. *J. Med. Food, 13*, 1415–1423.

Mazzanti, G., & Di Giacomo, S., (2016). Curcumin and resveratrol in the management of cognitive disorders: What is the clinical evidence? *Molecules, 21*, 1243.

Minamoto, T., Mai, M., & Ronai, Z., (1999). Environmental factors as regulators and effectors of multistep carcinogenesis. *Carcinogenesis, 20*, 519–527.

Miura, D., Miura, Y., & Yagasaki, K., (2003). Hypolipidemic action of dietary resveratrol, a phytoalexin in grapes and red wine, in hepatoma-bearing rats. *Life Sci., 73*, 1393–1400.

Molino, S., Dossena, M., Buonocore, D., Ferrari, F., Venturini, L., Ricevuti, G., & Verri, M., (2016). Polyphenols in dementia: From molecular basis to clinical trials. *Life Sci., 161*, 69–77.

Mondal, A., & Bennett, L. L., (2016). Resveratrol enhances the efficacy of sorafenib mediated apoptosis in human breast cancer MCF7 cells through ROS, cell cycle inhibition, caspase 3 and PARP cleavage. *Biomed. Pharmacother., 84*, 1906–1914.

Moran, B. W., Anderson, F. P., Devery, A., Cloonan, S., Butler, W. E., Varughese, S., Draper, S. M., & Kenny, P. T., (2009). Synthesis, structural characterization, and biological evaluation of fluorinated analogs of resveratrol. *Bioorg. Med. Chem., 17*, 4510–4522.

Nelson, A. R., Fingleton, B., Rothenberg, M. L., & Matrisian, L. M., (2000). Matrix metalloproteinases: Biologic activity and clinical implications. *J. Clin. Oncol., 18*, 1135–1149.

Newman, D. J., & Cragg, G. M., (2016). Natural products as sources of new drugs from 1981 to 2014. *J. Nat. Prod., 79*, 629–661.

Okimoto, R. A., & Bivona, T. G., (2014). Recent advances in personalized lung cancer medicine. *Pers. Med., 11*, 309–321.

Pacardo, D. B., Ligler, F. S., & Gu, Z., (2015). Programmable nanomedicine, synergistic and sequential drug delivery systems. *Nanoscale, 7*, 3381–3391.

Peng, T. L., Chen, J., Mao, W., Song, X., & Chen, M. H., (2009). Aryl hydrocarbon receptor pathway activation enhances gastric cancer cell invasiveness likely through a c-Jun-dependent induction of matrix metalloproteinase-9. *BMC Cell Boil., 10*, 27.

Prasannan, R., Kalesh, K. A., Shanmugam, M. K., Nachiyappan, A., Ramachandran, L., Nguyen, A. H., Kumar, A. P., et al., (2012). Key cell signaling pathways modulated by zerumbone: Role in the prevention and treatment of cancer. *Biochem. Pharmacol., 84*, 1268–1276.

Provinciali, M., Re, F., Donnini, A., Orlando, F., Bartozzi, B., Di Stasio, G., & Smorlesi, A., (2005). Effect of resveratrol on the development of spontaneous mammary tumors in HER-2/neu transgenic mice. *Int. J. Cancer, 115*, 36–45.

Rashid, A., Liu, C., Sanli, T., Tsiani, E., Singh, G., Bristow, R. G., Dayes, I., et al., (2011). Resveratrol enhances prostate cancer cell response to ionizing radiation. Modulation of the AMPK, Akt and mTOR pathways. *Radiat. Oncol., 6*, 144.

Ratan, H. L., Steward, W. P., Gescher, A. J., & Mellon, J., (2002). Resveratrol—a prostate cancer chemo preventive agent? *Urologic Oncology, 7*(6), 223–227.

Ray, P. S., Maulik, G., Cordis, G. A., Bertelli, A. A., Bertelli, A., & Das, D. K., (1999). The red wine antioxidant resveratrol protects isolated rat hearts from ischemia reperfusion injury. *Free Radic. Boil. Med., 27*, 160–169.

Renaud, S., & De Lorgeril, M., (1992). Wine, alcohol, platelets, and the French paradox for coronary heart disease. *Lancet, 339*, 1523–1526.

Safavy, A., Raisch, K. P., Mantena, S., Sanford, L. L., Sham, S. W., Krishna, N. R., & Bonner, J. A., (2007). Design and development of water-soluble curcumin conjugates as potential anticancer agents. *J. Med. Chem., 50*, 6284–6288.

Sahu, A., Kasoju, N., Goswami, P., & Bora, U., (2011). Encapsulation of curcumin in Pluronic block copolymer micelles for drug delivery applications. *J. Biomater. Appl., 25*, 619–639.

Sanna, V., Siddiqui, I. A., Sechi, M., & Mukhtar, H., (2013). Resveratrol-loaded nanoparticles based on poly epsilon caprolactone and poly-D,L-lacticco-glycolic acid-polyethylene glycol blend for prostate cancer treatment. *Mol. Pharm., 10*, 3871–3881.

Saxena, V., & Hussain, M. D., (2013). Polymeric mixed micelles for delivery of curcumin to multidrug resistant ovarian cancer. *J. Biomed. Nanotechnol., 9*, 1146–1154.

Sethi, G., & Tergaonkar, V., (2009). Potential pharmacological control of the NF-kB pathway. *Trends Pharmacol. Sci., 30*, 313–321.

Sethi, G., Shanmugam, M. K., Ramachandran, L., Kumar, A. P., & Tergaonkar, V., (2012). Multifaceted link between cancer and inflammation. *Biosci. Rep., 32*, 1–15.

Sexton, E., Van, T. C., LeBlanc, K., Parent, S., Lemoine, P., & Asselin, E., (2006). Resveratrol interferes with AKT activity and triggers apoptosis in human uterine cancer cells. *Mol. Cancer, 5*, 45.

Sgambato, A., Ardito, R., Faraglia, B., Boninsegna, A., Wolf, F. I., & Cittadini, A., (2001). Resveratrol, a natural phenolic compound, inhibits cell proliferation and prevents oxidative DNA damage. *Mutat. Res., 496*, 171–180.

Shanmugam, M. K., Arfuso, F., Kumar, A. P., Wang, L., Goh, B. C., Ahn, K. S., Bishayee, A., & Sethi, G., (2018). Modulation of diverse oncogenic transcription factors by thymoquinone, an essential oil compound isolated from the seeds of *Nigella sativa* Linn. *Pharmacol. Res., 129*, 357–364.

Shanmugam, M. K., Kannaiyan, R., & Sethi, G., (2011). Targeting cell signaling and apoptotic pathways by dietary agents: Role in the prevention and treatment of cancer. *Nutr. Cancer, 63*, 161–173.

Shanmugam, M. K., Lee, J. H., Chai, E. Z., Kanchi, M. M., Kar, S., Arfuso, F., Dharmarajan, A., Kumar, A. P., Ramar, P. S., Looi, C. Y., et al., (2016). Cancer prevention and therapy through the modulation of transcription factors by bioactive natural compounds. *Semin. Cancer Biol., 40, 41*, 35–47.

Shanmugam, M. K., Nguyen, A. H., Kumar, A. P., Tan, B. K., & Sethi, G., (2012). Targeted inhibition of tumor proliferation, survival, and metastasis by pentacyclic triterpenoids: Potential role in prevention and therapy of cancer. *Cancer Lett., 320*, 158–170.

Shanmugam, M. K., Rane, G., Kanchi, M. M., Arfuso, F., Chinnathambi, A., Zayed, M. E., Alharbi, S. A., et al., (2015). The multifaceted role of curcumin in cancer prevention and treatment. *Molecules, 20*, 2728–2769.

Shanmugam, M. K., Warrier, S., Kumar, A. P., Sethi, G., & Arfuso, F., (2017). Potential role of natural compounds as anti-angiogenic agents in cancer. *Curr. Vasc. Pharmacol., 15*, 503–519.

Shih, A., Zhang, S., Cao, H. J., Boswell, S., Wu, Y. H., Tang, H. Y., Lennartz, M. R., et al., (2004). Inhibitory effect of epidermal growth factor on resveratrol-induced apoptosis in prostate cancer cells is mediated by protein kinase C-α. *Molecular Cancer Therapeutics, 3*(11), 355–1363.

Shrimali, D., Shanmugam, M. K., Kumar, A. P., Zhang, J., Tan, B. K., Ahn, K. S., & Sethi, G., (2013). Targeted abrogation of diverse signal transduction cascades by emodin for the treatment of inflammatory disorders and cancer. *Cancer Lett., 341*, 139–149.

Siddiqui, I. A., Adhami, V. M., Chamcheu, C. J., & Mukhtar, H., (2012). Impact of nanotechnology in cancer, emphasis on nanochemoprevention. *Int. J. Nanomed., 7*, 591–605.

Sinha, D., Sarkar, N., Biswas, J., & Bishayee, A., (2016). Resveratrol for breast cancer prevention and therapy: Preclinical evidence and molecular mechanisms. *Semin. Cancer Boil., 40, 41*, 209–232.

Soleas, G. J., Grass, L., Josephy, P. D., Goldberg, D. M., & Diamandis, E. P., (2002). A comparison of the anticarcinogenic properties of four red wine polyphenols. *Clin. Biochem., 35*, 119–124.

Stagos, D., Amoutzias, G. D., Matakos, A., Spyrou, A., Tsatsakis, A. M., & Kouretas, D., (2012). Chemoprevention of liver cancer by plant polyphenols. *Food Chem. Toxicol., 50*, 2155–2170.

Stagos, D., Portesis, N., Spanou, C., Mossialos, D., Aligiannis, N., Chaita, E., Panagoulis, C., Reri, E., Skaltsounis, L., Tsatsakis, A. M., et al., (2012). Correlation of total polyphenolic content with antioxidant and antibacterial activity of 24 extracts from Greek domestic *Lamiaceae* species. *Food Chem. Toxicol., 50*, 4115–4124.

Stylianopoulos, T., & Jain, R. K., (2015). Design considerations for nanotherapeutics in oncology. *Nanomed. Nanotechnol. Biol. Med., 11*, 1893–1907.

Sun, L., Zhang, C., & Li, P., (2014). Copolymeric micelles for delivery of EGCG and cyclopamine to pancreatic cancer cells. *Nutr. Cancer, 66*, 896–903.

Tang, C. H., Sethi, G., & Kuo, P. L., (2014). Novel medicines and strategies in cancer treatment and prevention. *BioMed. Res. Int.,* 474078.

Tsan, M. F., White, J. E., Maheshwari, J. G., Bremner, T. A., & Sacco, J., (2000). Resveratrol induces Fas signaling-independent apoptosis in THP-1 human monocytic leukemia cells. *Br. J. Haematol., 109*, 405–412.

Van, G. P. R., Yan, M. B., Bhattacharya, S., Polans, A. S., & Kenealey, J. D., (2015). Natural products induce a G protein-mediated calcium pathway activating p53 in cancer cells. *Toxicol. Appl. Pharmacol., 288*, 453–462.

Wadsworth, T. L., & Koop, D. R., (1999). Effects of the wine polyphenolics quercetin and resveratrol on pro-inflammatory cytokine expression in RAW264.7 macrophages. *Biochem. Pharmacol., 57*, 941–949.

Wang, H., Zhang, H., Tang, L., Chen, H., Wu, C., Zhao, M., Yang, Y., Chen, X., & Liu, G., (2013). Resveratrol inhibits TGF-1-induced epithelial-to-mesenchymal transition and suppresses lung cancer invasion and metastasis. *Toxicology, 303*, 139–146.

Wang, S., Chen, R., Morott, J., Repka, M. A., Wang, Y., & Chen, M., (2015). MPEG-b-PCL/ TPGS mixed micelles for delivery of resveratrol in overcoming resistant breast cancer. *Expert Opin. Drug Deliv., 12*, 361–373.

Wang, W., Zhang, L., Le, Y., Chen, J. F., Wang, J., & Yun, J., (2016). Synergistic effect of PEGylated resveratrol on delivery of anticancer drugs. *Int. J. Pharm., 498*, 134–141.

Wang, X., Chen, Y., Dahmani, F. Z., Yin, L., Zhou, J., & Yao, J., (2014). Amphiphilic carboxymethyl chitosan-quercetin conjugates with P-gp inhibitory properties for oral delivery of paclitaxel. *Biomaterials, 35*, 7654–7665.

Weng, C. J., Wu, C. F., Huang, H. W., Wu, C. H., Ho, C. T., & Yen, G. C., (2010). Evaluation of anti-invasion effect of resveratrol and related methoxy analogs on human hepatocarcinoma cells. *J. Agric. Food Chem., 58*, 2886–2894.

Whitsett, T., Carpenter, M., & Lamartiniere, C. A., (2006). Resveratrol, but not EGCG, in the diet suppresses DMBA-induced mammary cancer in rats. *J. Carcinog., 5*, 15.

Windmill, K. F., McKinnon, R. A., Zhu, X., Gaedigk, A., Grant, D. M., & McManus, M. E., (1997). The role of xenobiotic metabolizing enzymes in arylamine toxicity and carcinogenesis: Functional and localization studies. *Mutat. Res., 376*, 153–160.

Wolter, F., Akoglu, B., Clausnitzer, A., & Stein, J., (2001). Down regulation of the cyclin D1/ Cdk4 complex occurs during resveratrol-induced cell cycle arrest in colon cancer cell lines. *J. Nutr., 131*, 2197–2203.

Yang, S. F., Weng, C. J., Sethi, G., & Hu, D. N., (2013). Natural bioactives and phytochemicals serve in cancer treatment and prevention. *Evid. Based Complement. Altern. Med.*, 698190.

CHAPTER 13

Thymoquinone-Loaded Nanocarriers for Healthcare Applications

RUQAIYAH KHAN,[1] HIMANI NAUTIYAL,[2] and SHAKIR SALEEM[1]

[1]*Chitkara College of Pharmacy, Chitkara University, Punjab, India,
E-mails: shakirsaleem@gmail.com*; shakir.saleem@chitkara.edu.in
(*S. Saleem*)

[2]*Siddhartha Institute of Pharmacy, Dobachi, Dehradun,
Uttarakhand, India*

ABSTRACT

Nano drug delivery system deals with the enhancement of bioavailability of orally administered therapeutic agents, target-specific drug delivery, and prolonged half-life of parenteral. Thymoquinone (TQ) is the chief active ingredient of *Nigella sativa* and has been incorporated in innumerable nano-formulations to assess its diverse pharmacological activity against many human illnesses including cancer, hypertension (HTN), diabetes, allergies, eczema, and immunogenic disorders. The major problem in developing TQ based nanoformulation is its highly hydrophobic nature which limits its solubility and its bioavailability. However, the emergence of surface engineering of the nanoparticle carrier systems has fixed this problem for TQ and hence, several nanoformulations have been developed and evaluated. This chapter briefly discusses the health applications of TQ based nanoformulations prepared through different techniques.

13.1 INTRODUCTION

Over the last couple of decades, remarkable progress has been envisaged in the field of nanotechnology-related to therapeutics and radio-imaging agents thereby minimizing the interventions (Martins et al., 2013). Nanotherapeutics aims to provide maximum pharmacological efficacy and minimum side effects by lowering the frequency of administration. Several nano-formulations like dendrimers, nanocrystals, nanoemulsions, liposomes, solid lipid nanoparticles (SLN), nano micelles, and polymeric nanoparticles have been developed to achieve better therapeutic compliance (Onoue et al., 2014). In the year 1996, the first nano-drug, Doxil, was approved by the FDA, hence laying the foundation of nano-drug delivery system. It was then followed by cascade of approvals including but not limited to oxaliplatin nanoparticles, nanoparticle comprising rapamycin and albumin as an anticancer agent, calcipotriol monohydrate nanocrystals, liposomes comprising docetaxel, nanoemulsion of 5-aminolevulinic acid and treatment of systemic fungal infections with phospholipid particles encapsulating polyene antibiotics (Krukemeyer et al., 2015).

Recently, various approaches involving polymer-based nanoparticles for oral administration of the drug has been undertaken for the treatment of cancer and several other diseases (Cho et al., 2008; Ravindran et al., 2010). Polymer-based nanoparticles have also been employed to deliver natural products like coenzyme Q10 (Ankola et al., 2007), estradiol (Hariharan et al., 2006), ellagic acid (Bala et al., 2006), curcumin (Bisht et al., 2007), and chemotherapeutic agents as paclitaxel (Mu et al., 2003) and doxorubicin (DOX) (Vasey et al., 1999).

13.2   THYMOQUINIONE AS A PROMINENT PHYTOMEDICINE

Bioactive compounds are one of the best alternative sources which can be employed in the prevention and treatment of various kinds of diseases including cancer (Shanmugam et al., 2018). *Nigella sativa*, also known as Black cumin, is an ancient herbal drug which is traditionally used to cure several conditions like asthma, bronchitis, inflammation, eczema, fever, influenza, hypertension (HTN), cough, headache, dizziness (Schneider et al., 2014; Ballout et al., 2018). Additionally, recent researches have revealed that black cumin can also be used to alleviate ailments like diabetes, renal, and liver malfunction, nervous system problems, rheumatic diseases, cancer, inflammatory diseases, gastrointestinal problems, and also for overall general wellness (Banerjee et al., 2010; Asaduzzaman et al., 2017).

Nigella sativa L. (Family-Ranunculaceae) contains Thymoquinone (TQ), which is the main bioactive component in the essential oil (EO) extracted from its seeds (Figure 13.1).

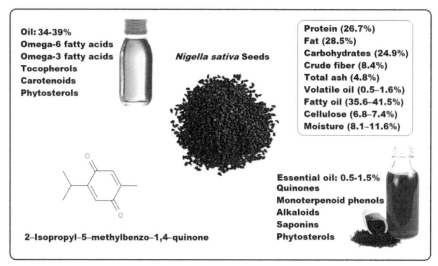

FIGURE 13.1 The seeds of *Nigella sativa*, its chemical structure, and its constituents.

Nigella sativa has been anciently used and is extensively reported as a folk medicine for numerous therapeutic applications like allergic rhinitis, eczema, HTN, diuretic, immunomodulation, analgesic, antioxidant, hepatoprotective, and renal protective agent (Salem et al., 2005; Ahmad et al., 2013) (see Table 13.1).

TABLE 13.1 The Therapeutic Areas Covered by Thymoquinone

Sl. No.	Therapeutic Use	References
1.	Anti-allergic	Aziz et al., 2011
2.	Anti-bacterial	Chaieb et al., 2011
3.	Anti-inflammatory	Inci et al., 2013
4.	Antioxidant activity	Inci et al., 2013
5.	Anti-depressant	Aquib et al., 2015
6.	Anti-anxiety	Gilhotra et al., 2011
7.	Anti-tumor	Zhang et al., 2016
8.	Anti-diabetic	El-Mahmoudy et al., 2005; Sangi et al., 2015
9.	Neuroprotective	Ramachandran et al., 2016
10.	Hepatoprotective	Oguz et al., 2012
11.	Anti-cancer drug-induced toxicity	Alenzi et al., 2010
12.	Hemorrhagic cystitis	Gore et al., 2016

TABLE 13.1   *(Continued)*

Sl. No.	Therapeutic Use	References
13.	Gastric ulcer	Magdy et al., 2012
14.	Streptozotocin-induced diabetes	Abdelmeguid et al., 2010

Thymoquinone, chemically named as 2-isopropyl-5-methylbenzo-1,4-quinone, is a promising candidate with significant potential for the treatment of several diseases (Figure 13.2) including anti-inflammation, anti-oxidation, anti-bacterial, and anti-cancer (Ballout et al., 2018; Liou et al., 2019). TQ has remarkable efficacy and selectivity against cancer cells and has no toxicity against normal cells (Mohammadabadi et al., 2018).

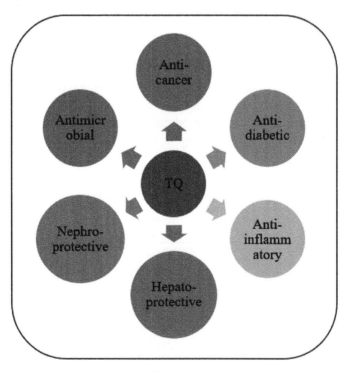

FIGURE 13.2   The major therapeutic activity of thymoquinone (TQ).

TQ, despite being of so much therapeutic significance is characterized with hydrophobicity which leads to poor solubility in aqueous media and hence limits its bioavailability. Moreover, the high index lipophilicity has been leading into poor formulation characteristics (Odeh et al., 2012). Most of the therapeutic agents, especially the hydrophobic compounds, with poor efficacy and safety measures have failed in the human clinical trials. Additionally, these drawbacks may also be a consequence of the ineffectual bioavailability associated with the compound's hydrophobicity (Ravindran et al., 2010). This has greatly hampered the development of the formulation of several clinically used natural compounds.

There are many glitches in delivering therapeutic agents to tumor cells *in vivo*, the major ones are enlisted as under (Brigger et al., 2002):

1. Drug resistance at the tumor level due to physiological barriers (noncellular based mechanisms);
2. Drug resistance at the cellular level (cellular mechanisms);
3. Distribution, biotransformation, and clearance of anti-cancer drugs in the body.

Nanoparticle drug delivery systems are now becoming one of the most preferred technology for developing therapeutics as they enhance the pharma-cokinetics (PKs) of the drugs and increased patient compliance by achieving quicker recovery (Kumar et al., 2016, 2017; Chauhan et al., 2017). Several natural polymers like albumin, alginate, chitosan (CS), dextran, starch, carboxy-methyl cellulose, gelatin, and gums have been used widely for the development of nanoparticles. There have been multiple reports for the use of anionic polymers namely gum Arabic (Rani et al., 2015), gum tragacanth (Ranjbar et al., 2016), guar gum (Sarmah et al., 2014), gellan gum (Kumar et al., 2017; Dahiya et al., 2017) and xanthan gum (Cai et al., 2016). Gum rosin has been established as a novel material for target-specific and sustained release formulations, additionally it is a non-toxic, biodegradable, and inexpensive polymer. All these properties make gum rosin a preferable and suitable nanocarrier for the encapsulation and sustained release of drugs (Rani et al., 2018).

Development of TQ into suitable formulation has been rigorously worked upon and several carrier systems have been engaged by now to attain high therapeutic concentrations in human illnesses especially in case of tumors. These formulations include microspheres (Chaurasia et al., 2006; Cheung et al., 2006), niosomes (Uchegbu et al., 1998, 2000), nanoparticles (Azarmi et al., 2006; Sun et al., 2008), dendrimers (Lin et al., 2018; Cai et al., 2017), SLNs (Wong et al., 2007; Chirio et al., 2018), micelles (Parida et al., 2017; Debele et al., 2017), liposomes (Shen et al., 2017; Cao et al., 2017) and nanoliposomes (Razazan et al., 2017; Sharma et al., 2017; Haghiralsadat et al., 2018).

The emergence of surface engineering of the nanoparticle carrier systems has led to the development of folate-decorated nanoparticles or polymer-linked vesicles like PEGylated liposomes. These carriers have enhanced circulation time and hence carrier-drug complex has greater possibility in reaching the target tissue (Figure 13.3). These surface-engineered micro- and nano-carriers can be employed to target tumor antigens, cancer-specific receptors, and the vasculatures of tumors with high affinity and precision, namely monoclonal antibodies or tumor-specific ligands (Mozafari et al., 2009).

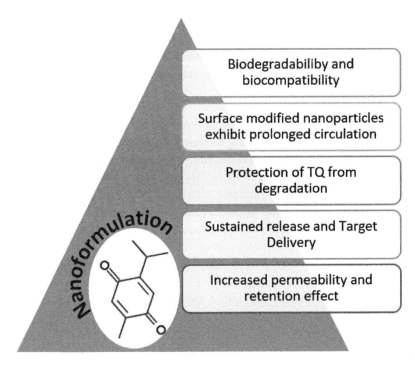

FIGURE 13.3   Advantages of TQ nanoformulations.

Many studies have been carried out to improve the bioavailability of TQ, especially for the oral route administration, which includes micelle nanoparticles, CS nanoparticles, and liposomes (Ganea et al., 2010; Alam et al., 2012; Odeh et al., 2012). Nano-TQ has better photostability, and its bioavailability is six times more than the free TQ solution and therefore liquid formulations of TQ meant for oral administration has improved solubility and bioavailability and is protected from photodegradation (Salmani et al., 2014; Nihei et al., 2016). In addition, Tubesha et al. (2013), reported in their study that nanoemulsion containing TQ has a stability of almost six months. In this chapter, we have focused more on the effect of TQ containing nanoformulations and their efficacy in different human diseases.

13.3   BIOLOGICAL ACTIVITIES OF THYMOQUINONE NANOFORMULATION

13.3.1   ANTICANCER ACTIVITY

TQ has a great potential for anticancer activity through its regulation of the diversity of cell signaling pathways and its interference with other cell components (see Figure 13.4) (El-Far et al., 2015).

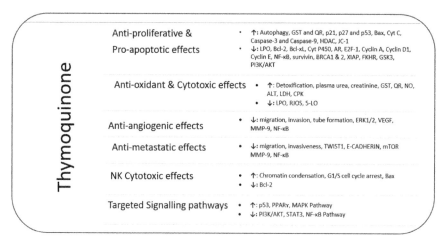

FIGURE 13.4   A brief summary of the TQ cellular and molecular activity; where ↑ means upregulation and ↓ means downregulation.

Source: Figure adapted from Majdalawieh et al. (2017).

Nanoformulation of TQ has been found to potentiate the anticancer activity (see Table 13.2) significantly, e.g., TQ, and Topotecan were loaded together in poly (D,L-lactide-co-glycolide) (PLGA) nanomatrix where TQ was loaded into the organic phase whereas the topotecan was dissolved in the inner aqueous phase of the double emulsion. The resulting nanomatrix enabled mutual drug delivery of both topotecan and TQ and enhanced the anticancer effect of this nanomatrix formulation (Verma et al., 2017).

TABLE 13.2 Illustrating Preparation of TQ Nanoformulation Using Different Techniques and Their Outcomes

Overview of Anticancer Effect of Various TQ Nanoformulation

Class of Particle	Materials	Methods	Pharmacological Effects	References
Polymer carriers	PLGA	Emulsification solvent evaporation	• Synergism between TQ and paclitaxel. • Improves anticancer activity of TQ as compared to free drugs against MCF-7 breast cancer cells.	Soni et al., 2015
			• Antioxidant and antibacterial activity against *E. coli*, *S. aureus*, and *S. typhi*.	Ilaiyaraja et al., 2013
	PHA-mPEG		• Non-toxic to neuronal hippocampal and fibroblast cells of prenatal rats.	Shah et al., 2010
	β-cyclodextrin	Self-assembly	• Enhances anticancer activity of TQ on MCF-7 breast cancer cell line. • Non-toxic to periodontal fibroblasts.	Abu-Dahab et al., 2013
	PEGylated	Nanoprecipitation	• Non-toxic to normal peripheral blood mononuclear cells. • Diminishes migration rate of MCF-7 and HBL-100 cells. • Interrupts cytoskeletal actin polymerization through upregulation of miR-34a.	Bhattacharya et al., 2015
Lipid-based	Nanostructured lipid carriers	High-pressure homogenization	• Inhibits the formation of ethanol-induced ulcers. • Heat shock protein 70 modulation. • No toxicity to normal human liver cells.	Abdelwahab et al., 2013

Overview of Anticancer Effect of Various TQ Nanoformulation

Class of Particle	Materials	Methods	Pharmacological Effects	References
		High speed homogenization followed by ultrasonication	• Lower toxicity than pure TQ administered orally to mice • 2–3 times increased bioavailability of TQ. • TQ-nanoformulation shows hepatoprotective and antioxidant efficacy.	Ong et al., 2016 Elmowafy et al., 2016
	Liposomes	Thin film hydration	• Inhibits the cancerous growth of MCF-7 and T47D.	Odeh et al., 2012
	Gold niosomes	Click chemistry	• Inhibits the bioavailability of tamoxifen resistant and AKT over proliferating breast cancer cells.	Rajput et al., 2015
	Solid-lipid nanoparticles	Ultrasonication or solvent injection	• Improved bioavailability, and distribution of drug.	Pathan et al., 2011; Singh et al., 2013
	Chitosan	Ionic gelation	• Enhanced drug targeting to brain cells.	Alam et al., 2012
Chitosan based	Myristic acid-chitosan	Self-assembly	• Proliferation of MCF-7 breast cancer cells decreases.	Dehghani et al., 2015

TQ loaded PLGA nanoparticles were found to be more efficacious than free TQ in restricting the proliferation of MDA-MB-231 breast cancer cells (Ganea et al., 2010). In another study, it was reported that the preparation of dual drug (TQ and paclitaxel) loaded nanoparticles by emulsion solvent-evaporation method using PVA as the stabilizer showed better effect in breast cancer cells even at lower doses (Soni et al., 2015). Similarly, there are many other studies enlisted in Table 13.2, which are assertive of the enhance effectiveness of TQ when loaded into a nanoformulation. These also suggest the possibility of using TQ-loaded PLGA nanoparticles in the clinical studies.

13.3.2   ANTIDIABETIC ACTIVITY

Diabetes, one of the rapidly growing metabolic disorders is mediated by abnormal insulin secretion or action or both. It is characterized by hyperglycemia which ultimately causes oxidative stress and damages different organs (American Diabetes Association, 2009). TQ is a potential antidiabetic compound which alleviates almost every diabetic complication remarkably (see Figure 13.5) (AbuKhader et al., 2012; Atta et al., 2017).

A study (Rani et al., 2018) investigated the antidiabetic potential of TQ loaded nanoparticle in streptozotocin-nicotinamide induced type-2 diabetes in rats and against metformin as the standard treatment. It was observed that TQ- and metformin-loaded nanocapsules (NCs) possessed a sustained release ability, and also decreased the blood glucose and glycated hemoglobin levels significantly in a dose-dependent manner accompanied with improvement in the serum lipid profile. This study strongly asserted that nanoformulation of TQ enhanced its antidiabetic activity remarkably. Further investigations are mandatory to determine the molecular mechanisms of TQ nano preparation's anti-diabetic properties. Determination of the role of nanoformulations loaded with TQ in pancreatic cell regeneration, insulin secretion and sensitivity will provide more therapeutic indications for diabetes management in the future.

13.3.3   CENTRAL NERVOUS SYSTEM PROTECTIVE ACTIVITY

The presence of different kinds of pollutants and chemical molecules in the environment increases the probability of inflammatory diseases in the CNS. There are numerous reports on the CNS protective activity of TQ for conditions like Alzheimer's, Parkinson's diseases, and glioblastoma (Ebrahimi et al., 2017; Abulfadl et al., 2018; Chowdhury et al., 2018). Effect of TQ-loaded solid lipid nanoparticles (TQ-SLN) on the brain of rats was evaluated in a study using tail suspension test, modified forced swim test, and locomotor activities (Alam et al., 2018). The study revealed that TQ-SLN enhanced the delivery of TQ to brain cells and it was also faster than free TQ, as demonstrated by the determination of monoamine and SOD levels in the brain (Figure 13.5). Thus, it was concluded that TQ-SLN is a potent formulation that can be employed to improve the efficiency of TQ, enhance its delivery, and mitigate the oxidative stress in CNS diseases.

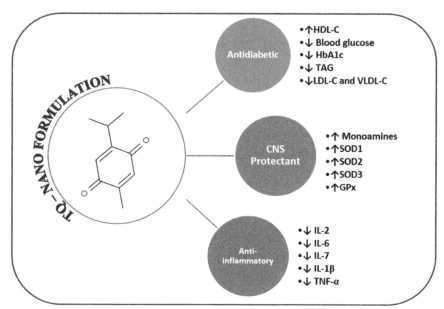

FIGURE 13.5 Illustrates the biological activities of TQ nanoformulations. HDL-C: high-density lipoprotein-cholesterol, HbA1c: glycated hemoglobin, IL: interleukin, LDL-C: low-density lipoprotein-cholesterol, VLDL-C: very low-density lipoprotein-cholesterol, SOD1: Copper, zinc-dependent superoxide dismutase (cytosolic), SOD2: manganese-dependent superoxide dismutase (mitochondrial), SOD3: Copper, zinc-dependent superoxide dismutase (extracellular), TAG: triacylglycerol, TNF-α:Tumor necrosisfactor-α, GPx: Glutathione peroxidase.

13.3.4 ANTI-INFLAMMATORY ACTIVITY

TQ has been traditionally used as an anti-inflammatory agent and this has been established by several studies in animal models (Rifaioglu et al., 2013; Atta et al., 2017). In a study, TQ containing liposomes were prepared and used as an anti-psoriatic drug. RAW 264.7 murine macrophage cell lines was used for testing the TQ lipospheres and it was found to decrease the levels of nitric oxide (NO) and prostaglandins like IL-2, IL-6, IL-1β and TNF-α (Figure 13.5). There are also other reports of TQ-nanoformulation when used topically it elucidates better efficacy and it also has a better stability.

13.3.5 HEPATOPROTECTIVE ACTIVITY

Liver is a vital organ and has a principal role in the physiological metabolism and xenobiotic detoxifications. Generally, oxidative stress is the prime cause of liver injuries. And, TQ has been found to possess hepatoprotective potential against injuries induced by several mechanisms including free radical scavenging (Farkhondeh et al., 2018). In a study, different self-nanoemulsifying drug delivery system (SNEDDS) formulations containing TQ were prepared for assessing hepatoprotective activity in rats (Kalam et al., 2017). TQ-SNEDDS formulations were found to have better absorption and enhanced bioavailability which protected the liver better than TQ suspension.

Similarly, TQ loaded in nanostructured lipid carriers (NLCs) also exhibited increased bioavailability in a male rat model when administered orally (Elmowafy et al., 2015). In another report, TQ-SLN was prepared, characterized, and evaluated for the treatment of paracetamol-induced liver cirrhosis, and compared with free TQ and SILYBON®. The investigators found that TQ-SLN formulations showed more stability than free TQ-suspension, as the serum glutamate oxaloacetate transaminase (SGOT), serum glutamate pyruvate transaminase (SGPT), and alkaline phosphatase (ALP) were significantly reduced (Figure 13.6) (Singh et al., 2013). The antioxidant potential of TQ was increased by the SLN formulation and hence remarkable hepatoprotection was observed.

13.3.6 ANTIMICROBIAL ACTIVITY OF NANO-TQ

Multi-drug resistance is one of the most horrifying clinical health problems in the upcoming time. It serves as an adamant challenge to the health professional and is a serious concern which if not dealt judiciously can create havoc. Multi-drug resistance is the resultant of the irrational use of antibiotics in the treatment of infectious diseases (Fernández et al., 2016). Hence, the investigators have started looking for the alternative herbal source of antimicrobial drugs (El-Far et al., 2014). There have been multiple records emphasizing on the antibacterial role of TQ, especially the nanoformulations, which may help in standing against the bacterial resistance (Bakal et al., 2017). Another study intended to explore the antifungal activity of nanoparticles loaded with amphotericin-B, ketoconazole, and TQ against *Candida albicans* yeasts and *Candida biofilm*. The study revealed that the fungal strains were disinfected 2–4 times more effectively by the nanoparticles loaded with TQ, ketoconazole, and amphotericin-B (Randhawa et al., 2015) (Figure 13.6). Thus, it can be deduced that TQ nanoformulations have better antibacterial and antifungal activity than its free forms. However, further citations are needed.

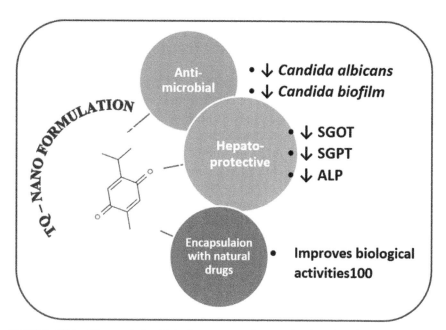

FIGURE 13.6 The antimicrobial, hepatoprotective, and other health application of TQ-nanoformulation.

13.3.7 APPLICATIONS OF TQ NANOFORMULATIONS

13.3.7.1 NANO-TQ COSMETICS

Liposomes can retain the encapsulated nutrients safe from the environment and are also capable of enhancing the solubility of hydrophobic nutrients in semi-solid or liquid form; therefore, liposomes were one of the first nanoformulations to be launched in the market. Moreover, liposomes also have better topical bioavailability as they have good dermal permeation

(Mu et al., 2010; Raj et al., 2012; Lohani et al., 2014) (Figure 13.7). TQ as mentioned earlier has potent antioxidant and anti-apoptotic activity and is reported to possess an anti-aging effect in mice (Sharoudi et al., 2017). Characterization of nano-TQ reveals high physical stability at a wider range of storage temperatures (Al-Haj et al., 2010). Also, TQ-SLN formulations prepared by high-pressure homogenization have exhibited activities like anti-aging, moisturizing, and protective for cosmeceuticals. However, further research needs to be carried out to ensure the safety of nano-TQ for application on human skin (Zolnik et al., 2010; Raj et al., 2012).

13.3.7.2 HEALTH AND NUTRITIONAL SUPPLEMENT

A number of health and nutritional supplements are in the market which is prepared using nanotechnology like beta-carotene, lutein, lycopene, CoQ10, and omega-3 fatty acids. TQ when loaded in nanoformulation has good bioavailability and has potent hepatoprotective, antioxidant, anti-inflammatory, anticarcinogenic, and many more other therapeutic effects that make it a suitable candidate for being a health and nutritional supplement (Table 13.1 and Figure 13.7). TQ was commonly used as a nutritional supplement in the Middle East by cancer patients undergoing chemotherapy (Jazieh et al., 2012). Nano-TQ, if used as a nutritional supplement may improve the therapeutic index and minimize the toxic effect of chemotherapy.

Conclusively, though TQ has a high potential of healing several critical health problems however, its low aqueous stability may be a challenge in the large-scale nanomanufacturing process. It may not be possible to maintain batch to batch reproducibility and the purification, lyophilization, and/or sterilization process of nano-TQ may be affected. To meet these problems and to omit the clinical translation gap, fervent collaborations between academic labs, research labs, and pharmaceutical companies need to be established.

13.4 CONCLUSIONS

Nanoformulations loaded with TQ enhance the pharmacological activity and efficacy of TQ by improving its bioavailability and by decreasing the doses required for elucidating the therapeutic effect. Incorporation of TQ into nanoformulations like nanocosmetics, nanocreams, health, and nutritional drinks should be more frequent to explore the hidden potentials of TQ and for finding its application in human disease.

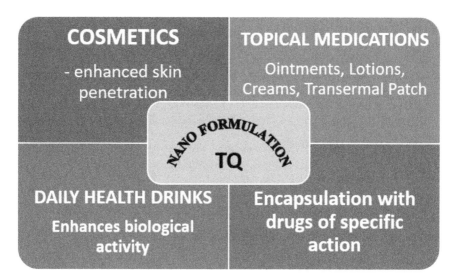

FIGURE 13.7   Application of TQ loaded nanoformulations.

CONFLICTS OF INTEREST

The authors declare no conflict of interest.

KEYWORDS

- **bioavailability**
- **black cumin**
- **nanoformulation**
- **nanoparticle**
- ***Nigella sativa***
- **phytomedicine**
- **thymoquinone**

REFERENCES

Abdelmeguid, N. E., Fakhoury, R., Kamal, S. M., & Al Wafai, R. J., (2010). Effects of *Nigella sativa* and thymoquinone on biochemical and subcellular changes in pancreatic β-cells of streptozotocin-induced diabetic rats. *J. Diabetes., 2*(4), 256–266.

Abdelwahab, S. I., Sheikh, B. Y., Taha, M. M. E., How, C. W., Abdullah, R., Yagoub, U., & Eid, E., (2013). Thymoquinone-loaded nanostructured lipid carriers: Preparation, gastro protection, *in vitro* toxicity, and pharmacokinetic properties after extra vascular administration. *Int. J. Nanomed., 8,* 2163–2172.

Abu-Dahab, R., Odeh, F., Ismail, S. I., Azzam, H., & AI-Bawab, A., (2013). Preparation, characterization, and antiproliferative activity of thymoquinone-beta-cyclodextrin self-assembling nanoparticles. *Pharmazie, 68,* 939–944.

AbuKhader, M. M., (2012). Thymoquinone: A promising antidiabetic agent. *Int. J. Diabetes Dev. Ctries., 32,* 65–68.

Abulfadl, Y. S., El-Maraghy, N. N., Ahmed, A. E., Nofal, S., Abdel-Mottaleb, Y., & Badary, O. A., (2018). Thymoquinone alleviates the experimentally induced Alzheimer's disease inflammation by modulation of TLRs signaling. *Hum. Exp. Toxicol., 37,* 1092–1104.

Ahmad, A., Husain, A., Mujeeb, M., Khan, S. A., Najmi, A. K., Siddique, N. A., Damanhouri, Z. A., & Anwar, F., (2013). A review on therapeutic potential of *Nigella sativa*: A miracle herb. *Asian Pac. J. Trop. Biomed., 3*(5), 337–352.

Alam, M., Najmi, A. K., Ahmad, I., Ahmad, F. J., Akhtar, M. J., Imam, S. S., & Akhtar, M., (2018). Formulation and evaluation of nano lipid formulation containing CNS acting drug: Molecular docking, *in-vitro* assessment and bioactivity detail in rats. *Artif. Cells Nanomed. Biotechnol.,* 1–12.

Alam, S., Khan, Z. I., Mustafa, G., Kumar, M., Islam, F., Bhatnagar, A., & Ahmad, F. J., (2012). Development and evaluation of thymoquinone-encapsulated chitosan nanoparticles for nose-to-brain targeting: A pharmacoscintigraphic study. *Int. J. Nanomed., 7,* 5705–5718.

Alenzi, F. Q., El-Bolkiny, Y. S., & Salem, M. L., (2010). Protective effects of *Nigella sativa* oil and thymoquinone against toxicity induced by the anticancer drug cyclophosphamide. *Br. J. Biomed. Sci., 67*(1), 20–28.

Al-Haj, N. A., Shamsudin, M. N., Alipiah, N. M., Zamri, H. F., Bustamam, A., Ibrahim, S., & Abdullah, R., (2010). Characterization of *Nigella sativa* L. Essential oil-loaded solid lipid nanoparticles. *Am. J. Pharmacol. Toxicol., 5,* 52–57.

American Diabetes Association, (2009). Diagnosis and classification of diabetes mellitus. *Diabetes Care, 33,* S62–S69.

Ankola, D. D., Viswanad, B., Bhardwaj, V., Ramarao, P., & Kumar, M. N., (2007). Development of potent oral nanoparticulate formulation of coenzyme Q10 for treatment of hypertension: Can the simple nutritional supplements be used as first line therapeutic agents for prophylaxis/therapy? *Eur. J. Pharm. Biopharm., 67,* 361–369.

Aquib, M., Najmi, A. K., & Akhtar, M., (2015). Antidepressant effect of thymoquinone in animal models of depression. *Drug Res. (Stuttg), 65*(09), 490–494.

Atta, M., Almadaly, E., El-Far, A., Saleh, R. M., Assar, D. H., Al Jaouni, S. K., & Mousa, S. A., (2017). Thymoquinone defeats diabetes-induced testicular damage in rats targeting antioxidant, inflammatory and aromatase expression. *Int. J. Mol. Sci., 18,* 919.

Azarmi, S., Huang, Y., Chen, H., McQuarrie, S., Abrams, D., Roa, W., Finlay, W. H., Miller, G. G., & Löbenberg, R., (2006). Optimization of a two-step desolvation method for preparing gelatin nanoparticles and cell uptake studies in 143B osteosarcoma cancer cells. *J. Pharm. Pharm. Sci., 9,* 124–132.

Aziz, A. E., Sayed, N. S. E., & Mahran, L. G., (2011). Anti-asthmatic and anti-allergic effects of thymoquinone on airway-induced hypersensitivity in experimental animals. *JAPS, 1*(8), 109–117.

Bakal, S. N., Bereswill, S., & Heimesaat, M. M., (2017). Finding novel antibiotic substances from medicinal plants-Antimicrobial properties of *Nigella sativa* directed against multidrug-resistant bacteria. *Eur. J. Microbiol. Immunol., 7*, 92–98.

Bala, I., Bhardwaj, V., Hariharan, S., & Kumar, M. N., (2006). Analytical methods for assay of ellagic acid and its solubility studies. *J. Pharmaceut. Biomed. Anal., 40*, 206–210.

Ballout, F., Habli, Z., Rahal, O. N., Fatfat, M., Gali-Muhtasib, H., (2018). Thymoquinone-based nanotechnology for cancer therapy: Promises and Challenges. *Drug Discov. Today, 23*, 5.

Banerjee, S., Azmi, A. S., Padhye, S., Singh, M. W., Baruah, J. B., Philip, P. A., Sarkar, F. H., & Mohammad, R. M., (2010). Structure-activity studies on therapeutic potential of thymoquinone analogs in pancreatic cancer. *Pharm. Res., 27*, 1146–1158.

Bhattacharya, S., Ahir, M., Patra, P., Mukherjee, S., Ghosh, S., Mazumdar, M., Chattopadhyay, S., et al., (2015). PEGylated-thymoquinone-nanoparticle mediated retardation of breast cancer cell migration by deregulation of cytoskeletal actin polymerization through miR-34a. *Biomaterials, 51*, 91–107.

Bisht, S., Feldmann, G., Soni, S., Ravi, R., Karikar, C., Maitra, A., & Maitra, A., (2007). Polymeric nanoparticle-encapsulated curcumin (nanocurcumin): A novel strategy for human cancer therapy. *J. Nanobiotechnol., 5*, 3.

Brigger, I., Dubernet, C., & Couvreur, P., (2002). Nanoparticles in cancer therapy and diagnosis. *Adv. Drug Del. Rev., 54*, 631–651.

Cai, X. J., Mesquida, P., & Jones, S. A., (2016). Investigating the ability of nanoparticle-loaded hydroxypropyl methylcellulose and xanthan gum gels to enhance drug penetration into the skin. *Int. J. Pharm., 513*(1/2), 302–308.

Cai, X., Zhu, H., Zhang, Y., & Gu, Z., (2017). Highly efficient and safe delivery of VEGF siRNA by bioreducible fluorinated peptide dendrimers for cancer therapy. *ACS App. Mat. Interfaces, 9*, 9402–9415.

Cao, Y., Yi, J., Yang, X., Liu, L., Yu, C., Huang, Y., Sun, L., Bao, Y., & Li, Y., (2017). Efficient cancer regression by a thermosensitive liposome for photoacoustic imaging-guided photothermal/chemo combinatorial therapy. *Biomacromolecules, 18*, 2306–2314.

Chaieb, K., Kouidhi, B., Jrah, H., Mahdouani, K., & Bakhrouf, A., (2011). Antibacterial activity of thymoquinone, an active principle of *Nigella sativa* and its potency to prevent bacterial biofilm formation. *BMC Complement. Altern. Med., 11*, 29.

Chauhan, N., Dilbaghi, N., Gopal, M., Kumar, R., Kim, K. H., & Kumar, S., (2017). Development of chitosan nanocapsules for the controlled release of hexaconazole. *Int. J. Biol. Macromol., 97*, 616–624.

Chaurasia, M., Chourasia, M. K., Jain, N. K., Jain, A., Soni, V., Gupta, Y., & Jain, S. K., (2006). Cross-linked guargum microspheres: A viable approach for improved delivery of anticancer drugs for the treatment of colorectal cancer. *AAPS Pharm. Sci. Tech., 7*, E143.

Cheung, R. Y., Rauth, A. M., Ronaldson, P. T., Bendayan, R., & Wu, X. Y., (2006). *In vitro* toxicity to breast cancer cells of microsphere-delivered mitomycin C and its combination with doxorubicin. *Eur. J. Pharm. Biopharm., 62*, 321–331.

Chirio, D., Peira, E., Battaglia, L., Ferrara, B., Barge, A., Sapino, S., Giordano, S., & Dianzani, C., Gallarate, M., (2018). Lipophilic prodrug of floxuridine loaded into solid lipid nanoparticles: *In vitro* cytotoxicity studies on different human cancer cell lines. *J. Nanoscience Nanotech., 18*, 556–563.

Cho, K., Wang, X., Nie, S., Chen, Z. G., & Shin, D. M., (2008). Therapeutic nanoparticles for drug delivery in cancer. *Clin Cancer Res., 14*, 1310–1316.

Chowdhury, F. A., Hossain, M. K., Mostofa, A. G. M., Akbor, M. M., & Bin, S. M. S., (2018). Therapeutic potential of thymoquinone in glioblastoma treatment: Targeting major gliomagenesis signaling pathways. *Biomed. Res. Int.,* 1–15.

Dahiya, S., Rani, R., Kumar, S., Dhingra, D., & Dilbaghi, N., (2017). Chitosan-gellan gum bipolymeric nanohydrogels: A potential nanocarrier for the delivery of epigallocatechin gallate. *Bio Nano Science, 7*(3), 508–520.

Debele, T. A., Lee, K. Y., Hsu, N. Y., Chiang, Y. T., Yu, L. Y., Shen, Y. A., & Lo, C. L., (2017). A pH sensitive polymeric micelle for co-delivery of doxorubicin and α-TOS for colon cancer therapy. *J. Materials Chem. B., 5,* 5870–5880.

Dehghani, H., Hashemi, M., Entezari, M., & Mohsenifar, A., (2015). The comparison of anticancer activity of thymoquinone and nanothymoquinone on human breast adenocarcinoma. *Iran. J. Pharm. Res., 14,* 539–546.

Ebrahimi, S. S., Oryan, S., Izadpanah, E., & Hassanzadeh, K., (2017). Thymoquinone exerts neuroprotective effect in animal model of Parkinson's disease. *Toxicol. Lett., 276,* 108–114.

El-Far, A. H., Korshom, M. A., Mandour, A. A., El-Bessoumy, A. A., & El-Sayed, Y. S., (2017). Hepatoprotective efficacy of *Nigella sativa* seeds dietary supplementation against lead acetate-induced oxidative damage in rabbit-purification and characterization of glutathione peroxidase. *Biomed. Pharmacother., 89,* 711–718.

El-Far, A., Bazh, E. K., & Moharam, M., (2014). Antioxidant and antinematodal effects of *Nigella sativa* and *Zingiber officinale* supplementations in ewes. *Int. J. Pharm. Sci. Rev. Res., 26,* 222–227.

El-Mahmoudy, A., Shimizu, Y., Shiina, T., Matsuyama, H., El-Sayed, M., Takewaki, T., (2005). Successful abrogation by thymoquinone against induction of diabetes mellitus with streptozotocin via nitric oxide inhibitory mechanism. *Int. Immunopharmacol., 5*(1), 195–207.

Elmowafy, M., Samy, A., Raslan, M. A., Salama, A., Said, R. A., Abdelaziz, A. E., El-Eraky, W., et al., (2015). Enhancement of bioavailability and pharmacodynamic effects of thymoquinone via nanostructured lipid carrier (NLC) formulation. *AAPS Pharm. Sci. Tech., 17,* 663–672.

Elmowafy, M., Samy, A., Raslan, M. A., Salama, A., Said, R. A., Abdelaziz, A. E., El-Eraky, W., et al., (2016). Enhancement of bioavailability and pharmacodynamic effects of thymoquinone via nanostructured lipid carrier (NLC) formulation. *AAPS Pharm. Sci. Tech., 17,* 663–672.

Farkhondeh, T., Noorbakhsh, M. F., Hayati, F., Samarghandian, S., & Shaterzadeh-Yazdi, H., (2018). An overview on hepatoprotective effects of thymoquinone. *Recent Pat. Food Nutr. Agric., 9,* 14–22.

Fernández, J., Bert, F., & Nicolas-Chanoine, M. H., (2016). The challenges of multi-drug-resistance in hepatology. *J. Hepatol., 65,* 1043–1054.

Ganea, G. M., Fakayode, S. O., Losso, J. N., Van, N. C. F., Sabliov, C. M., & Warner, I. M., (2010). Delivery of phytochemical thymoquinone using molecular micelle modified poly(D,L-lactide-co-glycolide) (PLGA) nanoparticles. *Nanotechnology, 21,* 285104.

Gilhotra, N., & Dhingra, D., (2011). Thymoquinone produced antianxiety like effects in mice through modulation of GABA and NO levels. *Pharmacol. Rep., 63*(3), 660–669.

Gore, P. R., Prajapati, C. P., Mahajan, U. B., Goyal, S. N., Belemkar, S., Ojha, S., & Patil, C. R., (2016). Protective effect of thymoquinone against cyclophosphamide-induced hemorrhagic cystitis through inhibiting DNA damage and up regulation of Nrf2 Expression. *Int. J. Biol. Sci., 12*(8), 944–953.

Haghiralsadat, F., Amoabediny, G., Naderinezhad, S., Forouzanfar, T., Helder, M. N., & Zandieh-Doulabi, B., (2018). Preparation of PEGylated cationic nanoliposome-siRNA complexes for cancer therapy. *Art. Cells Nanomed. Biotech., 23*, 1–9.

Hariharan, S., Bhardwaj, V., Bala, I., Sitterberg, J., Bakowsky, U., & Ravi-Kumar, M. N., (2006). Design of estradiol loaded PLGA nanoparticulate formulations: A potential oral delivery system for hormone therapy. *Pharmaceutical Research, 23*, 184–195.

IlaiyarajaNallamuthu, A. P., & Khanum, F., (2013). Thymoquinone-loaded PLGA nanoparticles: Antioxidant and anti-microbial properties. *Int. Curr. Pharm. J., 2*, 202–207.

Inci, M., Davarci, M., Inci, M., Motor, S., Yalcinkaya, F. R., Nacar, E., Aydin, M., et al., (2013). Anti-inflammatory and antioxidant activity of thymoquinone in a rat model of acute bacterial prostatitis. *Hum. Exp. Toxicol., 32*(4), 354–361.

Jain, A., Pooladanda, V., Bulbake, U., Doppalapudi, S., Rafeeqi, T. A., Godugu, C., & Khan, W., (2017). Liposphere mediated topical delivery of thymoquinone in the treatment of psoriasis. *Nanomedicine, 13*, 2251–2262.

Jazieh, A. R., Al-Sudairy, R., Abulkhair, O., Alaskar, A., Al Safi, F., Sheblaq, N., Young, S., Issa, M., & Tamim, H., (2012). Use of complementary and alternative medicine by patients with cancer in Saudi Arabia. *J. Altern. Complement. Med., 18*, 1045–1049.

Kalam, M. A., Raish, M., Ahmed, A., Alkharfy, K. M., Mohsin, K., Alshamsan, A., Al-Jenoobi, F. I., et al., (2017). Oral bioavailability enhancement and hepatoprotective effects of thymoquinone by self-nanoemulsifying drug delivery system. *Mater. Sci. Eng. C. Mater. Biol. Appl., 76*, 319–329.

Khan, M. A., Tania, M., Fu, S., & Fu, J., (2017). Thymoquinone, as an anticancer molecule: From basic research to clinical investigation. *Oncotarget., 8*, 51907–51919.

Krukemeyer, M. G., Krenn, V., Huebner, F., Wagner, W., & Resch, R., (2015). History and possible uses of nanomedicine based on nanoparticles and nanotechnological progress. *J. Nanomed. Nanotechnol., 6*, 6.

Kumar, S., Bhanjana, G., Kumar, A., Taneja, K., Dilbaghi, N., & Kim, K. H., (2016). Synthesis and optimization of ceftriaxone-loaded solid lipid nanocarriers. *Chem. Phys. Lipids., 200*, 126–132.

Kumar, S., Bhanjana, G., Verma, R. K., Dhingra, D., Dilbaghi, N., & Kim, K. H., (2017). Metformin-loaded alginate nanoparticles as an effective antidiabetic agent for controlled drug release. *J. Pharm. Pharmacol., 69*(2), 143–150.

Kumar, S., Rani, R., Dilbaghi, N., Tankeshwar, K., & Kim, K. H., (2017). Carbon nanotubes: A novel material for multifaceted applications in human healthcare. *Chem. Soc. Rev., 46*, 158–196.

Lin, J., Hu, W., Gao, F., Qin, J., Peng, C., & Lu, X., (2018). Folic acid-modified diatrizoic acid-linked dendrimer-entrapped gold nanoparticles enable targeted CT imaging of human cervical cancer. *J. Cancer, 9*, 564–577.

Liou, Y. F., Hsieh, Y. S., Hung, T. W., Chen, P. N., Chang, Y. Z., Kao, S. H., & Chang, H. R., (2019). Thymoquinone inhibits metastasis of renal cell carcinoma cell 786-O-SI3 associating with downregulation of MMP-2 and u-PA and suppression of PI3K/Src signaling. *Int. J. Med. Sci., 16*(5), 686–695.

Lohani, A., Verma, A., Joshi, H., Yadav, N., & Karki, N., (2014). Nanotechnology-based cosmeceuticals. *ISRN Dermatol., 843687*.

Magdy, M. A., Hanan, E. A., & Nabila, E. M., (2012). Thymoquinone: Novel gastroprotective mechanisms. *Eur. J. Pharmacol., 697*(1–3), 126–131.

Majdalawieh, A. F., Fayyad, M. W., & Nasrallah, G. K., (2017). Anti-cancer properties and mechanisms of action of thymoquinone, the major active ingredient of *Nigella sativa*. *Crit. Rev. Food Sci. Nutr., 57*(18), 3911–3928.

Martins, P., Rosa, D., Fernandes, R. A., & Baptista, V. P., (2013). Nanoparticles drug delivery system: Recent patents and applications in nanomedicine. *Recent Patents on Nanomed., 3*(2), 1e14.

Mohammadabadi, M. R., & Mozafari, M. R., (2018). Enhanced efficacy and bioavailability of thymoquinone using nanoliposomal dosage form. *J. Drug Del. Sci. Technol., 47*, 445–453.

Mozafari, M. R., Pardakhty, A., Azarmi, S., Jazayeri, J. A., Nokhodchi, A., & Omri, A., (2009). Role of nanocarrier systems in cancer nanotherapy. *J. Liposome Res., 19*, 310–321.

Mu, L., & Feng, S. S., (2003). A novel controlled release formulation for the anticancer drug paclitaxel (Taxol): PLGA nanoparticles containing vitamin E TPGS. *J Control Release, 86*, 33–48.

Mu, L., & Sprando, R. L., (2010). Application of nanotechnology in cosmetics. *Pharm. Res., 27*, 1746–1749.

Nihei, T., Suzuki, H., Aoki, A., Yuminoki, K., Hashimoto, N., Sato, H., Seto, Y., & Onoue, S., (2016). Development of a novel nanoparticle formulation of thymoquinone with a cold wet-milling system and its pharmacokinetic analysis. *Int. J. Pharm., 511*, 455–461.

Odeh, F., Ismail, S. I., Abu-Dahab, R., Mahmoud, I. S., & Al-Bawab, A., (2012). Thymoquinone in liposomes: A study of loading efficiency and biological activity towards breast cancer. *Drug Deliv., 19*, 371–377.

Oguz, S., Kanter, M., Erboga, M., & Erenoglu, C., (2012). Protective effects of thymoquinone against cholestatic oxidative stress and hepatic damage after biliary obstruction in rats. *J. Mol. Histol., 43*(2), 151–159.

Ong, Y. S., Yazan, L. S., Ng, W. K., Noordin, M. M., Sapuan, S., Foo, J. H., & Tor, Y. S., (2016). Acute and subacute toxicity profiles of thymoquinone-loaded nanostructured lipid carriers in BALB/c mice. *Int. J. Nanomed., 11*, 5905–5915.

Onoue, S., Yamada, S., & Kim, H. C., (2014). Nanodrugs: Pharmacokinetics and safety. *Int. J. Nanomed., 9*, 1025e37.

Parida, S., Maiti, C., Rajesh, Y., Dey, K. K., Pal, I., Parekh, A., Patra, R., et al., (2017). Gold nanorod embedded reduction responsive block copolymer micelletriggered drug delivery combined with photothermal ablation for targeted cancer therapy. *Biochim. Biophys. Acta(BBA)-General Subjects, 1861*, 3039–3052.

Pathan, S. A., Jain, G. K., Zaidi, S. M., Akhter, S., Vohora, D., Chander, P., Kole, P. L., Ahmad, F. J., & Khar, R. K., (2011). Stability- indicating ultra-performance liquid chromatography method for the estimation of thymoquinone and its application in biopharmaceutical studies. *Biomed. Chromatogr., 25*, 613–620.

Raj, S., Jose, S., Sumod, U. S., & Sabitha, M., (2012). Nanotechnology in cosmetics: Opportunities and challenges. *J. Pharm. Bioallied Sci., 4*, 186–193.

Rajput, S., Puvvada, N., Kumar, B. N., Sarkar, S., Konar, S., Bharti, R., Dey, G., et al., (2015). Overcoming Akt induced therapeutic resistance in breast cancer through siRNA and thymoquinone encapsulated multilamellar gold niosomes. *Mol. Pharm., 12*, 4214–4225.

Ramachandran, S., & Thangarajan, S., (2016). A novel therapeutic application of solid lipid nanoparticles encapsulated thymoquinone (TQ-SLNs) on 3-nitroproponic acid-induced Huntington's disease-like symptoms in Wistar rats. *Chem. Biol. Interact., 256*, 25–36.

Randhawa, M. A., Gondal, M. A., Al-Zahrani, A. H. J., Rashid, S. G., & Ali, A., (2015). Synthesis, morphology, and antifungal activity of nano-particulated amphotericin-b, ketoconazole and thymoquinone against Candida albicans yeasts and Candida biofilm. *J. Environ. Sci. Health Part A Toxic Hazard. Subst. Environ. Eng., 50*, 119–124.

Rani, R., Dahiya, S., Dhingra, D., Dilbaghi, N., Kim, K. H., & Kumar, S., (2018). Improvement of antihyperglycemic activity of nano-thymoquinone in rat model of type-2 diabetes. *Chem. Biol. Interact., 295*, 119–132.

Rani, R., Dilbaghi, N., Dhingra, D., & Kumar, S., (2015). Optimization and evaluation of bioactive drug-loaded polymeric nanoparticles for drug delivery. *Int. J. Biol. Macromol., 78*, 173–179.

Ranjbar-Mohammadi, M., & Bahrami, S. H., (2016). Electrospun curcumin loaded poly(ε-caprolactone)/gum tragacanthnanofibers for biomedical application. *Int. J. Biol. Macromol., 84*, 448–456.

Ravindran, J., Nair, H. B., Sung, B., Prasad, S., Tekmal, R. R., & Aggarwal, B. B., (2010). Thymoquinone poly(lactide-co-glycolide) nanoparticles exhibit enhanced anti-proliferative, anti-inflammatory, and chemo sensitization potential. *Biochem Pharmacol., 79*(11), 1640–1647.

Razazan, A., Behravan, J., Arab, A., Barati, N., Arabi, L., Gholizadeh, Z., Hatamipour, M., et al., (2017). Conjugated nanoliposome with the HER2/neu-derived peptide GP2 as an effective vaccine against breast cancer in mice xenograft model. *PloS One, 12*, e0185099.

Rifaioglu, M. M., Nacar, A., Yuksel, R., Yonden, Z., Karcioglu, M., Zorba, O. U., Davarci, I., & Sefil, N. K., (2013). Antioxidative and anti-inflammatory effect of thymoquinone in an acute Pseudomonas prostatitis rat model. *Urol. Int., 91*, 474–481.

Salem, M. L., (2005). Immunomodulatory and therapeutic properties of the *Nigella sativa* L. seed. *Int. Immunopharmacol., 5*, 1749–1770.

Salmani, J. M., Asghar, S., Lv, H. X., & Zhou, J. P., (2014). Aqueous solubility and degradation kinetics of the phytochemical anticancer thymoquinone; probing the effects of solvents, pH and light. *Molecules, 19*, 5925–5939.

Sangi, S. M., Sulaiman, M. I., El-Wahab, M. F., Ahmedani, E. I., & Ali, S. S., (2015). Antihyperglycemic effect of thymoquinone and oleuropein, on streptozotocin-induced diabetes mellitus in experimental animals. *Pharmacogn. Mag., 11*(2), S251–S257.

Sarmah, J. K., Bhattacharjee, S. K., Roy, S., Mahanta, R., & Mahanta, R., (2014). Biodegradable guar gum nanoparticles as carrier for tamoxifen citrate in treatment of breast cancer. *J. Biomater. Nanobiotechnol., 5*, 220–228.

Schneider-Stock, R., Fakhoury, I. H., Zaki, A. M., El-Baba, C. O., Gali-Muhtasib, H. U., (2014). Thymoquinone: Fifty years of success in the battle against cancer models. *Drug Discov. Today, 19*, 18–30.

Shah, M., Naseer, M. I., Choi, M. H., Kim, M. O., & Yoon, S. C., (2010). Amphiphilic PHA-mPEG copolymeric nanocontainers for drug delivery: Preparation, characterization and *in vitro* evaluation. *Int. J. Pharm., 400*, 165–175.

Shahroudi, M. J., Mehri, S., & Hosseinzadeh, H., (2017). Anti-aging effect of *Nigella sativa* fixed oil on D-galactose-induced aging in mice. *J. Pharmacopunct., 20*, 29–35.

Shanmugam, M. K., Arfuso, F., Kumar, A. P., Wang, L., Goh, B. C., Ahn, K. S., Bishayee, A., & Sethi, G., (2018). Modulation of diverse oncogenic transcription factors by thymoquinone, an essential oil compound isolated from the seeds of *Nigella sativa* Linn. *Pharmacol. Res., 129*, 357–364.

Sharma, R., Mody, N., Kushwah, V., Jain, S., & Vyas, S. P., (2017). C-Type lectin receptor(s)-targeted nanoliposomes: An intelligent approach for effective cancer immunotherapy. *Nanomedicine, 12*, 1945–1959.

Shen, J., Kim, H. C., Wolfram, J., Mu, C., Zhang, W., Liu, H., Xie, Y., et al., (2017). A liposome encapsulated ruthenium polypyridine complex as a theranostic platform for triple-negative breast cancer. *Nano Lett., 17*, 2913–2920.

Singh, A., Ahmad, I., Akhter, S., Jain, G. K., Iqbal, Z., Talegaonkar, S., & Ahmad, F. J., (2013). Nanocarrier based formulation of thymoquinone improves oral delivery: Stability assessment, *in vitro* and *in vivo* studies. *Colloids Surf. B Biointerfaces, 102*, 822–832.

Soni, P., Kaur, J., & Tikoo, K., (2015). Dual drug-loaded paclitaxel-thymoquinone nanoparticles for effective breast cancer therapy. *J. Nanopart. Res., 17*(18).

Sun, B., Ranganathan, B., & Feng, S. S., (2008). Multifunctional poly(D,L-lactide-coglycolide)/montmorillonite (PLGA/MMT) nanoparticles decorated by trastuzumab for targeted chemotherapy of breast cancer. *Biomaterials, 29*, 475–486.

Tubesha, Z., Abu-Bakar, Z., & Ismail, M., (2013). Characterization and stability evaluation of thymoquinone nanoemulsions prepared by high-pressure homogenization. *J. Nanomater, 2013*.

Uchegbu, I. F., & Vyas, S. P., (1998). Non-ionic surfactant-based vesicles (niosomes) in drug delivery. *Int. J. Pharm., 172*, 33–70.

Uchegbu, I. F., (2000). Niosomes and other synthetic surfactant vesicles with antitumor drugs. In: Uchegbu, I. F., (ed.), *Synthetic Surfactant Vesicles* (pp. 115–133). Harwood Academic: The Netherlands.

Vasey, P. A., Kaye, S. B., Morrison, R., Twelves, C., Wilson, P., Duncan, R., Thomson, A. H., et al., (1999). Phase I clinical and pharmacokinetic study of PK1 [N-(2-hydroxypropyl) methacrylamide copolymer doxorubicin]: First member of a new class of chemotherapeutic agents-drug-polymer conjugates. Cancer Research Campaign Phase I/II Committee. *Clin Cancer Res., 5*, 83–94.

Verma, D., Thakur, P. S., Padhi, S., Khuroo, T., Talegaonkar, S., & Iqbal, Z., (2017). Design expert assisted nanoformulation design for co-delivery of topotecan and thymoquinone: Optimization, *in vitro* characterization and stability assessment. *J. Mol. Liq., 242*, 382–394.

Wong, H. L., Bendayan, R., Rauth, A. M., Li, Y., & Wu, X. Y., (2007). Chemotherapy with anticancer drugs encapsulated in solid lipid nanoparticles. *Adv. Drug Deliv. Rev., 59*, 491–504.

Zhang, L., Bai, Y., & Yang, Y., (2016). Thymoquinone chemo sensitizes colon cancer cells through inhibition of NF-κB. *Oncol. Lett., 12*(4), 2840–2845.

Zolnik, B. S., González-Fernández, A. F., Sadrieh, N., & Dobrovolskaia, M. A., (2010). Mini review: Nanoparticles and the immune system. *Endocrinology, 151*, 458–465.

Index

Printed and bound by CPI Group (UK) Ltd, Croydon, CR0 4YY

23/10/2024

01777701-0008